Immune System Disorders

SOURCEBOOK

Third Edition

Third Edition

Immune System Disorders SOURCEBOOK

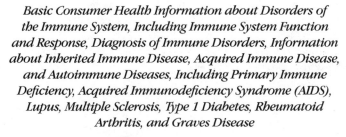

Basic Consumer Health Information about Disorders of the Immune System, Including Immune System Function and Response, Diagnosis of Immune Disorders, Information about Inherited Immune Disease, Acquired Immune Disease, and Autoimmune Diseases, Including Primary Immune Deficiency, Acquired Immunodeficiency Syndrome (AIDS), Lupus, Multiple Sclerosis, Type 1 Diabetes, Rheumatoid Arthritis, and Graves Disease

Along with Treatments, Tips for Coping with Immune Disorders, a Glossary, and a Directory of Additional Resources

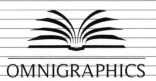

OMNIGRAPHICS

615 Griswold, Ste. 901, Detroit, MI 48226

Bibliographic Note
Because this page cannot legibly accommodate all the copyright notices, the Bibliographic
Note portion of the Preface constitutes an extension of the copyright notice.

* * *

Health Reference Series
Keith Jones, *Managing Editor*
***

OMNIGRAPHICS
A PART OF RELEVANT INFORMATION
***

Copyright © 2017 Omnigraphics
ISBN 978-0-7808-1468-4
E-ISBN 978-0-7808-1467-7

Library of Congress Cataloging-in-Publication Data

Title: Immune system disorders sourcebook: basic consumer health information
about disorders of the immune system, including immune system function and
response, diagnosis of immune disorders, information about inherited immune
disease, acquired immune disease, and autoimmune diseases, including primary
immune deficiency, acquired immunodeficiency syndrome (AIDS), lupus, multiple
sclerosis, type 1 diabetes, rheumatoid arthritis, and graves disease along with
treatments, tips for coping with immune disorders, a glossary, and a directory
of additional resources. Other titles: Basic consumer health information about
disorders of the immune system ...

Description: Third edition. I Detroit, MI: Omnigraphics, [2017] I Series: Health
reference series I Includes bibliographical references and index.

Identifiers: LCCN 2016039929 (print) I LCCN 2016041460 (ebook) I ISBN
9780780814684 (hardcover: alk. paper) I ISBN 9780780814677 (ebook) I ISBN
9780780814677 (eBook)

Subjects: LCSH: Immunologic diseases--Popular works.

Classification: LCC RC582.I4626 2017 (print) I LCC RC582 (ebook) I DDC
616.07/9--dc23

LC record available at https://lccn.loc.gov/2016039929

Table of Contents

Part III: Inherited Immune Deficiency Diseases

Part IV: Acquired Immune Deficiency Diseases

Part V: Autoimmune Diseases

Part VI: Other Altered Immune Responses

Part VII: Treatments for Immune Deficiencies and Diseases

Part VIII: Coping with Immune Disease

Part IX: Additional Help and Information

Preface

About This Book

The body's immune system usually works efficiently to ward off disease, but things can go wrong. Sometimes dysfunctions result from inherited conditions. Sometimes they are caused when bacteria or viruses, such as the human immunodeficiency virus (HIV), slip past normal immune system defenses. Sometimes, for reasons poorly understood, the immune system begins to attack normal body cells; this can result in an autoimmune disease. According to the National Institutes of Health (NIH), autoimmune diseases afflict over 23 million Americans and annual direct healthcare costs associated with AD are in the range of $100 billion. The NIH research plan also states that "Research discoveries of the last decade have made autoimmune research one of the most promising areas of new discovery."

Immune System Disorders Sourcebook, Third Edition, provides information about immune system function and related disorders. Readers will learn about inherited, acquired, and autoimmune diseases, including primary immune deficiency, acquired immunodeficiency syndrome (AIDS), lupus, multiple sclerosis, type 1 diabetes, rheumatoid arthritis, and Graves disease. Information about symptoms and treatments is included along with tips for coping with an immune disorder, suggestions for caregivers, glossaries of terms and diseases, and a directory of additional resources.

How to Use This Book

This book is divided into parts and chapters. Parts focus on broad areas of interest. Chapters are devoted to single topics within a part.

Part I: Immune System Overview describes how the immune system works and explains both natural and acquired immunity. It summarizes the types of disorders that affect the immune system and describes factors that influence its function. Research initiatives to help better understand the immune system and learn how it can be manipulated to produce health benefits are also described.

Part II: Diagnosis of Immune System Disorders provides information for people concerned about the diagnostic challenges involved in identifying immune disorders. Facts about the tests most commonly used, including blood, gene, and allergy tests, are provided.

Part III: Inherited Immune Deficiency Diseases explains the symptoms, diagnosis, and treatment of diseases that result when genetic defects cause essential parts of the immune system to be missing or to malfunction. Inherited immune deficiency diseases include primary immune deficiency (PID), ataxia-telangiectasia, hyper-immunoglobulin M (hyper-IgM) syndromes, and severe combined immunodeficiency (SCID). Rare primary immunodeficiency diseases such as common variable immunodeficiency (CVID), and leukocyte adhesion deficiency (LAD) are also discussed.

Part IV: Acquired Immune Deficiency Diseases describes immune system diseases that are not present at birth but that are acquired later. These can result from exposure to the human immunodeficiency virus (HIV), opportunistic infections, or the body's response to a transplant.

Part V: Autoimmune Diseases explains the symptoms, diagnosis, and treatment of diseases caused when immune cells mistake the body's own cells as invaders and attack them. Individual chapters cover diseases alphabetically from Addison disease to vitiligo.

Part VI: Other Altered Immune Responses describes immune system reactions to environmental triggers and medical treatments. Topics include allergies and asthma, blood transfusion reaction, transplant rejection, and anaphylaxis.

Part VII: Treatments for Immune Deficiencies and Diseases contains information about drug and gene therapies, and stem cell transplantation. Treatments used for specific immune diseases are also described.

Part VIII: Coping with Immune Disease provides tips for individuals and families living with an autoimmune or immune system disease, including, immunization recommendations, and suggestions for students and travelers with immune system disorders.

Part IX: Additional Help and Information offers glossaries of immune system terms and autoimmune diseases and a directory of resources.

Bibliographic Note

This volume contains documents and excerpts from publications issued by the following U.S. government agencies: AIDS.gov; Centers for Disease Control and Prevention (CDC); Environmental Protection Agency (EPA); Genetic and Rare Diseases Information Center (GARD); Genetics Home Reference (GHR); National Cancer Institute (NCI); National Eye Institute (NEI); National Heart, Lung, and Blood Institute (NHLBI); National Institute of Allergy and Infectious Diseases (NIAID); National Institute of Arthritis and Musculoskeletal and Skin Diseases (NIAMS); National Institute of Diabetes and Digestive and Kidney Diseases (NIDDK); National Institute of Mental Health (NIMH); National Institute of Neurological Disorders and Stroke (NINDS); National Institute on Alcohol Abuse and Alcoholism (NIAAA); National Institutes of Health (NIH); Office on Women's Health (OWH); and U.S. Department of Health and Human Services (HHS).

In addition, this volume contains copyrighted documents from the following organizations:

American Association for Clinical Chemistry (AACC)
The Nemours Foundation

It may also contain original material produced by Omnigraphics and reviewed by medical consultants.

About the Health Reference Series

The *Health Reference Series* is designed to provide basic medical information for patients, families, caregivers, and the general public. Each volume takes a particular topic and provides comprehensive coverage. This is especially important for people who may be dealing with a newly diagnosed disease or a chronic disorder in themselves or in a family member. People looking for preventive guidance, information about disease warning signs, medical statistics, and risk factors for health problems will also find answers to their questions in the

Health Reference Series. The *Series*, however, is not intended to serve as a tool for diagnosing illness, in prescribing treatments, or as a substitute for the physician/patient relationship. All people concerned about medical symptoms or the possibility of disease are encouraged to seek professional care from an appropriate health care provider.

A Note about Spelling and Style

Health Reference Series editors use *Stedman's Medical Dictionary* as an authority for questions related to the spelling of medical terms and the *Chicago Manual of Style* for questions related to grammatical structures, punctuation, and other editorial concerns. Consistent adherence is not always possible, however, because the individual volumes within the *Series* include many documents from a wide variety of different producers, and the editor's primary goal is to present material from each source as accurately as is possible. This sometimes means that information in different chapters or sections may follow other guidelines and alternate spelling authorities.

Medical Review

Omnigraphics contracts with a team of qualified, senior medical professionals who serve as medical consultants for the *Health Reference Series*. As necessary, medical consultants review reprinted and originally written material for currency and accuracy. Citations including the phrase, "Reviewed (month, year)" indicate material reviewed by this team. Medical consultation services are provided to the *Health Reference Series* editors by:

Dr. Senthil Selvan, MBBS, DCH, MD
Dr. K. Sivanandham, MBBS, DCH, MS (Research), PhD

Our Advisory Board

We would like to thank the following board members for providing initial guidance on the development of this series:

- Dr. Lynda Baker, Associate Professor of Library and Information Science, Wayne State University, Detroit, MI

- Nancy Bulgarelli, William Beaumont Hospital Library, Royal Oak, MI

- Karen Imarisio, Bloomfield Township Public Library, Bloomfield Township, MI

- Karen Morgan, Mardigian Library, University of Michigan-Dearborn, Dearborn, MI

- Rosemary Orlando, St. Clair Shores Public Library, St. Clair Shores, MI

Health Reference Series *Update Policy*

The inaugural book in the *Health Reference Series* was the first edition of *Cancer Sourcebook* published in 1989. Since then, the *Series* has been enthusiastically received by librarians and in the medical community. In order to maintain the standard of providing high-quality health information for the layperson the editorial staff at Omnigraphics felt it was necessary to implement a policy of updating volumes when warranted.

Medical researchers have been making tremendous strides, and it is the purpose of the *Health Reference Series* to stay current with the most recent advances. Each decision to update a volume is made on an individual basis. Some of the considerations include how much new information is available and the feedback we receive from people who use the books. If there is a topic you would like to see added to the update list, or an area of medical concern you feel has not been adequately addressed, please write to:

Managing Editor
Health Reference Series
Omnigraphics
615 Griswold, Ste. 901
Detroit, MI 48226

Part One

Immune System Overview

Chapter 1

Understanding the Immune System: How It Works

The immune system is a network of cells, tissues, and organs that work together to defend the body against attacks by foreign invaders. These are primarily microbes (germs)—tiny, infection-causing organisms such as bacteria, viruses, parasites, and fungi. Because the human body provides an ideal environment for many microbes, they try to break in. It is the immune system's job to keep them out, or failing that, to seek out and destroy them. When the immune system hits the wrong target or is crippled, it can unleash a torrent of diseases, including allergy, arthritis, or acquired immunodeficiency syndrome (AIDS).

The immune system is amazingly complex. It can recognize and remember millions of different enemies, and it can produce secretions and cells to match up with and wipe out each one of them. The secret to its success is an elaborate and dynamic communications network. Millions and millions of cells, organized into sets and subsets, gather like clouds of bees swarming around a hive and pass information back and forth. Once immune cells receive the alarm, they undergo tactical changes and begin to produce powerful chemicals. These substances allow the cells to regulate their own growth and behavior, enlist their fellows, and direct new recruits to trouble spots.

This chapter includes text excerpted from "Understanding the Immune System: How It Works," National Institute of Allergy and Infectious Diseases (NIAID), NIH Publication No. 03–5423, December 19, 2011. Reviewed October 2016.

Self and Non-Self

The key to a healthy immune system is its remarkable ability to distinguish between the body's own cells (self), and foreign cells (non-self). The body's immune defenses normally coexist peacefully with cells that carry distinctive self marker molecules. But when immune defenders encounter cells or organisms carrying markers that are foreign, they quickly launch an attack.

Anything that can trigger this immune response is called an antigen. An antigen can be a microbe such as a virus, or even a part of a microbe. Tissues or cells from another person (except an identical twin) also carry foreign markers and act as antigens. This explains why tissue transplants may be rejected.

In abnormal situations, the immune system can mistake cells as foreign and launch an attack against the body's own cells or tissues. The result is called an autoimmune disease. Some forms of arthritis and diabetes are autoimmune diseases. In other cases, the immune system responds to a seemingly harmless foreign substance such as ragweed pollen. The result is allergy, and this kind of antigen is called an allergen.

The Structure of the Immune System

The organs of the immune system are positioned throughout the body. They are called lymphoid organs because they are home to lymphocytes, small white blood cells that are the key players in the immune system.

Bone marrow, the soft tissue in the hollow center of bones, is the ultimate source of all blood cells, including white blood cells destined to become immune cells.

The thymus is an organ that lies behind the breastbone; lymphocytes known as T lymphocytes, or just T cells, mature in the thymus.

The spleen is a flattened organ at the upper left of the abdomen. Like the lymph nodes, the spleen contains specialized compartments where immune cells gather and work, and serves as a meeting ground where immune defenses confront antigens.

Clumps of lymphoid tissue are found in many parts of the body, especially in the linings of the digestive tract and the airways and lungs—territories that serve as gateways to the body. These tissues include the tonsils, adenoids, and appendix.

Lymphatic vessels carry lymph, a clear fluid that bathes the body's tissues. Lymphocytes can travel throughout the body using the blood vessels. The cells can also travel through a system of lymphatic vessels that closely parallels the body's veins and arteries. Cells and fluids are exchanged between blood and lymphatic vessels, enabling the lymphatic system to monitor the body for invading microbes.

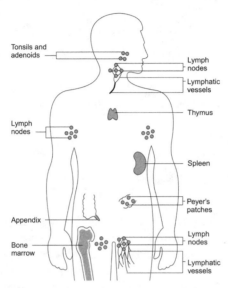

Figure 1.1. *Organs of the Immune System*

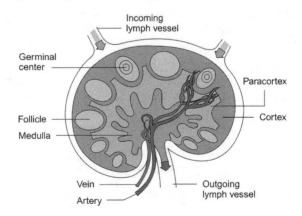

Figure 1.2. *Lymph Node*

The lymph node contains numerous specialized structures. T cells concentrate in the paracortex, B cells in and around the germinal centers, and plasma cells in the medulla.

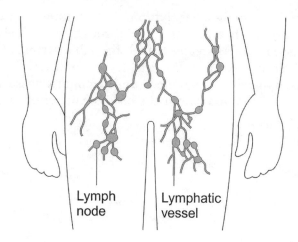

Figure 1.3. *Lymphatic Vessels*

Immune cells and foreign particles enter the lymph nodes via incoming lymphatic vessels or the lymph nodes' tiny blood vessels.

Lymph nodes—small, bean-shaped nodes—are laced along the lymphatic vessels, with clusters in the neck, armpits, abdomen, and groin. Each lymph node contains specialized compartments where immune cells congregate, and where they can encounter antigens. All lymphocytes exit lymph nodes through outgoing lymphatic vessels. Once in the bloodstream, they are transported to tissues throughout the body. They patrol everywhere for foreign antigens, then gradually drift back into the lymphatic system, to begin the cycle all over again.

Immune Cells and Their Products

The immune system stockpiles a huge arsenal of cells, not only lymphocytes, but also cell-devouring phagocytes and their relatives. Some immune cells take on all comers, while others are trained on highly specific targets. To work effectively, most immune cells need the cooperation of their comrades. Sometimes immune cells communicate by direct physical contact, sometimes by releasing chemical messengers.

The immune system stores just a few of each kind of the different cells needed to recognize millions of possible enemies. When an antigen appears, those few matching cells multiply into a full-scale army. After their job is done, they fade away, leaving sentries behind to watch for future attacks.

All immune cells begin as immature stem cells in the bone marrow. They respond to different cytokines and other signals to grow into specific immune cell types, such as T cells, B cells, or phagocytes. Because stem cells have not yet committed to a particular future, they are an interesting possibility for treating some immune system disorders. Researchers are investigating if a person's own stem cells can be used to regenerate damaged immune responses in autoimmune diseases and immune deficiency diseases.

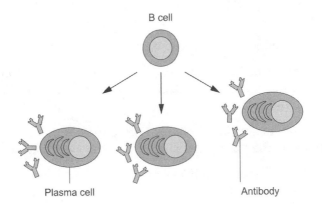

Figure 1.4. *B Cell*

B cells mature into plasma cells that produce antibodies.

B Lymphocytes

B cells and T cells are the main types of lymphocytes. B cells work chiefly by secreting substances called antibodies into the body's fluids. Antibodies ambush antigens circulating the bloodstream. However, they are powerless to penetrate cells. The job of attacking target cells— either cells that have been infected by viruses or cells that have been distorted by cancer—is left to T cells or other immune cells.

Each B cell is programmed to make one specific antibody. For example, one B cell will make an antibody that blocks a virus that causes the common cold, while another produces an antibody that attacks a bacterium that causes pneumonia.

When a B cell encounters its triggering antigen, it gives rise to many large cells known as plasma cells. Every plasma cell is essentially a factory for producing an antibody. Each of the plasma cells descended from a given B cell manufactures millions of identical antibody molecules and pours them into the bloodstream.

An antigen matches an antibody much as a key matches a lock. Some match exactly; others fit more like a skeleton key. But whenever antigen and antibody interlock, the antibody marks the antigen for destruction.

Antibodies belong to a family of large molecules known as immunoglobulins. Different types play different roles in the immune defense strategy.

- Immunoglobulin (Ig) G, or IgG, works efficiently to coat microbes, speeding their uptake by other cells in the immune system.

- IgM is very effective at killing bacteria.

- IgA concentrates in body fluids—tears, saliva, the secretions of the respiratory tract, and the digestive tract—guarding the entrances to the body.

- IgE, whose natural job probably is to protect against parasitic infections, is the villain responsible for the symptoms of allergy.

- IgD remains attached to B cells and plays a key role in initiating early B cell response.

T Cells

Unlike B cells, T cells do not recognize free-floating antigens. Rather, their surfaces contain specialized antibody-like receptors that see fragments of antigens on the surfaces of infected or cancerous cells. T cells contribute to immune defenses in two major ways: some direct and regulate immune responses; others directly attack infected or cancerous cells.

Helper T cells, or Th cells, coordinate immune responses by communicating with other cells. Some stimulate nearby B cells to produce antibodies, others call in microbe gobbling cells called phagocytes, still others activate other T cells.

Killer T cells—also called cytotoxic T lymphocytes (CTLs)—perform a different function. These cells directly attack other cells carrying certain foreign or abnormal molecules on their surfaces. CTLs are especially useful for attacking viruses because viruses often hide from other parts of the immune system while they grow inside infected cells. CTLs recognize small fragments of these viruses peeking out from the cell membrane and launch an attack to kill the cell.

In most cases, T cells only recognize an antigen if it is carried on the surface of a cell by one of the body's own major histocompatibility complex (MHC) molecules. MHC molecules are proteins recognized by T cells when distinguishing between self and non-self. A self MHC molecule provides a recognizable scaffolding to present a foreign antigen to the T cell.

Although MHC molecules are required for T cell responses against foreign invaders, they also pose a difficulty during organ transplantations. Virtually every cell in the body is covered with MHC proteins, but each person has a different set of these proteins on his or her cells. If a T cell recognizes a foreign MHC molecule on another cell, it will destroy the cell. Therefore, doctors must match organ recipients with donors who have the closest MHC makeup. Otherwise the recipient's T cells will likely attack the transplanted organ, leading to graft rejection.

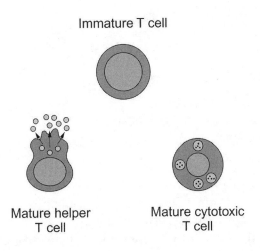

Immature T cell

Mature helper
T cell

Mature cytotoxic
T cell

Figure 1.5. *Types of T Cells*

Natural killer (NK) cells are another kind of lethal white cell, or lymphocyte. Like killer T cells, NK cells are armed with granules filled with potent chemicals. But while killer T cells look for antigen fragments bound to self-MHC molecules, NK cells recognize cells lacking self-MHC molecules. Thus NK cells have the potential to attack many types of foreign cells.

Both kinds of killer cells slay on contact. The deadly assassins bind to their targets, aim their weapons, and then deliver a lethal burst of chemicals.

9

Phagocytes and Their Relatives

Phagocytes are large white cells that can swallow and digest microbes and other foreign particles. Monocytes are phagocytes that circulate in the blood. When monocytes migrate into tissues, they develop into macrophages. Specialized types of macrophages can be found in many organs, including lungs, kidneys, brain, and liver.

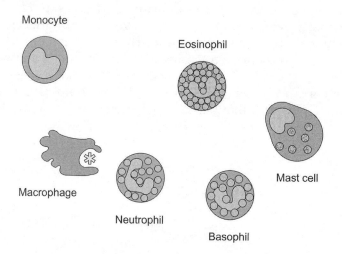

Figure 1.6. *Phagocytes and Their Relative Cells*

Phagocytes, granulocytes, and mast cells, all with different methods of attack, demonstrate the immune system's versatility.

Macrophages play many roles. As scavengers, they rid the body of worn-out cells and other debris. They display bits of foreign antigen in a way that draws the attention of matching lymphocytes. And they churn out an amazing variety of powerful chemical signals, known as monokine, which are vital to the immune responses.

Granulocytes are another kind of immune cell. They contain granules filled with potent chemicals, which allow the granulocytes to destroy microorganisms. Some of these chemicals, such as histamine, also contribute to inflammation and allergy.

One type of granulocyte, the neutrophil, is also a phagocyte; it uses its prepackaged chemicals to break down the microbes it ingests. Eosinophils and basophils are granulocytes that spray their chemicals onto harmful cells or microbes nearby.

The mast cell is a twin of the basophil, except that it is not a blood cell. Rather, it is found in the lungs, skin, tongue, and linings of the nose and intestinal tract, where it is responsible for the symptoms of allergy.

A related structure, the blood platelet, is a cell fragment. Platelets, too, contain granules. In addition to promoting blood clotting and wound repair, platelets activate some of the immune defenses.

Cytokines

Components of the immune system communicate with one another by exchanging chemical messengers called cytokines. These proteins are secreted by cells and act on other cells to coordinate an appropriate immune response. Cytokines include a diverse assortment of interleukins, interferons, and growth factors. Some cytokines are chemical switches that turn certain immune cell types on and off.

One cytokine, interleukin 2 (IL-2), triggers the immune system to produce T cells. IL-2's immunity-boosting properties have traditionally made it a promising treatment for several illnesses. Clinical studies are ongoing to test its benefits in other diseases such as cancer, hepatitis C, human immunodeficiency virus (HIV) infection, and AIDS. Other cytokines also are being studied for their potential clinical benefit.

Other cytokines chemically attract specific cell types. These so-called chemokines are released by cells at a site of injury or infection and call other immune cells to the region to help repair the damage or fight off the invader. Chemokines often play a key role in inflammation and are a promising target for new drugs to help regulate immune responses.

Complement

The complement system is made up of about 25 proteins that work together to complement the action of antibodies in destroying bacteria. It also helps to rid the body of antibody-coated antigens (antigen-antibody complexes). Complement proteins, which cause blood vessels to become dilated and then leaky, contribute to the redness, warmth, swelling, pain, and loss of function that characterize an inflammatory response.

Complement proteins circulate in the blood in an inactive form. When the first protein in the complement series is activated—typically by antibody that has locked onto an antigen—it sets in motion a domino effect. Each component takes its turn in a precise chain of steps known as the complement cascade. The end product is a cylinder inserted into and puncturing a hole in the cell's wall. With fluids and molecules flowing in and out, the cell swells and bursts. Other components of the complement system make bacteria more susceptible to phagocytosis or beckon other cells to the area.

Chapter 2

Immunity Types

Immunity to a disease is achieved through the presence of **anti-bodies** to that disease in a person's system. Antibodies are proteins produced by the body to neutralize or destroy toxins or disease-carrying organisms. Antibodies are disease-specific. For example, measles antibody will protect a person who is exposed to measles disease, but will have no effect if he or she is exposed to mumps.

There are two types of immunity: active and passive.

Active Immunity

Active immunity results when exposure to a disease organism triggers the immune system to produce antibodies to that disease. Exposure to the disease organism can occur through infection with the actual disease (resulting in **natural immunity**), or introduction of a killed or weakened form of the disease organism through vaccination (**vaccine-induced immunity**). Either way, if an immune person comes into contact with that disease in the future, their immune system will recognize it and immediately produce the antibodies needed to fight it.

Active immunity is long-lasting, and sometimes life-long.

Passive Immunity

Passive immunity is provided when a person is given antibodies to a disease rather than producing them through his or her own immune system.

This chapter includes text excerpted from "Vaccines and Immunizations," Centers for Disease Control and Prevention (CDC), May 19, 2014.

A newborn baby acquires passive immunity from its mother through the placenta. A person can also get passive immunity through anti-body-containing blood products such as **immune globulin**, which may be given when immediate protection from a specific disease is needed. This is the major advantage to passive immunity; protection is immediate, whereas active immunity takes time (usually several weeks) to develop.

However, passive immunity lasts only for a few weeks or months. Only active immunity is long-lasting.

Chapter 3

Features of an Immune Response

An immune response is generally divided into innate and adaptive immunity. Innate immunity occurs immediately, when circulating innate cells recognize a problem. Adaptive immunity occurs later, as it relies on the coordination and expansion of specific adaptive immune cells. Immune memory follows the adaptive response, when mature adaptive cells, highly specific to the original pathogen, are retained for later use.

Innate Immunity

Innate immune cells express genetically encoded receptors, called Toll-like receptors (TLRs), which recognize general danger- or pathogen-associated patterns. Collectively, these receptors can broadly recognize viruses, bacteria, fungi, and even non-infectious problems. However, they cannot distinguish between specific strains of bacteria or viruses.

There are numerous types of innate immune cells with specialized functions. They include neutrophils, eosinophils, basophils, mast cells, monocytes, dendritic cells, and macrophages. Their main feature is the ability to respond quickly and broadly when a problem arises, typically leading to inflammation. Innate immune cells also are important for

This chapter includes text excerpted from "Immune System Research," National Institute of Allergy and Infectious Diseases (NIAID), January 16, 2014.

activating adaptive immunity. Innate cells are critical for host defense, and disorders in innate cell function may cause chronic susceptibility to infection.

Adaptive Immunity

Adaptive immune cells are more specialized, with each adaptive B or T cell bearing unique receptors, B-cell receptors (BCRs) and T-cell receptors (TCRs), that recognize specific signals rather than general patterns. Each receptor recognizes an antigen, which is simply any molecule that may bind to a BCR or TCR. Antigens are derived from a variety of sources including pathogens, host cells, and allergens. Antigens are typically processed by innate immune cells and presented to adaptive cells in the lymph nodes.

The genes for BCRs and TCRs are randomly rearranged at specific cell maturation stages, resulting in unique receptors that may potentially recognize anything. Random generation of receptors allows the immune system to respond to new or unforeseen problems. This concept is especially important because environments may frequently change, for instance when seasons change or a person relocates, and pathogens are constantly evolving to survive. Because BCRs and TCRs are so specific, adaptive cells may only recognize one strain of a particular pathogen, unlike innate cells, which recognize broad classes of pathogens. In fact, a group of adaptive cells that recognize the same strain will likely recognize different areas of that pathogen.

If a B or T cell has a receptor that recognizes an antigen from a pathogen and also receives cues from innate cells that something is wrong, the B or T cell will activate, divide, and disperse to address the problem. B cells make antibodies, which neutralize pathogens, rendering them harmless. T cells carry out multiple functions, including killing infected cells and activating or recruiting other immune cells. The adaptive response has a system of checks and balances to prevent unnecessary activation that could cause damage to the host. If a B or T cell is autoreactive, meaning its receptor recognizes antigens from the body's own cells, the cell will be deleted. Also, if a B or T cell does not receive signals from innate cells, it will not be optimally activated.

Immune memory is a feature of the adaptive immune response. After B or T cells are activated, they expand rapidly. As the problem resolves, cells stop dividing and are retained in the body as memory cells. The next time this same pathogen enters the body, a memory cell is already poised to react and can clear away the pathogen before it establishes itself.

Vaccination

Vaccination, or immunization, is a way to train your immune system against a specific pathogen. Vaccination achieves immune memory without an actual infection, so the body is prepared when the virus or bacterium enters. Saving time is important to prevent a pathogen from establishing itself and infecting more cells in the body.

An effective vaccine will optimally activate both the innate and adaptive response. An immunogen is used to activate the adaptive immune response so that specific memory cells are generated. Because BCRs and TCRs are unique, some memory cells are simply better at eliminating the pathogen. The goal of vaccine design is to select immunogens that will generate the most effective and efficient memory response against a particular pathogen. Adjuvants, which are important for activating innate immunity, can be added to vaccines to optimize the immune response. Innate immunity recognizes broad patterns, and without innate responses, adaptive immunity cannot be optimally achieved.

Chapter 4

Immune Cells

Granulocytes include basophils, eosinophils, and neutrophils. Basophils and eosinophils are important for host defense against parasites. They also are involved in allergic reactions. Neutrophils, the most numerous innate immune cell, patrol for problems by circulating in the bloodstream. They can phagocytose, or ingest, bacteria, degrading them inside special compartments called vesicles.

Mast cells also are important for defense against parasites. Mast cells are found in tissues and can mediate allergic reactions by releasing inflammatory chemicals like histamine.

Monocytes, which develop into *macrophages*, also patrol and respond to problems. They are found in the bloodstream and in tissues. Macrophages, "big eater" in Greek, are named for their ability to ingest and degrade bacteria. Upon activation, monocytes and macrophages coordinate an immune response by notifying other immune cells of the problem. Macrophages also have important non-immune functions, such as recycling dead cells, like red blood cells, and clearing away cellular debris. These "housekeeping" functions occur without activation of an immune response.

Dendritic cells (DC) are an important antigen-presenting cell (APC), and they also can develop from monocytes. Antigens are molecules from pathogens, host cells, and allergens that may be recognized by adaptive immune cells. APCs like DCs are responsible for processing large molecules into "readable" fragments (antigens) recognized by

This chapter includes text excerpted from "Immune Cells," National Institute of Allergy and Infectious Diseases (NIAID), January 17, 2014.

adaptive B or T cells. However, antigens alone cannot activate T cells. They must be presented with the appropriate major histocompatiblity complex (MHC) expressed on the APC. MHC provides a checkpoint and helps immune cells distinguish between host and foreign cells.

Natural killer (NK) cells have features of both innate and adaptive immunity. They are important for recognizing and killing virus-infected cells or tumor cells. They contain intracellular compartments called granules, which are filled with proteins that can form holes in the target cell and also cause apoptosis, the process for programmed cell death. It is important to distinguish between apoptosis and other forms of cell death like necrosis. Apoptosis, unlike necrosis, does not release danger signals that can lead to greater immune activation and inflammation. Through apoptosis, immune cells can discreetly remove infected cells and limit bystander damage. Researchers have shown in mouse models that NK cells, like adaptive cells, can be retained as memory cells and respond to subsequent infections by the same pathogen.

Adaptive Cells

B cells have two major functions: They present antigens to T cells, and more importantly, they produce antibodies to neutralize infectious microbes. Antibodies coat the surface of a pathogen and serve three major roles: neutralization, opsonization, and complement activation.

Neutralization occurs when the pathogen, because it is covered in antibodies, is unable to bind and infect host cells. In opsonization, an antibody-bound pathogen serves as a red flag to alert immune cells like neutrophils and macrophages, to engulf and digest the pathogen. Complement is a process for directly destroying, or lysing, bacteria.

Antibodies are expressed in two ways. The B-cell receptor (BCR), which sits on the surface of a B cell, is actually an antibody. B cells also secrete antibodies to diffuse and bind to pathogens. This dual expression is important because the initial problem, for instance a bacterium, is recognized by a unique BCR and activates the B cell. The activated B cell responds by secreting antibodies, essentially the BCR but in soluble form. This ensures that the response is specific against the bacterium that started the whole process.

Every antibody is unique, but they fall under general categories: IgM, IgD, IgG, IgA, and IgE. (Ig is short for immunoglobulin, which is another word for antibody.) While they have overlapping roles, IgM generally is important for complement activation; IgD is involved in activating basophils; IgG is important for neutralization, opsonization, and complement activation; IgA is essential for neutralization in the gastrointestinal tract; and IgE is necessary for activating mast cells in parasitic and allergic responses.

T cells have a variety of roles and are classified by subsets. T cells are divided into two broad categories: CD8+ T cells or CD4+ T cells, based on which protein is present on the cell's surface. T cells carry out multiple functions, including killing infected cells and activating or recruiting other immune cells.

CD8+ T cells also are called cytotoxic T cells or cytotoxic lymphocytes (CTLs). They are crucial for recognizing and removing virus-infected cells and cancer cells. CTLs have specialized compartments, or granules, containing cytotoxins that cause apoptosis, i.e., programmed cell death. Because of its potency, the release of granules is tightly regulated by the immune system.

The four major CD4+ T-cell subsets are TH1, TH2, TH17, and Treg, with "TH" referring to "T helper cell." TH1 cells are critical for coordinating immune responses against intracellular microbes, especially bacteria. They produce and secrete molecules that alert and activate other immune cells, like bacteria-ingesting macrophages. TH2 cells are important for coordinating immune responses against extracellular pathogens, like helminths (parasitic worms), by alerting B cells, granulocytes, and mast cells. TH17 cells are named for their ability to produce interleukin 17 (IL-17), a signaling molecule that activates immune and non-immune cells. TH17 cells are important for recruiting neutrophils.

Regulatory T cells (Tregs), as the name suggests, monitor and inhibit the activity of other T cells. They prevent adverse immune activation and maintain tolerance, or the prevention of immune responses against the body's own cells and antigens.

Communication

Immune cells communicate in a number of ways, either by cell-to-cell contact or through secreted signaling molecules. Receptors and ligands are fundamental for cellular communication. Receptors are protein structures that may be expressed on the surface of a cell or in intracellular compartments. The molecules that activate receptors are called ligands, which may be free-floating or membrane-bound.

Ligand-receptor interaction leads to a series of events inside the cell involving networks of intracellular molecules that relay the message. By altering the expression and density of various receptors and ligands, immune cells can dispatch specific instructions tailored to the situation at hand.

Cytokines are small proteins with diverse functions. In immunity, there are several categories of cytokines important for immune cell growth, activation, and function.

- Colony-stimulating factors are essential for cell development and differentiation.

- Interferons are necessary for immune-cell activation. Type I interferons mediate antiviral immune responses, and type II interferon is important for antibacterial responses.

- Interleukins, which come in over 30 varieties, provide context-specific instructions, with activating or inhibitory responses.

- Chemokines are made in specific locations of the body or at a site of infection to attract immune cells. Different chemokines will recruit different immune cells to the site needed.

- The tumor necrosis factor (TNF) family of cytokines stimulates immune-cell proliferation and activation. They are critical for activating inflammatory responses, and as such, TNF blockers are used to treat a variety of disorders, including some autoimmune diseases.

Toll-like receptors (TLRs) are expressed on innate immune cells, like macrophages and dendritic cells. They are located on the cell surface or in intracellular compartments because microbes may be found in the body or inside infected cells. TLRs recognize general microbial patterns, and they are essential for innate immune-cell activation and inflammatory responses.

B-cell receptors (BCRs) and *T-cell receptors* (TCRs) are expressed on adaptive immune cells. They are both found on the cell surface, but BCRs also are secreted as antibodies to neutralize pathogens. The genes for BCRs and TCRs are randomly rearranged at specific cell-maturation stages, resulting in unique receptors that may potentially recognize anything. Random generation of receptors allows the immune system to respond to unforeseen problems. They also explain why memory B or T cells are highly specific and, upon re-encountering their specific pathogen, can immediately induce a neutralizing immune response.

Major histocompatibility complex (MHC), or *human leukocyte antigen* (HLA), proteins serve two general roles.

MHC proteins function as carriers to present antigens on cell surfaces. MHC class I proteins are essential for presenting viral antigens and are expressed by nearly all cell types, except red blood cells. Any cell infected by a virus has the ability to signal the problem through MHC class I proteins. In response, CD8+ T cells (also called CTLs) will recognize and kill infected cells. MHC class II proteins are generally only expressed by antigen-presenting cells like dendritic cells and macrophages. MHC class II proteins are important for presenting antigens to CD4+ T cells. MHC class II antigens are varied and include both pathogen- and host-derived molecules.

MHC proteins also signal whether a cell is a host cell or a foreign cell. They are very diverse, and every person has a unique set of MHC proteins inherited from his or her parents. As such, there are similarities in MHC proteins between family members. Immune cells use MHC to determine whether or not a cell is friendly. In organ transplantation, the MHC or HLA proteins of donors and recipients are matched to lower the risk of transplant rejection, which occurs when the recipient's immune system attacks the donor tissue or organ. In stem cell or bone marrow transplantation, improper MHC or HLA matching can result in graft-versus-host disease, which occurs when the donor cells attack the recipient's body.

Complement refers to a unique process that clears away pathogens or dying cells and also activates immune cells. Complement consists of a series of proteins found in the blood that form a membrane-attack complex. Complement proteins are only activated by enzymes when a problem, like an infection, occurs. Activated complement proteins stick to a pathogen, recruiting and activating additional complement proteins, which assemble in a specific order to form a round pore or hole. Complement literally punches small holes into the pathogen, creating leaks that lead to cell death. Complement proteins also serve as signaling molecules that alert immune cells and recruit them to the problem area.

Chapter 5

Immune Tolerance

Features of Immune Tolerance

Tolerance is the prevention of an immune response against a particular antigen. For instance, the immune system is generally tolerant of self-antigens, so it does not usually attack the body's own cells, tissues, and organs. However, when tolerance is lost, disorders like autoimmune disease or food allergy may occur. Tolerance is maintained in a number of ways:

- When adaptive immune cells mature, there are several checkpoints in place to eliminate autoreactive cells. If a B cell produces antibodies that strongly recognize host cells, or if a T cell strongly recognizes self-antigen, they are deleted.

- Nevertheless, there are autoreactive immune cells present in healthy individuals. Autoreactive immune cells are kept in a non-reactive, or anergic, state. Even though they recognize the body's own cells, they do not have the ability to react and cannot cause host damage.

- Regulatory immune cells circulate throughout the body to maintain tolerance. Besides limiting autoreactive cells, regulatory cells are important for turning an immune response off after the problem is resolved. They can act as drains, depleting areas of

This chapter includes text excerpted from "Immune Tolerance," National Institute of Allergy and Infectious Diseases (NIAID), January 17, 2014.

essential nutrients that surrounding immune cells need for activation or survival.

• Some locations in the body are called immunologically privileged sites. These areas, like the eye and brain, do not typically elicit strong immune responses. Part of this is because of physical barriers, like the blood-brain barrier, that limit the degree to which immune cells may enter. These areas also may express higher levels of suppressive cytokines to prevent a robust immune response.

Fetomaternal tolerance is the prevention of a maternal immune response against a developing fetus. Major histocompatibility complex (MHC) proteins help the immune system distinguish between host and foreign cells. MHC also is called human leukocyte antigen (HLA). By expressing paternal MHC or HLA proteins and paternal antigens, a fetus can potentially trigger the mother's immune system. However, there are several barriers that may prevent this from occurring: The placenta reduces the exposure of the fetus to maternal immune cells, the proteins expressed on the outer layer of the placenta may limit immune recognition, and regulatory cells and suppressive signals may play a role.

Transplantation of a donor tissue or organ requires appropriate MHC or HLA matching to limit the risk of rejection. Because MHC or HLA matching is rarely complete, transplant recipients must continuously take immunosuppressive drugs, which can cause complications like higher susceptibility to infection and some cancers. Researchers are developing more targeted ways to induce tolerance to transplanted tissues and organs while leaving protective immune responses intact.

Chapter 6

Disorders of the Immune System

Complications arise when the immune system does not function properly. Some issues are less pervasive, such as pollen allergy, while others are extensive, such as genetic disorders that wipe out the presence or function of an entire set of immune cells.

Immune Deficiencies

Immune deficiencies may be temporary or permanent. Temporary immune deficiency can be caused by a variety of sources that weaken the immune system. Common infections, including influenza and mononucleosis, can suppress the immune system.

When immune cells are the target of infection, severe immune suppression can occur. For example, HIV specifically infects T cells, and their elimination allows for secondary infections by other pathogens. Patients receiving chemotherapy, bone marrow transplants, or immunosuppressive drugs experience weakened immune systems until immune cell levels are restored. Pregnancy also suppresses the maternal immune system, increasing susceptibility to infections by common microbes.

Primary immune deficiency diseases (PIDDs) are inherited genetic disorders and tend to cause chronic susceptibility to infection. There are over 150 PIDDs, and almost all are considered rare (affecting

This chapter includes text excerpted from "Disorders of the Immune System," National Institute of Allergy and Infectious Diesease (NIAID), January 17, 2014.

fewer than 200,000 people in the United States). They may result from altered immune signaling molecules or the complete absence of mature immune cells. For instance, X-linked severe combined immunodeficiency (SCID) is caused by a mutation in a signaling receptor gene, rendering immune cells insensitive to multiple cytokines. Without the growth and activation signals delivered by cytokines, immune cell subsets, particularly T and natural killer cells, fail to develop normally. The NIAID Primary Immune Deficiency Clinic was established with the goal of accepting all PIDD patients for examination to provide a disease diagnosis and better treatment recommendations.

Allergy

Allergies are a form of hypersensitivity reaction, typically in response to harmless environmental allergens like pollen or food. Hypersensitivity reactions are divided into four classes. Class I, II, and III are caused by antibodies, IgE or IgG, which are produced by B cells in response to an allergen. Overproduction of these antibodies activates immune cells like basophils and mast cells, which respond by releasing inflammatory chemicals like histamine. Class IV reactions are caused by T cells, which may either directly cause damage themselves or activate macrophages and eosinophils that damage host cells.

Autoimmune Diseases

Autoimmune diseases occur when self-tolerance is broken. Self-tolerance breaks when adaptive immune cells that recognize host cells persist unchecked. B cells may produce antibodies targeting host cells, and active T cells may recognize self-antigen. This amplifies when they recruit and activate other immune cells.

Autoimmunity is either organ-specific or systemic, meaning it affects the whole body. For instance, type I diabetes is organ-specific and caused by immune cells erroneously recognizing insulin-producing pancreatic β cells as foreign. However, systemic lupus erythematosus, commonly called lupus, can result from antibodies that recognize antigens expressed by nearly all healthy cells. Autoimmune diseases have a strong genetic component, and with advances in gene sequencing tools, researchers have a better understanding of what may contribute to specific diseases.

Sepsis

Sepsis may refer to an infection of the bloodstream, or it can refer to a systemic inflammatory state caused by the uncontrolled, broad release of cytokines that quickly activate immune cells throughout the body. Sepsis is an extremely serious condition and is typically triggered by an infection. However, the damage itself is caused by cytokines (the adverse response is sometimes referred to as a "cytokine storm"). The systemic release of cytokines may lead to loss of blood pressure, resulting in septic shock and possible multi-organ failure.

Cancer

Some forms of cancer are directly caused by the uncontrolled growth of immune cells. Leukemia is cancer caused by white blood cells, which is another term for immune cells. Lymphoma is cancer caused by lymphocytes, which is another term for adaptive B or T cells. Myeloma is cancer caused by plasma cells, which are mature B cells. Unrestricted growth of any of these cell types causes cancer.

In addition, an emerging concept is that cancer progression may partially result from the ability of cancer cells to avoid immune detection. The immune system is capable of removing infectious pathogens and dangerous host cells like tumors. Cancer researchers are studying how the tumor microenvironment may allow cancer cells to evade immune cells. Immune evasion may result from the abundance of suppressive, regulatory immune cells, excessive inhibitory cytokines, and other features that are not well understood.

Chapter 7

Understanding How Vaccines Work

Diseases that vaccines prevent can be dangerous, or even deadly. Vaccines greatly reduce the risk of infection by working with the body's natural defenses to safely develop immunity to disease. This chapter explains how the body fights infection and how vaccines work to protect people by producing immunity.

The Immune System—The Body's Defense against Infection

To understand how vaccines work, it is helpful to first look at how the body fights illness. When germs, such as bacteria or viruses, invade the body, they attack and multiply. This invasion is called an infection, and the infection is what causes illness. The immune system uses several tools to fight infection. Blood contains red blood cells, for carrying oxygen to tissues and organs, and white or immune cells, for fighting infection. These white cells consist primarily of B-lymphocytes, T-lymphocytes, and macrophages:

- **Macrophages** are white blood cells that swallow up and digest germs, plus dead or dying cells. The macrophages leave behind parts of the invading germs called antigens. The body identifies antigens as dangerous and stimulates the body to attack them.

This chapter includes text excerpted from "Understanding How Vaccines Work," Centers for Disease Control and Prevention (CDC), February 2013.

- **Antibodies** attack the antigens left behind by the macrophages. Antibodies are produced by defensive white blood cells called **B-lymphocytes**.

- **T-lymphocytes** are another type of defensive white blood cell. They attack cells in the body that have already been infected.

The first time the body encounters a germ, it can take several days to make and use all the germ-fighting tools needed to get over the infection. After the infection, the immune system remembers what it learned about how to protect the body against that disease.

The body keeps a few T-lymphocytes, called memory cells that go into action quickly if the body encounters the same germ again. When the familiar antigens are detected, B-lymphocytes produce antibodies to attack them.

How Vaccines Work

Vaccines help develop immunity by imitating an infection. This type of infection, however, does not cause illness, but it does cause the immune system to produce T-lymphocytes and antibodies. Sometimes, after getting a vaccine, the imitation infection can cause minor symptoms, such as fever. Such minor symptoms are normal and should be expected as the body builds immunity.

Once the imitation infection goes away, the body is left with a supply of "memory" T-lymphocytes, as well as B-lymphocytes that will remember how to fight that disease in the future. However, it typically takes a few weeks for the body to produce T-lymphocytes and B-lymphocytes after vaccination. Therefore, it is possible that a person who was infected with a disease just before or just after vaccination could develop symptoms and get a disease, because the vaccine has not had enough time to provide protection.

Types of Vaccines

Scientists take many approaches to designing vaccines. These approaches are based on information about the germs (viruses or bacteria) the vaccine will prevent, such as how it infects cells and how the immune system responds to it. Practical considerations, such as regions of the world where the vaccine would be used, are also important because the strain of a virus and environmental conditions, such as temperature and risk of exposure, may be different in various parts of the world. The vaccine delivery options available may also differ geographically. There are five main types of vaccines that infants and young children commonly receive:

- **Live, attenuated vaccines** fight viruses. These vaccines contain a version of the living virus that has been weakened so that it does not cause serious disease in people with healthy immune systems. Because live, attenuated vaccines are the closest thing to a natural infection, they are good teachers for the immune system. Examples of live, attenuated vaccines include measles, mumps, and rubella vaccine (MMR) and varicella (chickenpox) vaccine. Even though these vaccines are very effective, not everyone can receive them. Children with weakened immune systems—for example, those who are undergoing chemotherapy—cannot get live vaccines.

- **Inactivated vaccines** also fight viruses. These vaccines are made by inactivating, or killing, the virus during the process of making the vaccine. The inactivated polio vaccine is an example of this type of vaccine. Inactivated vaccines produce immune responses in different ways than live, attenuated vaccines. Often, multiple doses are necessary to build up and/or maintain immunity.

- **Toxoid vaccines** prevent diseases caused by bacteria that produce toxins (poisons) in the body. In the process of making these vaccines, the toxins are weakened so they cannot cause illness. Weakened toxins are called toxoids. When the immune system receives a vaccine containing a toxoid, it learns how to fight off the natural toxin. The DTaP vaccine contains diphtheria and tetanus toxoids.

- **Subunit vaccines** include only parts of the virus or bacteria, or subunits, instead of the entire germ. Because these vaccines contain only the essential antigens and not all the other molecules that make up the germ, side effects are less common. The pertussis (whooping cough) component of the DTaP vaccine is an example of a subunit vaccine.

- **Conjugate vaccines** fight a different type of bacteria. These bacteria have antigens with an outer coating of sugar-like substances called polysaccharides. This type of coating disguises the antigen, making it hard for a young child's immature immune system to recognize it and respond to it. Conjugate vaccines are effective for these types of bacteria because they connect (or conjugate) the polysaccharides to antigens that the immune system responds to very well. This linkage helps the immature immune system react to the coating and develop an immune response. An example of this type of vaccine is the Haemophilus influenzae type B (Hib) vaccine.

Vaccines Require More than One Dose

There are four reasons that babies—and even teens or adults for that matter—who receive a vaccine for the first time may need more than one dose:

- For some vaccines (primarily inactivated vaccines), the first dose does not provide as much immunity as possible. So, more than one dose is needed to build more complete immunity. The vaccine that protects against the bacteria Hib, which causes meningitis, is a good example.

- In other cases, such as the DTaP vaccine, which protects against diphtheria, tetanus, and pertussis, the initial series of four shots that children receive as part of their infant immunizations helps them build immunity. After a while, however, that immunity begins to wear off. At that point, a "booster" dose is needed to bring immunity levels back up. This booster dose is needed at 4 years through 6 years old for DTaP. Another booster against these diseases is needed at 11 years or 12 years of age. This booster for older children—and teens and adults, too—is called Tdap.

- For some vaccines (primarily live vaccines), studies have shown that more than one dose is needed for everyone to develop the best immune response. For example, after one dose of the MMR vaccine, some people may not develop enough antibodies to fight off infection. The second dose helps make sure that almost everyone is protected.

- Finally, in the case of the flu vaccine, adults and children (older than 6 months) need to get a dose every year. Children 6 months through 8 years old who have never gotten the flu vaccine in the past or have only gotten one dose in past years need two doses the first year they are vaccinated against flu for best protection. Then, annual flu shots are needed because the disease-causing viruses may be different from year to year. Every year, the flu vaccine is designed to prevent the specific viruses that experts predict will be circulating.

The Bottom Line

Some people believe that naturally acquired immunity—immunity from having the disease itself—is better than the immunity provided by vaccines. However, natural infections can cause severe complications and be deadly. This is true even for diseases that most people consider mild, like chickenpox. It is impossible to predict who will get serious infections that may lead to hospitalization. Vaccines, like any medication, can cause side effects. The most common side effects are mild. However, many vaccine-preventable disease symptoms can be serious, or even deadly. Although many of these diseases are rare in this country, they do circulate around the world and can be brought into the United States, putting unvaccinated children at risk. Even with advances in healthcare, the diseases that vaccines prevent can still be very serious—and vaccination is the best way to prevent them.

Chapter 8

Influence of Alcohol on Immune Response

Alcohol affects many organs, including the immune system, with even moderate amounts of alcohol influencing immune responses. Although alcohol can alter the actions of all cell populations involved in the innate and adaptive immune responses, the effect in many cases is a subclinical immunosuppression that becomes clinically relevant only after a secondary insult (e.g., bacterial or viral infection or other tissue damage). Alcohol's specific effects on the innate immune system depend on the pattern of alcohol exposure, with acute alcohol inhibiting and chronic alcohol accelerating inflammatory responses. The proinflammatory effects of chronic alcohol play a major role in the pathogenesis of alcoholic liver disease and pancreatitis, but also affect numerous other organs and tissues. In addition to promoting proinflammatory immune responses, alcohol also impairs anti-inflammatory cytokines. Chronic alcohol exposure also interferes with the normal functioning of all aspects of the adaptive immune response, including both cell-mediated and humoral responses. All of these effects enhance the susceptibility of chronic alcoholics to viral and bacterial infections and to sterile inflammation.

Alcohol has been the most common substance of use and abuse in human history. Moderate amounts of alcohol are enjoyed for its anxiolytic effects; however, its addictive properties can lead to chronic, excessive alcohol use and alcohol use disorder. In addition to its

This chapter includes text excerpted from "Alcohol's Effect on Host Defense," National Institute on Alcohol Abuse and Alcoholism (NIAAA), 2015.

commonly recognized behavioral effects, alcohol affects many organs, including the immune system that controls the body's defense against infectious pathogens (e.g., bacteria and viruses) and other harmful agents. Chronic alcohol use is associated with significant alterations in the immune system that predispose people to viral and bacterial infections and cancer development. In general, severe chronic alcoholics are considered immunocompromised hosts. Although moderate alcohol use has less obvious clinical effects on the immune system, both in vitro and in vivo studies indicate that even moderate amounts of alcohol and binge drinking modulate host immune responses.

This chapter gives a general overview of the immune effects of alcohol. However, it is important to realize that many aspects of alcohol consumption and its effects on immunity and host defense have not yet been fully elucidated. For example, the pattern of alcohol consumption (e.g., occasional binge drinking versus chronic heavy drinking) may affect the immune system in different ways that are yet to be explored.

Overview of the Immune System

The immune system serves to defend the host from pathogens and to prevent unwanted immune reactions to self. This defense involves coordinated complex interactions between two arms of the immune system—the innate and the adaptive immune responses. Innate immunity provides immediate responses to pathogen-derived or nonpathogen-associated (i.e., sterile) danger signals and results in activation of proinflammatory cytokines and/or Type I interferons, regardless of the underlying cause and without the body having encountered the pathogen before. Adaptive immunity, in contrast, which only sets in after a certain delay, is specific to the pathogen or antigen and requires an initial encounter with the pathogen or antigen to activate the response.

Alcohol's Effects on the Immune System

Alcohol can modulate the activities of all of these cell populations by affecting the frequency, survival, and function of most of these cells, thereby interfering with pivotal immune responses. However, unlike other mechanisms that cause classical immunocompromised states, such as HIV or tuberculosis infection, alcohol use typically results in a subclinical immunosuppression that becomes clinically significant only in case of a secondary insult. For example, chronic alcohol consumption increases the risk and severity of chronic infections with HIV; hepatitis C virus (HCV); or *Mycobacterium tuberculosis*, the bacterium that causes tuberculosis, and promotes posttrauma immunosuppression.

Emerging evidence also suggests that alcohol may affect immune functions by altering the balance and interactions between the host immune system and the entirety of microorganisms found in the host (i.e., the host microbiome). This microbiome is composed of the normal microorganisms found in and on the body (i.e., commensal microorganisms), which are needed for the body's normal functioning, and disease-causing pathogens. Increasing evidence suggests that alcohol may modulate the composition of pathogenic and commensal organisms in the microbiome of the gut, oral cavity, skin, and other mucosal surfaces. These alcohol-induced changes could have clinical significance because the composition of the microbiome sends important pathogenic as well as homeostatic signals for the functions of host immunity. For example, chronic alcohol use is associated with changes in the gut microbiome, both increasing the microbial content in the first part of the large intestine (i.e., cecum) and changing the abundance of different types of microorganisms in the gut. This may alter the levels of lipopolysaccharides (LPS) released by certain types of bacteria in the gut, which can contribute to inflammation in alcoholic liver disease as well as in liver cancer (i.e., hepatocellular carcinoma).

Alcohol-Induced Modulation of the Host Defense against Different Pathogens

It has been known for decades that chronic alcoholic individuals have increased susceptibility to infections. This increased susceptibility to both viral and bacterial infections has been attributed to alcohol's general immunosuppressive effects, and animal models of chronic alcohol use and infections repeatedly have confirmed this. In addition, chronic alcoholics seem to be vulnerable to inflammatory reactions not associated with pathogenic infections (i.e., sterile inflammation).

Viral Infections

Most evidence for alcohol-associated increases in susceptibility to infection comes from studies of human viral infections, such as HCV, hepatitis B virus (HBV), HIV, and pulmonary viral infections. Such investigations have yielded the following findings:

- The prevalence of HCV infection is higher in individuals with chronic alcohol use than in the general population. Alcohol exposure and HCV interact at several levels. For example, alcohol exposure augments HCV replication by altering the levels of a molecule that supports HCV replication (i.e., microRNA-122) in liver cells (i.e., hepatocytes). Moreover, alcohol and HCV synergistically impair antiviral immunity by interfering with the function of antigen-presenting cells, altering the activity and frequency of Treg cells, and modifying production of Type-I interferons. In patients with liver disease caused by chronic HCV infection, chronic alcohol use is an independent risk factor for development of advanced liver disease and cirrhosis.

• Chronic HBV infection affects about 240 million people worldwide. Research has shown that alcohol use accelerates the progression of liver disease caused by chronic HBV infection to liver fibrosis and hepatocellular cancer. However, the cellular and molecular mechanisms by which alcohol and HBV interact still await further investigations.

• Studies on the effect of alcohol on HIV infectivity in humans have yielded conflicting results. However, the combined immunosuppressive effects of alcohol use and advanced HIV infection (AIDS) are well established.

• In pulmonary viral infections, it is unclear whether alcohol increases susceptibility to influenza infections or adversely affects the outcome of established infections. However, in animal models of pulmonary infections, alcohol administration is associated with adverse clinical parameters and increased lung damage.

Bacterial Infections

Bacterial infections can be either systemic or localized to a specific organ, such as the lungs. Alcohol use has negative effects on all types of pulmonary bacterial infections. For example, infections with *Mycobacterium tuberculosis* are more severe in chronic alcoholics, and alcohol use is associated with systemic dissemination of tuberculosis. Furthermore, infections with *Klebsiella pneumoniae* and *Streptococcus pneumoniae*, common causes of pneumonia in humans, are more common in alcoholics compared with the nonalcoholic general population. Alcohol-induced dysfunction of specific immune cells contributes to severe pneumonias in this population. For example, the function of alveolar macrophages is impaired because of alcohol-induced changes in cytokine profiles as well as in the levels of reactive oxygen species (ROS) and antioxidants that result in oxidative stress. Recruitment and function of neutrophils in alcoholic individuals also are increased, resulting in increased tissue damage in the lung alveoli.

Not only chronic alcohol abuse but also acute alcohol exposure can impair immune response to pulmonary infections. For example, acute intoxication in humans with blood alcohol levels of 0.2 percent can severely disrupt neutrophil functioning and their ability to destroy bacteria. Studies in laboratory animals have confirmed the adverse effects of acute alcohol exposure on pulmonary infections. Thus, acute alcohol exposure in animals that were then infected with *S. pneumoniae* impaired lung chemokine activity in response to the infection, which resulted in reduced recruitment of immune cells into the lungs, decreased bacterial clearance from the lungs, and increased mortality.

Sterile Inflammation

Inflammatory reactions (i.e., innate immune responses) can be induced not only by invading pathogens but also by danger signals resulting from damage to the body's own cells. Elucidation of the immune processes occurring in response to damaged self also may offer a better understanding of the proinflammatory effects of alcohol in various organs (e.g., liver or brain). One example of this is the relationship between gut-derived bacterial LPS, alcohol exposure, and inflammatory reactions. Although gut-derived LPS clearly has a role in alcoholic liver disease, it is equally clear that LPS alone does not cause alcoholic liver disease. Many other conditions associated with increased levels of gut-derived LPS in the systemic circulation, such as HIV infection or inflammatory bowel disease, do not involve liver disease. Furthermore, inflammatory reactions can occur in the brain after alcohol use, even in the absence of detectable LPS in the brain. These observations suggest that although gut-derived LPS can promote tissue inflammation, another alcohol-induced component is required as well. Thus, it seems that alcohol exposure directly leads to the release of sterile danger signals from parenchymal cells in different tissues, which in turn result in the activation of inflammatory cells via toll-like receptors (TLRs) and nod-like receptors (NLRs). These alcohol-induced sterile danger signals include a wide variety of molecules, such as high-mobility-group protein B1 (HMGB1), heat shock proteins, adenosine triphosphate (ATP), and potassium ions.

It is now thought that alcohol-induced sterile danger signals contribute to the proinflammatory cytokine activation seen after chronic alcohol use in various organs (e.g., liver, intestine, and brain). This hypothesis also is supported by findings that in hepatocytes, alcohol

41

exposure results in a rapid induction of apoptosis, which precedes induction of inflammatory cytokines. Additional evidence for the role of sterile inflammatory signals in alcohol-induced inflammation and tissue damage comes from findings that HMGB1 is increased both in the liver and brain after chronic alcohol exposure. Finally, NLRs, specifically NLRP3 and NLRP4, have been found to be involved in alcoholic liver inflammation. Given the role of NLRs in sensing endogenous danger molecules, this observation further supports the notion that alcohol-induced tissue inflammations is caused at least partially by alcohol-induced danger signals.

Chapter 9

Immune System Research

Antibodies are made by B cells, and each antibody recognizes a unique molecule. This specificity makes antibodies a powerful research, diagnostic, and therapeutic tool. Antibodies are used by researchers for a variety of reasons, but they are mainly used for labeling, in one form or another. For instance, scientists studying a protein, like a cytokine, need a way to isolate this protein from samples. With an antibody specific for the protein, they may easily separate the protein through binding assays.

Scientists also may want to visualize a protein on a cell to understand how it works. Antibodies coupled with other tags, like a fluorescent label, allow researchers to image a cell and see how the protein is expressed. This concept also is useful for separating cells. For example, scientists studying T cells need to isolate T cells from all others. By identifying proteins expressed only on T cells, an antibody specific for this protein allows researchers to pull T cells out of a sample.

Antibodies are used clinically and are the subject of numerous clinical trials. Conceptually, antibodies may be used to soak up or block harmful proteins in a disease setting. For instance, tumor necrosis factor (TNF) is an inflammatory cytokine that may worsen symptoms in several diseases, like Crohn's disease and rheumatoid arthritis. There are several U.S. Food and Drug Administration (FDA)-approved drugs that target TNF, and these drugs are actually antibodies that block TNF and alleviate disease symptoms. Antibodies also are used in cancer

This chapter includes text excerpted from "Immune System Research," National Institute of Allergy and Infectious Diseases (NIAID), June 16, 2014.

therapy. Proteins that suppress immune cells may be targeted by antibodies, so that immune cells remain active to clear away cancer cells.

Genetic Engineering

Genetic engineering is another useful research tool. In model systems, scientists can study and manipulate genes, in animals ranging from fruit flies to mice, to understand what causes various diseases and how to treat them. Gene therapy has been studied in clinical trials to treat diseases. For instance, patients with genetic immune disorders, like severe combined immunodeficiency (SCID), may receive a copy of the gene they are missing, to potentially restore healthy immune function. Gene therapy studies are ongoing, to understand long-term effectiveness and side effects.

Epigenetics

Epigenetics is the study of gene expression, particularly factors unrelated to changes in gene sequence that may turn it "on" or "off." Genes are DNA blueprints that code for RNA, which is translated into protein, like a cytokine. When an immune cell activates and needs to produce cytokines to signal other cells, the cytokine gene needs to be in an "on" state for this to occur. If the gene is in an "off" state, it cannot be stimulated, no matter what cues are present around the cell.

Scientists study how gene status is regulated through epigenetic processes that alter the on/off state, generally by regulating how tightly DNA is packed around proteins in the nucleus. Tightly wound DNA is inaccessible and "off," while loosely wound DNA is accessible and "on." Understanding epigenetic mechanisms may lead to new therapy, and drugs that target epigenetic processes are currently being studied in clinical trials. Instead of blocking a harmful protein with antibodies, a drug that targets epigenetic mechanisms may potentially prevent that harmful protein from being made in the first place.

Immunotherapy

Immunotherapy is the manipulation of the immune system to solve a health problem. There are many clinical trials examining immunotherapy for cancer by directing the patient's own immune system to attack cancer cells. Researchers have examined the potential of innate and adaptive cells to fight cancer. Similar to how vaccines induce memory responses against a particular microbe, cancer immunotherapy is an attempt to induce effective immune responses against a specific cancer.

Immunotherapy may be used to treat food allergy, another focus of clinical trials. Oral immunotherapy is feeding small, increasing amounts of a food allergen—milk, egg, or peanut—to an allergic person over time. Studies show that this can decrease sensitivity to an allergen, but it must be done under the supervision of a physician. New clinical trials are testing other routes, like a skin patch, to deliver immunotherapy for allergies.

Metabolism

In recent years, scientists have focused on the role of the immune system in regulating metabolism. The activity of immune cells, like macrophages, may influence a variety of diseases including diabetes, obesity, and atherosclerosis. For example, signals secreted by macrophages may affect the activity and size of adipocytes, which are the cells that store fat as energy. More research must be done to understand how the immune system and inflammatory responses contribute to metabolic disorders.

Microbiome

The human microbiome is the trillions of relatively harmless microorganisms (bacteria, fungi, and viruses) that reside on and in the human body. These resident microbes also are referred to as commensals. Scientists are beginning to understand the essential role of the microbiome in human health. Without commensals, the immune system fails to develop properly.

Studies in animal models have shown that commensals play an important role in altering the activity of immune cells, which may lead to different outcomes in disease settings. More work is needed however, to understand how different commensals skew immune responses and how these changes may affect various human diseases.

Part Two

Diagnosis of Immune System Disorders

Chapter 10

Getting a Proper Diagnosis of Autoimmune Disease

Problems with Diagnosing Autoimmune Diseases

People with autoimmune diseases face significant difficulty in getting an accurate diagnosis. The symptoms of many autoimmune diseases, such as fatigue, fever, depression, and difficulty concentrating, tend to be very general in nature and easily attributed to other illnesses. And sometimes doctors attribute the varied symptoms to stress, worry, or other conditions.

More than 80 autoimmune diseases exist, and the diagnosis is only slightly different for each of them. Determination is made even more difficult by the fact that autoimmune diseases often arrive unpredictably, and testing for them can be a lengthy and complicated process.

What Are Autoimmune Diseases?

In all autoimmune disorders the immune system turns on itself and begins attacking the body's own cells. Rather than making antibodies that fight infection, the body begins producing autoantibodies, which attack body tissue. The localization of the attack determines the disorder and associated symptoms.

"Getting a Proper Diagnosis of Autoimmune Disease," © 2017 Omnigraphics. Reviewed October 2016.

49

Many autoimmune diseases are thought to be triggered when the body is exposed to foreign agents. These can range from infections to foods, such as iodine and gluten, to toxins like smoke, drugs, hair dyes, and chemicals in the home or at the work place.

Symptoms of Autoimmune Diseases

The symptoms of autoimmune disorders are often nonspecific and may linger for a considerable length of time. They can include:

- fatigue

- weakness

- muscle and joint pain

- low-grade fever

- rashes

- weight loss

- difficulty concentrating

- heart palpitations

- shortness of breath

- miscarriage

Autoimmune diseases are generally chronic and not fatal. The objective of treatment is to control the disease and not necessarily to cure it.

Why Autoimmune Diseases Are Difficult to Diagnose

Reasons that autoimmune diseases can be very difficult to diagnose include:

- Symptoms may be delayed or completely absent. For example, symptoms of celiac disease may be present in children as young as nine months of age or remain latent until well into adulthood.

- Many symptoms are common to a number of autoimmune diseases, as well as other disorders. Joint pain is one such common symptom, but some diseases are systemic and can cause pain anywhere in the body.

- One autoimmune condition can mask another, which increases the difficulty of making a diagnosis.

- Some people tend to disregard pain and avoid consulting a doctor, thinking that their symptoms are too mild or that they are too young to be afflicted with such conditions as rheumatoid arthritis.

- Autoimmune diseases mimic one another. For instance, multiple sclerosis looks similar to lupus and other neurological conditions. This makes it difficult to rule out one or the other.

- Autoimmune disease symptoms present differently in different individuals, so doctors cannot depend on symptoms alone to make a correct diagnosis.

Methods of Diagnosis

The diagnosis of autoimmune disorders involves an array of blood tests, urinalysis, assessment of symptoms, medical history review, and physical examinations. Diagnostic tests can help in making a diagnosis but are often not definitive on their own.

Blood tests primarily detect the presence of autoantibodies that are responsible for attacking the body's own tissues. An antinuclear antibody (ANA) test is one such test. Since some autoimmune diseases affect the internal organs, a variety of organ-function tests and inflammation tests are carried out to determine whether or not these body parts are working properly.

How to Help Ensure An Accurate Diagnosis

There are some things a patient can do to help the doctor make an accurate diagnosis. These include the following.

Know your family's medical history: Autoimmune diseases are known to be inherited, but the diseases can overlap, and there is a chance that you may have a different disease than another person in your family. Talk to your relatives and gather information to see if someone in the family had a history of autoimmune disease. Let your doctor know about it so he or she can take the genetic factors into consideration when making a diagnosis.

Maintain a journal of symptoms: Autoimmune diseases come with numerous symptoms, and you may not remember them in detail when you see your doctor. Although symptoms may seem unrelated, the combination could be important in making a diagnosis. So keep a diary and note all the symptoms you experienced, the time they occurred, the food and drink you had, and the medications you were taking. And don't forget to take the journal with you when you visit the doctor.

Find a knowledgeable physician: Ask your friends and relatives for recommendations to good physicians who will be able to make an accurate diagnosis. Go to a health agency and community health meetings, and discuss your symptoms with healthcare professionals. Agencies that specialize in autoimmune diseases maintain referral lists, which can help you find the right doctor. "Autoimmunology" as a medical specialty does not exist, so it may take some work to identify a physician who will be able to treat your major symptoms under his or her area of specialization.

Get an exhaustive clinical examination: A thorough physical exam, along with a complete patient history and various tests, are carried out and analyzed in order to diagnose an autoimmune disease. During the examination, the patient can ask questions and relate concerns regarding tests, such as cost, alternatives, preparation, discomfort, and insurance options. It is important to understand that test results can be uncertain at times, so additional testing and long-term observation may be required.

Get a second opinion: If your doctor is unable to pinpoint the cause of symptoms, consider making an appointment with another physician. Get a referral to a doctor who is skilled at dealing with conditions that are particularly difficult to diagnose. Be sure to take your test results when seeing a second physician. And if you are referred to a psychologist by a doctor who dismisses your symptoms as stress-related, and you feel you are not under undue stress, it would be wise to consult another physician.

Consult a specialist: If your doctor thinks you may have an autoimmune disease, ask him or her to refer you to a physician who specializes in treating your primary symptoms. Although diagnosis may still not be easy or fast, a specialist is the best person to diagnose the disease based on the specific symptoms you are experiencing.

Consider other disorders: There is a chance that you may have more than one autoimmune condition. If the treatment is ineffective, talk to your doctor about making a fresh diagnosis. Or consult another physician and, after providing your complete history and test results, ask him or her to begin investigating other illnesses.

Understand that the road to diagnosis is challenging: A survey conducted by the American Autoimmune Related Disease Association

(AARDA) concluded that the majority of patients who were diagnosed with autoimmune diseases faced significant problems in obtaining a proper diagnosis. Many were incorrectly diagnosed with other conditions, due to the absence of specific blood tests, and patients were often told they were stressed and were imagining their symptoms. The survey revealed that 45 percent of the respondents were initially labeled as chronic complainers who were unnecessarily concerned about their health.

Finally, since the symptoms associated with autoimmune diseases can be varied, unrelated, and inconclusive, it is important to be aware that diagnosis can be a long and sometimes arduous process. The AARDA survey found that the average time it took for respondents to receive the correct identification of an autoimmune disorder was four years. So patience may be required, but with the proper attention from knowledgeable medical professionals effective diagnosis and treatment can be achieved.

References

1. McCoy, Krisha. "Diagnosing an Autoimmune Disorder," Everyday Health Media, 2016.

2. Lawrence, Jean. "Life with an Autoimmune Disease," WebMD, 2003.

3. Marshall, Amy Sarah. "The Detective Work of Autoimmune Disease," Healthy Balance, October 31, 2014.

4. Khairallah, Ramzi. "Autoimmune Disease: Can't Get a Diagnosis? Here's What to Do," My Family Doctor, February, 2016.

5. "Tips for Getting a Proper Diagnosis of an Autoimmune Disease," American Autoimmune Related Disease Association, September 1, 2013.

Chapter 11

Immune Function Blood Tests

The primary function of the immune system is to defend the body against foreign invaders, such as bacteria, viruses, fungi, germs, and allergens, which can cause infections and diseases. A doctor will analyze various symptoms of these illnesses, as well as the patient's medical and family history, to determine which lab tests would be the most appropriate to assess immune system function. The following are some of the blood tests that are commonly used to diagnose underlying health conditions and to initiate or monitor treatment.

Complete Blood Count (CBC)

A complete blood count (CBC) is ordered by a physician to assess the immune system function and overall health of a patient. This test measures the number and physical characteristics of the three major components of blood: red blood cells (RBCs), white blood cells (WBCs), and plasma. If the numbers of any of these components fall outside the healthy range, the person may require further medical assessment.

A doctor will generally order a CBC test when the patient exhibits symptoms like inflammation, bleeding, bruising, fatigue, or weakness. The test can help detect a number of conditions, such as vitamin or mineral deficiencies, infections, bone marrow disorders, anemia, and leukemia, and can also monitor a medical condition after its diagnosis.

It may also be used to ensure the effectiveness of treatment being provided for a blood-related disorder or to monitor treatment that can affect blood-cell count, such as chemotherapy or radiation therapy.

CBC test results will include:

- **Red blood cell, hemoglobin, and hematocrit count.** These can indicate anemia, nutritional deficiency, or chronic kidney disease if RBC level is below normal, or such conditions as polycythemia vera (PCV), lung disease, or dehydration if the level is above normal.

- **White blood cell count.** If low, this can reveal issues such as autoimmune disorder, sepsis, dietary deficiencies, or cancer, and if high it can indicate conditions like infection, inflammation, allergies, or asthma. If WBC count is either high or low, it can be a sign of bone marrow disease or reaction to certain medications.

- **Platelet count.** Low platelet count can be an indicator of such disorders as viral infection, cirrhosis, sepsis, or response to chemo or radiation therapy, while a high count may reveal conditions like cancer, anemia, rheumatoid arthritis, or inflammatory bowel disease.

A CBC is not considered a definitive test by itself but is typically ordered along with other diagnostic tests. Sometimes, depending on the CBC report, the doctor may order additional tests as a follow-up. A number of conditions can affect the CBC count, including factors such as the age of the patient and a recent blood transfusion.

Immunoglobulin Test

This test provides a measurement of immunoglobulins (antibodies) in the blood serum. Immunoglobulins are produced in plasma cells in response to foreign particles, such as bacteria, fungi, viruses, cancer cells, or animal dander. They are of five major types: IgA antibodies, which protect body surfaces exposed to foreign particles; IgG antibodies, found in all body fluids to fight bacterial and viral infections; IgM antibodies, which are found in blood and lymph fluid and are first produced in response to an infection; IgE antibodies, found in the lungs, skin, and mucous membranes, and are responsible for allergic reactions; and IgD antibodies; found in small amounts in the tissues that line the stomach or chest.

The test helps to identify the presence of immunoglobulins in the blood, which if detected implies that the body is reacting to some foreign invader. Each of its types is produced to fight a specific condition, so identification of these immunoglobulins helps to detect underlying disorders, such as infection, autoimmune diseases, allergies, and certain types of cancer. Test results can also be used to monitor treatment for *H. pylori* bacteria or certain cancers that affect the bone marrow, or to check the body's response to immunizations.

Some of the conditions that are detected through an immunoglobulin test include:

- **IgA.** If low, this can be a sign of some types of leukemia, kidney damage (nephrotic syndrome), enteropathy, or ataxia-telangiectasia. High levels may be a sign of monoclonal gammopathy of unknown significance (MGUS), multiple myeloma, autoimmune diseases, or liver diseases.

- **IgG.** Low IgG could can be an indication of conditions like macroglobulinemia, certain types of leukemia, or kidney damage (nephrotic syndrome), while a high reading might be a warning of chronic infections, such as HIV and hepatitis, as well as multiple myeloma or multiple sclerosis (MS).

- **IgM.** Some types of leukemia, multiple myeloma, or certain inherited types of immune diseases may cause low levels of IgM, and high results could indicate macroglobulinemia, parasite infection, mononucleosis, early viral hepatitis, rheumatoid arthritis, or nephrotic syndrome.

- **IgD.** High levels of IgD may be an indicator of multiple myeloma, although this is much less common than IgA or IgG multiple myeloma.

- **IgE.** A low IgE reading could be a warning sign of ataxia-telangiectasia (a rare inherited disease that affects muscle coordination), while high levels might indicate allergic reactions, asthma, parasitic infection, atopic dermatitis, certain autoimmune diseases, some types of cancer, or in rare cases, multiple myeloma.

A number of factors can affect the results of an immunoglobulin test, so it is important that the doctor ordering the test be informed about:

- blood transfusions, if any, in the last six months

- vaccinations in the last six months, particularly those with booster doses

- drugs such as those used for heart failure, rheumatoid arthritis, seizures, or birth control

- radiation and chemotherapy for cancer
- radioactive scan, if any, in the last three days
- the use of alcohol or illegal drugs

Complement Test

A complement test is done to analyze the activity of a group of blood serum proteins in the immune system. This group of nine major proteins (labeled C1 to C9) forms the complement system and helps antibodies fight against foreign microorganisms. Autoimmune disorders, too, will sometimes activate the antibodies, and in such cases they will fight against the body's own tissues, which it considers to be foreign invaders.

When a patient shows symptoms of such conditions as cryoglobulinemia, rheumatoid arthritis, lupus, kidney disease, myasthenia gravis, or an infectious disease like meningitis, the doctor may order a total complement measurement, or one or all of the more targeted tests (C1, C3, and C4). The doctor can then assess the underlying condition's progression by examining the test results for the activity of specific complement proteins and, additionally, monitor the effectiveness of its treatment. A total complement test may also be used to detect some infectious diseases and cancers or may be ordered when a patient has a family history of complement deficiency.

A complement test will show low activity for health conditions that include autoimmune disorders, like lupus, or a flare-up of an autoimmune disease, cirrhosis, hepatitis, glomerulonephritis (kidney disease), or hereditary angioedema (rapid swelling that affects face, limbs, or some internal organs). Low complement activity can also be a sign of malnutrition, an underlying infection, or rejection of a transplanted kidney. Disorders identified through a higher-than-normal measure of complement activity include thyroiditis, sarcoidosis, myocardial infarction, juvenile rheumatoid arthritis, cancer, or ulcerative colitis (inflammatory bowel disease).

Typically, a lack of early complement proteins (C1 through C4) make the individual more susceptible to infections, particularly those caused by fungi, and to some parasitic infections, like malaria, identified when C3 levels are low. Insufficient late complement proteins (C5 through C9), on the other hand, may make the person more prone to infections caused by *Neisseria* bacteria, a group that includes the bacteria that cause meningitis and gonorrhea. A complement test does not indicate precisely what condition the patient has; it only gives an indication that the immune system is involved and narrows down the possible causes. The doctor will need to order additional diagnostic tests to determine the underlying disorder.

Lymphocyte Transformation Test (LTT)

The lymphocyte transformation test (LTT) is performed to assess the function of lymphocytes taken from blood. Lymphocytes are a sub-type of white blood cells that are further divided into two types: B cells and T cells, specialized defender cells that help the immune system fight off infection and disease. B cells do this by producing antibodies, which attack invasive antigens (foreign substances), while T cells can work in a variety of different ways, such as killing invaders directly, sending chemical messages to parts of the immune system, or helping B cells produce antibodies.

When a B-lymphocyte makes contact with certain types of antigens, it initiates cell division that forms plasma cells, which then secrete antibodies that bind to specific antigens and label them for destruction, as well as memory cells that recognize the antigen when it is exposed to it again. The LTT uses this principle of antigen-specific initiation of cell division to its advantage. A positive reaction to the test will indicate the presence of antigen-specific memory cells. Based on this, the doctor will then perform further tests to identify and diagnose the underlying condition.

A physician will order an LTT when a patient exhibits symptoms of immune deficiency, such as poor resistance to infections, delay in time taken to recover after an infection, or problems with the healing of a wound. The LTT is primarily used to detect immunodeficiency, pathogens (such as chlamydia, *Borrelia*, and herpes viruses), and type IV allergy (allergic sensitization to medication, molds, environmental pollutants, or certain foods).

Some other conditions an LTT may help identify include:

- repeated infections in the upper respiratory tract
- bacterial infections
- infections like those caused by intestinal virus or *Candida*
- immune deficiency due to protein, vitamin, iron, or zinc deficiency
- immune deficiency as a complication of chronic inflammatory disease

LTT is also performed to assess a person's immunity before and after cancer treatment (surgical, radiation, or chemotherapy) and antiviral treatment for such conditions as HIV infection.

References

1. "Complement," American Association for Clinical Chemistry, September 15, 2014.

2. "Complete Blood Count (CBC)," Mayo Clinic, February 14, 2014.

3. "Complete Blood Count," American Association for Clinical Chemistry, September 8, 2016.

4. "Immunoglobulins," WebMD, September 9, 2014.

5. "Immune System," BiologyGuide, n.d.

6. "LTT Immune Function Test," Synevo Laboratories, n.d.

7. "Lymphocyte Transformation Test (LTT)," IMD Labor Berlin-Potsdam, n.d.

8. Pietrangelo, Ann. "Complement Test," HealthLine Media, December 18, 2015.

9. "What Are the Best Lab Tests for Immune System Function?" Bright Hub, July 13, 2010.

Chapter 12

Antibody Blood Tests

Chapter Contents

Section 12.1

Anti Nuclear Antibody (ANA) Test

Reprinted with permission from American Association for
Clinical Chemistry (AACC), producer of Lab Tests Online.
For more information, see labtestsonline.org/
understanding/analytes/ana/tab/test.

The Test

How Is It Used?

The antinuclear antibody (ANA) test is used as a primary test to help
evaluate a person for autoimmune disorders that affect many tissues
and organs throughout the body (systemic) and is most often used as
one of the tests to help diagnose systemic lupus erythematosus (SLE).

ANA are a group of autoantibodies produced by a person's immune
system when it fails to adequately distinguish between "self" and "non-
self." They target substances found in the nucleus of a cell and cause
organ and tissue damage.

Depending on a person's signs and symptoms and the suspected
disorder, ANA testing may be used along with or followed by other autoantibody tests. Some of these tests are considered subsets of the general
ANA test and detect the presence of autoantibodies that target specific
substances within cell nuclei, including anti-double stranded DNA (anti-
dsDNA), anti-centromere, anti-nucleolar, anti-histone and anti-RNA
antibodies. An ENA panel may also be used in follow up to an ANA.

These supplemental tests are used in conjunction with a person's
clinical history to help diagnose or rule out other autoimmune disorders, such as Sjögren syndrome, polymyositis and scleroderma.

Different laboratories may use different test methods to detect
ANA. Two common methods include immunoassay and indirect fluorescent antibody (IFA). IFA is considered the gold standard. Some
laboratories will use immunoassay to screen for ANA and use IFA to
confirm positive or equivocal results.

- Indirect fluorescent antibody (IFA)—this is a method in which
a person's blood sample is mixed with cells that are affixed to a

slide. Autoantibodies that may be present in the blood react with the cells. The slide is treated with a fluorescent antibody reagent and examined under a microscope. The presence (or absence) and pattern of fluorescence is noted.

- Immunoassays--these methods are usually performed on automated instrumentation but may be less sensitive than IFA in detecting ANA.

Other laboratory tests associated with the presence of inflammation, such as erythrocyte sedimentation rate (ESR) and/or C-reactive protein (CRP), may also be used to evaluate a person for SLE or other autoimmune disese.

When Is It Ordered?

The ANA test is ordered when someone shows signs and symptoms that are associated with a systemic autoimmune disorder. People with autoimmune disorders can have a variety of symptoms that are vague and non-specific and that change over time, progressively worsen, or alternate between periods of flare ups and remissions. Some examples of signs and symptoms include:

- low-grade fever
- persistent fatigue, weakness
- arthritis-like pain in one or more joints
- red rash (for lupus, one resembling a butterfly across the nose and cheeks)
- skin sensitivity to light
- hair loss
- muscle pain
- numbness or tingling in the hands or feet
- inflammation and damage to organs and tissues, including the kidneys, lungs, heart, lining of the heart, central nervous system, and blood vessels

What Does the Test Result Mean?

A positive ANA test result means that autoantibodies are present. In a person with signs and symptoms, this suggests the presence of an autoimmune disease, but further evaluation is required to assist in making a final diagnosis.

Tests for ANA

Amount of autoantibody present
Two types of tests are commonly performed to detect and measure ANA:

- Immunoassay (enzyme linked immunosorbent assay, ELISA, or enzyme immunoassay, EIA)—the results are usually reported as a number with an arbitrary unit of measure (abbreviated as a "U" on the report, for example).

- Indirect fluorescent antibody (IFA)—the results of this method are reported as a titer. Titers are expressed as ratios. For example, the result 1:320 means that one part blood sample was mixed with 320 parts of a diluting substance and ANA was still detectable.

Patterns of cellular fluorescence
In addition to a titer, positive results on IFA will include a description of the particular type of fluorescent pattern seen. Different patterns have been associated with different autoimmune disorders, although some overlap may occur. Some of the more common patterns include:

- Homogenous (diffuse)—associated with SLE, mixed connective tissue disease, and drug-induced lupus

- Speckled—associated with SLE, Sjögren syndrome, scleroderma, polymyositis, rheumatoid arthritis, and mixed connective tissue disease

- Nucleolar—associated with scleroderma and polymyositis

- Centromere pattern (peripheral)—associated with scleroderma and CREST (Calcinosis, Raynaud syndrome, Esophogeal dysmotility, Sclerodactyly, Telangiectasia)

A positive result from the ELISA or EIA method will be a number of units that is above the laboratory's reference number (cutoff) for the lowest possible value that is considered positive.

An example of a positive result using the IFA method would give the dilution titer and a description of the pattern, such as "Positive at 1:320 dilution with a homogenous pattern."

For either method, the higher the value reported, the more likely the result is a true positive.

ANA test results can be positive in people without any known autoimmune disease and thus need to be evaluated carefully in conjunction with an individual's signs and symptoms.

An ANA test may become positive before signs and symptoms of an autoimmune disease develop, so it may take time to tell the meaning of a positive ANA in a person who does not have symptoms.

Conditions Associated with a Positive ANA Test

The most common condition is SLE.

- SLE—ANA are most commonly seen with SLE. About 95 percent of those with SLE have a positive ANA test result. If someone also has symptoms of SLE, such as arthritis, a rash, and skin sensitivity to light, then the person probably has SLE. A positive anti-dsDNA and anti-SM (often ordered as part of an ENA panel) help confirm that the condition is SLE.

Other conditions in which a positive ANA test result may be seen include:

- Drug-induced lupus—a number of medications may trigger this condition, which is associated with SLE symptoms. When the drugs are stopped, the symptoms usually go away. Although many medications have been reported to cause drug-induced lupus, those most closely associated with this syndrome include hydralazine, isoniazid, procainamide, and several anticonvulsants. Because this condition is associated with the development of autoantibodies to histones, an anti-histone antibody test may be ordered to support the diagnosis.

- Sjögren syndrome—40–70 percent of those with this condition have a positive ANA test result. While this finding supports the diagnosis, a negative result does not rule it out. A health practitioner may want to test for two subsets of ANA: Anti-SS-A (Ro) and Anti-SS-B (La). About 90 percent or more of people with Sjögren syndrome have autoantibodies to SSA.

- Scleroderma (systemic sclerosis)—About 60–90 percent of those with scleroderma have a positive ANA. In people who may have this condition, ANA subset tests can help distinguish two forms of the disease, limited versus diffuse. The diffuse form is more severe. The limited form is most closely associated with the anti-centromere pattern of ANA staining (and the anticentromere test), while the diffuse form is associated with autoantibodies to Scl-70.

• Less commonly, ANA may occur in people with Raynaud syndrome, arthritis, dermatomyositis or polymyositis, mixed connective tissue disease, and other autoimmune conditions. For more on these, read the article on Autoimmune Diseases.

A health practitioner must rely on test results, clinical symptoms, and the person's history for diagnosis. Because symptoms may come and go, it may take months or years to show a pattern that might suggest SLE or any of the other autoimmune diseases.

A negative ANA result makes SLE an unlikely diagnosis. It usually is not necessary to immediately repeat a negative ANA test; however, due to the episodic nature of autoimmune diseases, it may be worthwhile to repeat the ANA test at a future date if symptoms recur.

Aside from rare cases, further autoantibody (subset) testing is not necessary if a person has a negative ANA result.

Is There Anything Else I Should Know?

ANA testing is not used to track or monitor the clinical course of SLE, thus serial ANA tests for diagnosed patients are not commonly ordered.

Use of a number of drugs, some infections, autoimmune hepatitis and primary biliary cirrhosis as well as other conditions mentioned above can give a positive result for the ANA test.

About 3–5 percent of healthy Caucasians may be positive for ANA, and it may reach as high as 10–37 percent in healthy individuals over the age of 65 because ANA frequency increases with age. These would be considered false-positive results because they are not associated with an autoimmune disease. Such instances are more common in women than men.

Section 12.2

C-Reactive Protein

What It Is

A C-reactive protein (CRP) blood test is used to identify inflammation or infection in the body.

C-reactive protein is released into the blood by the liver shortly after the start of an infection or inflammation. CRP is an early indicator of these problems and its levels can rise quickly.

Why It's Done

Doctors may order the C-reactive protein test if symptoms suggest any kind of inflammation, particularly related to inflammatory bowel disease (IBD), arthritis flare-ups, or an autoimmune disorder such as rheumatoid arthritis or lupus.

It may also be used to detect infections in vulnerable patients, such as those who've just had surgery or newborn babies. The CRP test also may help determine whether treatment for any of these conditions is working, because CRP levels drop quickly as inflammation subsides.

Preparation

No special preparations are needed for this test. Make sure to tell your doctor about any medications your child is taking because certain drugs might alter the test results.

On the day of the test, having your child wear a T-shirt or short-sleeved shirt can make things easier for your child and the technician who will be drawing the blood.

The Procedure

A health professional will usually draw the blood from a vein. For an infant, the blood may be obtained by puncturing the heel with a small needle (lancet). If the blood is being drawn from a vein, the skin surface is cleaned with antiseptic, and an elastic band (tourniquet) is placed around the upper arm to apply pressure and cause the veins to swell with blood. A needle is inserted into a vein (usually in the arm inside of the elbow or on the back of the hand) and blood is withdrawn and collected in a vial or syringe.

After the procedure, the elastic band is removed. Once the blood has been collected, the needle is removed and the area is covered with cotton or a bandage to stop the bleeding. Collecting blood for this test will only take a few minutes.

What to Expect

Either method (heel or vein withdrawal) of collecting a sample of blood is only temporarily uncomfortable and can feel like a quick pinprick. Afterward, there may be some mild bruising, which should go away in a few days.

Getting the Results

The blood sample will be processed by a machine. The results are commonly available after a few hours or the next day.

Generally, an elevated CRP level indicates an infection or inflammation somewhere in the body. But the CRP alone can't tell doctors where the problem is or what's causing it, so further testing may be necessary.

Risks

The C-reactive protein test is considered a safe procedure. However, as with many medical tests, some problems can occur with having blood drawn, such as:

- fainting or feeling lightheaded

- hematoma (blood accumulating under the skin causing a lump or bruise)

- pain associated with multiple punctures to locate a vein

Helping Your Child

Having a blood test is relatively painless. Still, many kids are afraid of needles. Explaining the test in terms your child can understand might help ease some of the fear.

Allow your child to ask the technician any questions he or she might have. Tell your child to try to relax and stay still during the procedure, as tensing muscles and moving can make it harder and more painful to draw blood. It also may help if your child looks away when the needle is being inserted into the skin.

If You Have Questions

If you have questions about the C-reactive protein test, speak with your doctor.

Section 12.3

Erythrocyte Sedimentation Rate (ESR)

Text in this section is excerpted from "Blood Test: Erythrocyte Sedimentation Rate (ESR)," © 1995–2016. The Nemours Foundation/ KidsHealth®. Reprinted with permission.

What Is An Erythrocyte Sedimentation Rate Test?

An erythrocyte sedimentation rate test (also called an ESR or sed rate test) measures the speed at which red blood cells fall to the bottom of an upright glass test tube. This measurement is important because when a person's blood has abnormal amounts of certain proteins in it, they cause red blood cells to clump together and sink more quickly.

Why Is It Done?

The ESR helps doctors detect inflammation or irritation in the body that may be caused by infection, some cancers, and certain autoimmune diseases such as rheumatoid arthritis, lupus, and Kawasaki disease. The ESR test alone can't be used to diagnose any specific disease, however.

Preparation

If your doctor asks you to get an ESR test, you won't need to do anything special beforehand to get ready. It can help to wear a T shirt or other short-sleeve top on the day of the test to make things faster and easier for the technician who will be drawing the blood.

The Procedure

A health professional will usually draw the blood from a vein in your arm—most often on the inside of the elbow, but sometimes on the back of the hand. The technician cleans the skin surface with antiseptic and ties an elastic band (tourniquet) around the upper arm so the veins swell with blood and are easy to see.

Next, it's time for the needle. It should feel like a quick pinprick. Occasionally, it can be hard to find a vein so a nurse, doctor, or technician might need to try more than once. That's not the norm, though—most people's veins are easy to find.

It's best to try to relax and stay still during the procedure since tensing muscles can make it harder and more painful to draw blood. And if you don't want to watch the needle being inserted or see the blood collecting, you don't have to. Look the other way and maybe relax by focusing on saying the alphabet backwards, doing some breathing exercises, thinking of a place that makes you happy, or listening to music.

The technician will draw the blood so it collects in a vial or syringe. Collecting blood will only take a few minutes. Once the technician has enough blood, he or she removes the needle and covers the area with cotton or a bandage to stop the bleeding.

After the test, you may notice some bruising—that's normal and it should go away in a few days. Don't be afraid to ask the technician if you have any questions about the blood draw.

Safety

A blood test is a safe procedure and there are no real risks. Some people may feel faint or lightheaded during a blood test. And while nobody really loves needles, a few teens have a strong fear of them. If that's you, talk to your doctor since there are things that can be done to make the procedure easier for you.

Results

It usually only takes a few hours or a day or so for your doctor to get the results of an ESR test. If the test seems to show problems, your doctor may want to do other tests to find out what the cause is.

Section 12.4

Rheumatoid Factor

Reprinted with permission from American Association for
Clinical Chemistry (AACC), producer of Lab Tests Online.
For more information, see labtestsonline.org/
understanding/analytes/rheumatoid/tab/test.

The Test

How Is It Used?

The rheumatoid factor (RF) test is primarily used to help diagnose
rheumatoid arthritis (RA) and to help distinguish RA from other forms
of arthritis or other conditions that cause similar symptoms.

While diagnosis of RA relies heavily on the clinical picture, some of
the signs and symptoms may not be present or follow a typical pattern,
especially early in the disease. Furthermore, the signs and symptoms
may not always be clearly identifiable since people with RA may also
have other connective tissue disorders or conditions, such as Raynaud
phenomenon, scleroderma, autoimmune thyroid disorders, and systemic lupus erythematosis, and display symptoms of these disorders
as well. The RF test is one tool among others that can be used to help
make a diagnosis when RA is suspected.

When Is It Ordered?

The test for RF may be ordered when a person has signs and symptoms of RA. Symptoms may include pain, warmth, swelling, and morning stiffness in the joints, nodules under the skin, and, if the disease
has progressed, evidence on X-rays of swollen joint capsules and loss
of cartilage and bone. An RF test may be repeated when the first test
is negative and symptoms persist.

A cyclic citrullinated peptide (CCP) antibody test can help diagnose
RA in someone who has joint inflammation with symptoms that suggest but do not yet meet the criteria of RA and may be ordered along
with RF or if the RF result is negative.

71

The RF test may also be ordered along with other autoimmune-related tests, such as an antinuclear antibody (ANA), and other markers of inflammation, such as a C-reactive protein (CRP) and erythrocyte sedimentation rate (ESR), as well as a complete blood count (CBC) to evaluate blood cells.

What Does the Test Result Mean?

The RF test must be interpreted in conjunction with a person's symptoms and clinical history.

In those with symptoms and clinical signs of rheumatoid arthritis, the presence of significant concentrations of RF indicates that it is likely that they have RA. Higher levels of RF generally correlate with more severe disease and a poorer prognosis.

A negative RF test does not rule out RA. About 20 percent of people with RA will have very low levels of or no detectable RF. In these cases, a CCP antibody test may be positive and used to confirm RA.

Positive RF test results may also be seen in 1–5 percent of healthy people and in some people with conditions such as: Sjögren syndrome, scleroderma, systemic lupus erythematosus (lupus), sarcoidosis, endocarditis, tuberculosis, syphilis, HIV/AIDS, hepatitis, infectious mononucleosis, cancers such as leukemia and multiple myeloma, parasitic infection, or disease of the liver, lung, or kidney. The RF test is not used to diagnose or monitor these other conditions.

Is There Anything Else I Should Know?

The 2010 Rheumatoid Arthritis Classification Criteria from the American College of Rheumatology (ACR) includes cyclic citrullinated peptide (CCP) antibody testing, along with RF, as part of its criteria for diagnosing rheumatoid arthritis. According to the ACR, CCP antibodies may be detected in about 50–60 percent of people with early RA, as early as 3–6 months after the beginning of symptoms. Early detection and diagnosis of RA allows health practitioners to begin aggressive treatment of the condition, minimizing the associated complications and tissue damage.

Section 12.5

Serum Angiotensin Converting Enzyme (SACE)

Reprinted with permission from American Association for
Clinical Chemistry (AACC), producer of Lab Tests Online.
For more information, see labtestsonline.org/
understanding/analytes/ace/tab/test.

The Test

How Is It Used?

The angiotensin-converting enzyme (ACE) test is primarily ordered
to help diagnose and monitor sarcoidosis. It is often ordered as part of
an investigation into the cause of a group of troubling chronic symptoms that are possibly due to sarcoidosis.

Sarcoidosis is a disorder in which small nodules called granulomas
may form under the skin and in organs throughout the body. The cells
surrounding granulomas can produce increased amounts of ACE and
the blood level of ACE may increase when sarcoidosis is present.

The blood level of ACE tends to rise and fall with disease activity.
If ACE is initially elevated in someone with sarcoidosis, the ACE test
can be used to monitor the course of the disease and the effectiveness
of corticosteroid treatment.

A health practitioner may order ACE along with other tests, such
as AFB tests that detect mycobacterial infections or fungal tests. This
may help to differentiate between sarcoidosis and another condition
causing granuloma formation.

When Is It Ordered?

An ACE test is ordered when someone has signs or symptoms that
may be due to sarcoidosis, such as:

- granulomas
- a chronic cough or shortness of breath

- red, watery eyes

- joint pain

This is especially true if the person is between 20 and 40 years of age, when sarcoidosis is most frequently seen.

When someone has been diagnosed with sarcoidosis and initial ACE levels were elevated, a health practitioner may order ACE testing at regular intervals to monitor the change in ACE over time as a reflection of disease activity.

What Does the Test Result Mean?

An increased ACE level in a person who has clinical findings consistent with sarcoidosis means that it is likely that the person has an active case of sarcoidosis, if other diseases have been ruled out. ACE will be elevated in 50–80 percent of those with active sarcoidosis. The finding of a high ACE level helps to confirm the diagnosis.

A normal ACE level cannot be used to rule out sarcoidosis because sarcoidosis can be present without an elevated ACE level. Findings of normal ACE levels in sarcoidosis may occur if the disease is in an inactive state, may reflect early detection of sarcoidosis, or may be a case where the cells do not produce increased amounts of ACE. ACE levels are also less likely to be elevated in cases of chronic sarcoidosis.

When monitoring the course of the disease, an ACE level that is initially high and then decreases over time usually indicates spontaneous or therapy-induced remission and a favorable prognosis. A rising level of ACE, on the other hand, may indicate either an early disease process that is progressing or disease activity that is not responding to therapy.

Is There Anything Else I Should Know?

ACE assists in the conversion of angiotensin I (an inactive protein) to angiotensin II. Angiotensin II functions as a strong vasopressor; it causes arteries to contract, making them temporarily narrower and increasing the pressure of the blood flowing through them. This conversion is a normal regulatory process in the body. The process has been targeted by the development of drugs called ACE inhibitors that are commonly used in treating hypertension and diabetes. These drugs inhibit the conversion process, keeping the blood vessels more dilated and the blood pressure lower. ACE inhibitors are useful in managing hypertension, but they are not monitored with ACE blood tests. They may, however, interfere with ACE measurements ordered for other reasons.

High and low levels of ACE may be seen in a variety of conditions other than sarcoidosis. The ACE test, however, is not routinely used to diagnose or monitor these conditions; it has not been shown to be clinically useful.

Decreased ACE levels may also be seen in people with:

- chronic obstructive pulmonary disease (COPD)

- lung diseases such as emphysema, lung cancer, cystic fibrosis

- starvation

- steroid drug therapy

- hypothyroidism

ACE has been found in moderately increased levels in a variety of diseases and disorders, such as:

- HIV

- histoplasmosis (fungal respiratory infection)

- diabetes mellitus

- hyperthyroidism

- lymphoma

- alcoholic cirrhosis

- Gaucher disease (a rare inherited lipid metabolism disorder)

- tuberculosis

- leprosy

Section 12.6

Protein Electrophoresis and Immunofixation Electrophoresis

Reprinted with permission from American Association for Clinical Chemistry (AACC), producer of Lab Tests Online. For more information, see labtestsonline.org/ understanding/analytes/electrophoresis/tab/test.

The Test

How Is It Used?

Protein electrophoresis is used to identify the presence of abnormal proteins, to identify the absence of normal proteins, and to determine when different groups of proteins are present in unusually high or low amounts in blood or other body fluids.

Proteins do many things in the body, including the transport of nutrients, removal of toxins, control of metabolic processes, and defense against invaders.

Protein electrophoresis separates proteins based on their size and electrical charge. This forms a characteristic pattern of bands of different widths and intensities on a test media and reflects the mixture of proteins present in the body fluid evaluated. The pattern is divided into five fractions, called albumin, alpha 1, alpha 2, beta, and gamma. In some cases, the beta fraction is further divided into beta 1 and beta 2.

Immunofixation electrophoresis (IFE) can be used as needed to further identify abnormal bands, in order to determine which type of antibody (immunoglobulin) is present.

The major plasma proteins and their functions are listed according to their electrophoretic group (the visible band that they are part of) in a table titled Protein Groups.

Alterations to the usual appearance of the patterns formed can help in the diagnosis of disease. The presence of an abnormality on a protein electrophorectic pattern is seldom diagnostic in itself. Instead, it provides a clue. Follow-up testing is then usually performed, based on that clue, to try to identify the nature of the underlying disease.

Follow-up tests may include, for example, albumin, immunoelec-trophoresis, serum free light chains, quantitative immunoglobuins, alpha-1 antitrypsin or cryoglobulins.

When Is It Ordered?

Protein electrophoresis may be ordered as a follow up to abnormal findings on other laboratory tests or as an initial test in evaluating a person's symptoms. Once a disease or condition has been diagnosed, electrophoresis may be ordered at regular intervals to monitor the course of the disease and the effectiveness of treatment. Some examples of when an electrophoresis test may be ordered are listed below.

Serum electrophoresis may be ordered:

- as a follow up to abnormal findings on other laboratory tests, such as total protein and/or albumin level, elevated urine protein levels, elevated calcium levels, or low white or red blood cell counts

- when symptoms suggest an inflammatory condition, an auto-immune disease, an acute or chronic infection, a kidney or liver disorder, or a protein-losing condition

- when a health practitioner is investigating symptoms that suggest multiple myeloma, such as bone pain, anemia, fatigue, unexplained fractures, or recurrent infections, to look for the presence of a characteristic band (monoclonal immunoglobulin) in the beta or gamma region; if a sharp band is seen, its identity as a monoclonal immunoglobulin is typically confirmed by immunofixation electrophoresis.

- to monitor treatment of multiple myeloma to see if the monoclonal band is reduced in quantity or disappears completely with treatment

Urine protein electrophoresis may be ordered:

- when protein is present in urine in higher than normal amounts to determine the source of the abnormally high protein; it may be used to determine whether the protein is escaping from the blood plasma (suggesting compromised kidney function) or is an abnormal protein coming from a different source (such as a plasma cell cancer like multiple myeloma).

- when multiple myeloma is suspected, to determine whether any of the monoclonal immunoglobulins or fragments of monoclonal immunoglobulin are escaping into the urine; if a sharp band suggestive of a monoclonal protein is observed, its identity is typically confirmed by immunofixation electrophoresis.

CSF protein electrophoresis may be ordered:

• to search for the characteristic banding seen in multiple sclerosis; the presence of multiple distinct bands in the cerebrospinal fluid (CSF) (that are not also present in serum) are referred to as oligoclonal bands. Most people with multiple sclerosis, as well as some other inflammatory conditions of the brain, have such oligoclonal bands.

• to evaluate people having headaches or other neurologic symptoms to look for proteins suggestive of inflammation or infection

Immunofixation electrophoresis may be ordered:

• when an abnormal band suggestive of a monoclonal immunoglobulin is seen on either a serum or a urine electrophoresis pattern

What Does the Test Result Mean?

Protein electrophoresis tests give a health practitioner a rough estimate of how much of each protein fraction is present and whether any abnormal proteins are present. The value of immunofixation electrophoresis is in the identification of the presence of a particular type of immunoglobulin. The laboratory report may include an interpretation of the results.

Serum Electrophoresis

Certain conditions or diseases may be associated with decreases or increases in various serum proteins, as reflected below.

Table 12.1. Serum Protein Levels in Certain Diseases and Conditions

Protein	May be decreased in:	May be increased in:
Albumin	• Malnutrition and malabsorption • Pregnancy • Kidney disease (especially nephrotic syndrome) • Liver disease • Inflammatory conditions • Protein-losing syndromes	• Dehydration
Alpha 1 globulin	• Congenital emphysema (alpha-1 antitrypsin deficiency, a rare genetic disease) • Severe liver disease	• Acute or chronic inflammatory diseases
Alpha 2 globulin	• Malnutrition • Severe liver disease • Hemolysis	• Kidney disease (nephrotic syndrome) • Acute or chronic inflammatory disease
Beta globulin	• Malnutrition • Cirrhosis	• High blood cholesterol (hypercholesterolemia) • Iron deficiency anemia • Some cases of multiple myeloma or monoclonal gammopathy of unknown significance MGUS)

Gamma globulin	• Variety of genetic immune disorders
	• Secondary immune deficiency
		• Polyclonal, antibody produced by or derived from different plasma cells:
		  • Chronic inflammatory disease
		  • Rheumatoid arthritis
		  • Lupus
		  • Cirrhosis
		  • Chronic liver disease
		  • Acute and chronic infection
		  • Recent immunization
		• Monoclonal, antibody produced by or derived from a single type (clone) of plasma cell:
		  • Malignancy
		  • Multiple myeloma
		  • Lymphoma
		  • Waldenstrom's macroglobulinemia

Urine Electrophoresis

Usually there is very little protein in urine. Typically, if a significant amount of protein is present, it appears in one of three main patterns.

- Normally, the glomeruli prevent protein from leaking into the urine. When the glomeruli are damaged, albumin and other plasma proteins may leak through and be detected in the urine.

- Normally, some very small proteins can pass through the glomeruli but are removed from the urine by the tubules. When the tubules are damaged, these proteins will appear in the urine.

- Some other small proteins are not normally present in significant amounts in serum, for example, free light chains, myoglobin and hemoglobin. When they are present in the serum, they can pass through the glomeruli and appear in the urine.

CSF Electrophoresis

- Presence of multiple bands in the gamma region (oligoclonal bands) that are not present in serum is indicative of multiple sclerosis.

- Presence of higher than normal polyclonal immunoglobulins, antibodies produced and secreted by many different plasma cells, suggests an infection.

Immunofixation Electrophoresis

Identifies the type of immunoglobulin protein(s) present in monoclonal bands on a protein electrophoresis pattern; typically immunofixation determines the presence of a heavy chain (IgG, IgM or IgA) and a light chain (kappa or lambda).

Is There Anything Else I Should Know?

Immunizations within the previous six months can increase immunoglobulins as can drugs such as phenytoin (Dilantin), procainamide, oral contraceptives, methadone, and therapeutic gamma globulin.

Aspirin, bicarbonates, chlorpromazine (Thorazine), corticosteroids, and neomycin can affect protein electrophoresis results.

Chapter 13

Genetic Testing

What Is Genetic Testing?

Genetic testing is a type of medical test that identifies changes in chromosomes, genes, or proteins. The results of a genetic test can confirm or rule out a suspected genetic condition or help determine a person's chance of developing or passing on a genetic disorder. More than 1,000 genetic tests are currently in use, and more are being developed.

Several methods can be used for genetic testing:

- Molecular genetic tests (or gene tests) study single genes or short lengths of DNA to identify variations or mutations that lead to a genetic disorder.

- Chromosomal genetic tests analyze whole chromosomes or long lengths of DNA to see if there are large genetic changes, such as an extra copy of a chromosome, that cause a genetic condition.

- Biochemical genetic tests study the amount or activity level of proteins; abnormalities in either can indicate changes to the DNA that result in a genetic disorder.

Genetic testing is voluntary. Because testing has benefits as well as limitations and risks, the decision about whether to be tested is a personal and complex one. A geneticist or genetic counselor can help

This chapter includes text excerpted from "Genetic Testing," Genetics Home Reference (GHR), National Institutes of Health (NIH), September 28, 2016.

by providing information about the pros and cons of the test and discussing the social and emotional aspects of testing.

What Are the Types of Genetic Tests?

Genetic testing can provide information about a person's genes and chromosomes. Available types of testing include:

Newborn Screening

Newborn screening is used just after birth to identify genetic disorders that can be treated early in life. Millions of babies are tested each year in the United States. All states currently test infants for phenylketonuria (a genetic disorder that causes intellectual disability if left untreated) and congenital hypothyroidism (a disorder of the thyroid gland). Most states also test for other genetic disorders.

Diagnostic Testing

Diagnostic testing is used to identify or rule out a specific genetic or chromosomal condition. In many cases, genetic testing is used to confirm a diagnosis when a particular condition is suspected based on physical signs and symptoms. Diagnostic testing can be performed before birth or at any time during a person's life, but is not available for all genes or all genetic conditions. The results of a diagnostic test can influence a person's choices about healthcare and the management of the disorder.

Carrier Testing

Carrier testing is used to identify people who carry one copy of a gene mutation that, when present in two copies, causes a genetic disorder. This type of testing is offered to individuals who have a family history of a genetic disorder and to people in certain ethnic groups with an increased risk of specific genetic conditions. If both parents are tested, the test can provide information about a couple's risk of having a child with a genetic condition.

Prenatal Testing

Prenatal testing is used to detect changes in a fetus's genes or chromosomes before birth. This type of testing is offered during pregnancy if there is an increased risk that the baby will have a genetic or chromosomal disorder. In some cases, prenatal testing can lessen a couple's uncertainty or help them make decisions about a pregnancy. It cannot identify all possible inherited disorders and birth defects, however.

Preimplantation Testing

Preimplantation testing, also called preimplantation genetic diagnosis (PGD), is a specialized technique that can reduce the risk of having a child with a particular genetic or chromosomal disorder. It is used to detect genetic changes in embryos that were created using assisted reproductive techniques such as in-vitro fertilization. In-vitro fertilization involves removing egg cells from a woman's ovaries and fertilizing them with sperm cells outside the body. To perform preimplantation testing, a small number of cells are taken from these embryos and tested for certain genetic changes. Only embryos without these changes are implanted in the uterus to initiate a pregnancy.

Predictive and Presymptomatic Testing

Predictive and presymptomatic types of testing are used to detect gene mutations associated with disorders that appear after birth, often later in life. These tests can be helpful to people who have a family member with a genetic disorder, but who have no features of the disorder themselves at the time of testing. Predictive testing can identify mutations that increase a person's risk of developing disorders with a genetic basis, such as certain types of cancer. Presymptomatic testing can determine whether a person will develop a genetic disorder, such as hereditary hemochromatosis (an iron overload disorder), before any signs or symptoms appear. The results of predictive and presymptomatic testing can provide information about a person's risk of developing a specific disorder and help with making decisions about medical care.

Forensic testing

Forensic testing uses DNA sequences to identify an individual for legal purposes. Unlike the tests described above, forensic testing is not used to detect gene mutations associated with disease. This type of testing can identify crime or catastrophe victims, rule out or implicate a crime suspect, or establish biological relationships between people (for example, paternity).

How Is Genetic Testing Done?

Once a person decides to proceed with genetic testing, a medical geneticist, primary care doctor, specialist, or nurse practitioner can order the test. Genetic testing is often done as part of a genetic consultation.

Genetic tests are performed on a sample of blood, hair, skin, amniotic fluid (the fluid that surrounds a fetus during pregnancy), or other tissue. For example, a procedure called a buccal smear uses a small brush or cotton swab to collect a sample of cells from the inside surface of the cheek. The sample is sent to a laboratory where technicians look for specific changes in chromosomes, DNA, or proteins, depending on the suspected disorder. The laboratory reports the test results in writing to a person's doctor or genetic counselor, or directly to the patient if requested.

Newborn screening tests are done on a small blood sample, which is taken by pricking the baby's heel. Unlike other types of genetic testing, a parent will usually only receive the result if it is positive. If the test result is positive, additional testing is needed to determine whether the baby has a genetic disorder.

Before a person has a genetic test, it is important that he or she understands the testing procedure, the benefits and limitations of the test, and the possible consequences of the test results. The process of educating a person about the test and obtaining permission is called informed consent.

How Can Consumers Be Sure a Genetic Test Is Valid and Useful?

Before undergoing genetic testing, it is important to be sure that the test is valid and useful. A genetic test is valid if it provides an accurate result. Two main measures of accuracy apply to genetic tests: analytical validity and clinical validity. Another measure of the quality of a genetic test is its usefulness, or clinical utility.

- Analytical validity refers to how well the test predicts the presence or absence of a particular gene or genetic change. In other words, can the test accurately detect whether a specific genetic variant is present or absent?

- Clinical validity refers to how well the genetic variant being analyzed is related to the presence, absence, or risk of a specific disease.

- Clinical utility refers to whether the test can provide information about diagnosis, treatment, management, or prevention of a disease that will be helpful to a consumer.

All laboratories that perform health-related testing, including genetic testing, are subject to federal regulatory standards called the Clinical Laboratory Improvement Amendments (CLIA) or even stricter state requirements. CLIA standards cover how tests are performed, the qualifications of laboratory personnel, and quality control and testing procedures for each laboratory. By controlling the quality of laboratory practices, CLIA standards are designed to ensure the analytical validity of genetic tests.

CLIA standards do not address the clinical validity or clinical utility of genetic tests. The U.S. Food and Drug Administration (FDA) requires information about clinical validity for some genetic tests. Additionally, the state of New York requires information on clinical validity for all laboratory tests performed for people living in that state. Consumers, health providers, and health insurance companies are often the ones who determine the clinical utility of a genetic test.

It can be difficult to determine the quality of a genetic test sold directly to the public. Some providers of direct-to-consumer genetic tests on page 11 are not CLIA-certified, so it can be difficult to tell whether their tests are valid. If providers of direct-to-consumer genetic tests offer easy-to-understand information about the scientific basis of their tests, it can help consumers make more informed decisions. It may also be helpful to discuss any concerns with a health professional before ordering a direct-to-consumer genetic test.

What Do the Results of Genetic Tests Mean?

The results of genetic tests are not always straightforward, which often makes them challenging to interpret and explain. Therefore, it is important for patients and their families to ask questions about the potential meaning of genetic test results both before and after the test is performed. When interpreting test results, healthcare professionals consider a person's medical history, family history, and the type of genetic test that was done.

A positive test result means that the laboratory found a change in a particular gene, chromosome, or protein of interest. Depending on the purpose of the test, this result may confirm a diagnosis, indicate that a person is a carrier of a particular genetic mutation, identify an increased risk of developing a disease (such as cancer) in the future, or suggest a need for further testing. Because family members have some genetic material in common, a positive test result may also have implications for certain blood relatives of the person undergoing testing. It is important to note that a positive result of a predictive or presymptomatic genetic test usually cannot establish the exact risk of developing a disorder. Also, health professionals typically cannot use a positive test result to predict the course or severity of a condition.

A negative test result means that the laboratory did not find a change in the gene, chromosome, or protein under consideration. This result can indicate that a person is not affected by a particular disorder, is not a carrier of a specific genetic mutation, or does not have an increased risk of developing a certain disease. It is possible, however, that the test missed a disease-causing genetic alteration because many tests cannot detect all genetic changes that can cause a particular disorder. Further testing may be required to confirm a negative result.

In some cases, a test result might not give any useful information. This type of result is called uninformative, indeterminate, inconclusive, or ambiguous. Uninformative test results sometimes occur because everyone has common, natural variations in their DNA, called polymorphisms, that do not affect health. If a genetic test finds a change in DNA that has not been associated with a disorder in other people, it can be difficult to tell whether it is a natural polymorphism or a disease-causing mutation. An uninformative result cannot confirm or rule out a specific diagnosis, and it cannot indicate whether a person has an increased risk of developing a disorder. In some cases, testing other affected and unaffected family members can help clarify this type of result.

What Is the Cost of Genetic Testing, and How Long Does It Take to Get the Results?

The cost of genetic testing can range from under $100 to more than $2,000, depending on the nature and complexity of the test. The cost increases if more than one test is necessary or if multiple family members must be tested to obtain a meaningful result. For newborn screening, costs vary by state. Some states cover part of the total cost, but most charge a fee of $15 to $60 per infant.

From the date that a sample is taken, it may take a few weeks to several months to receive the test results. Results for prenatal testing are usually available more quickly because time is an important consideration in making decisions about a pregnancy. The doctor or genetic counselor who orders a particular test can provide specific information about the cost and time frame associated with that test.

What Are the Benefits of Genetic Testing?

Genetic testing has potential benefits whether the results are positive or negative for a gene mutation. Test results can provide a sense of relief from uncertainty and help people make informed decisions about managing their healthcare. For example, a negative result can eliminate the need for unnecessary checkups and screening tests in some cases. A positive result can direct a person toward available prevention, monitoring, and treatment options. Some test results can also help people make decisions about having children. Newborn screening can identify genetic disorders early in life so treatment can be started as early as possible.

What Are the Risks and Limitations of Genetic Testing?

The physical risks associated with most genetic tests are very small, particularly for those tests that require only a blood sample or buccal smear (a procedure that samples cells from the inside surface of the cheek). The procedures used for prenatal testing carry a small but real risk of losing the pregnancy (miscarriage) because they require a sample of amniotic fluid or tissue from around the fetus.

Many of the risks associated with genetic testing involve the emotional, social, or financial consequences of the test results. People may feel angry, depressed, anxious, or guilty about their results. In some cases, genetic testing creates tension within a family because the results can reveal information about other family members in addition to the person who is tested. The possibility of genetic discrimination in employment or insurance is also a concern.

Genetic testing can provide only limited information about an inherited condition. The test often can't determine if a person will show symptoms of a disorder, how severe the symptoms will be, or whether the disorder will progress over time. Another major limitation is the lack of treatment strategies for many genetic disorders once they are diagnosed.

A genetics professional can explain in detail the benefits, risks, and limitations of a particular test. It is important that any person who is considering genetic testing understand and weigh these factors before making a decision.

Chapter 14

Allergen-Specific Immunoglobulin E (IgE) Blood Test

An allergen-specific immunoglobulin E (IgE) blood test is done to check whether a person is allergic to a particular substance.

An allergic reaction occurs when the immune system overreacts to something, often in the environment, that's harmless to most people. To protect the body from this perceived threat, or allergen, the immune system of an allergic person produces antibodies called immunoglobulin E.

IgE antibodies are found mostly in the lungs, skin, and mucous membranes. They cause mast cells (a type of cell involved in the body's immune response) to release chemicals, including histamine, into the bloodstream. It's these chemicals that bring on many of the allergy symptoms that affect a person's eyes, nose, throat, lungs, skin, or gastrointestinal tract.

Because IgE antibodies are unique to each allergen (for example, IgE produced in response to pollen differs from IgE produced after a bee sting), checking for specific variants in the blood can help determine if an allergy is present.

Common allergens that may be tested for by using the allergen-specific IgE test include:

- pollen
- mold
- animal dander
- dust mites
- foods (including peanuts, milk, eggs, or shellfish)
- cockroaches
- medications (such as penicillin)
- insect venom (from bee or wasp stings)
- latex (found in certain balloons or hospital gloves)

Your doctor also may order a group of these tests—sometimes called a mini-screen or mini-panel—to look for antibodies against a variety of suspected allergens.

Why It's Done

This test is performed to check for allergies to specific allergens. Doctors may order it when a child has symptoms of an allergy (include hives, itchy eyes or nose, sneezing, nasal congestion, throat tightness, or trouble breathing). Symptoms may be seasonal (as with allergies due to pollen or molds) or year-round (as with pet dander) and can range from mild to severe.

This test is especially useful in children who've had life-threatening reactions to a certain allergen and for whom a skin-prick test would be too dangerous. In some cases, the test may also be used to monitor the effectiveness of allergy treatments, or to see if a child has outgrown an allergy.

Preparation

No special preparations are needed for this test. On the day of the test, having your child wear a T-shirt or short-sleeved shirt can make things easier for your child and the technician who will be drawing the blood.

The Procedure

A health professional will usually draw the blood from a vein. For an infant, the blood may be obtained by puncturing the heel with a small needle (lancet). If the blood is being drawn from a vein, the skin surface is cleaned with antiseptic, and an elastic band (tourniquet) is placed around the upper arm to apply pressure and cause the veins to swell with blood. A needle is inserted into a vein (usually in the arm inside of the elbow or on the back of the hand) and blood is withdrawn and collected in a vial or syringe.

After the procedure, the elastic band is removed. Once the blood has been collected, the needle is removed and the area is covered with cotton or a bandage to stop the bleeding. Collecting blood for this test will only take a few minutes.

What to Expect

Either method (heel or vein withdrawal) of collecting a sample of blood is only temporarily uncomfortable and can feel like a quick pinprick. Afterward, there may be some mild bruising, which should go away in a few days.

Getting the Results

The blood sample will be processed by a machine, and the results are usually available within a few days.

Elevated levels of specific IgE antibodies may mean an allergy is present. However, the amount of IgE doesn't necessarily predict the severity of the reaction. For this reason, your doctor will interpret the results in comparison with your child's symptoms and other allergy tests.

Risks

The allergen-specific IgE test is considered a safe procedure. However, as with many medical tests, some problems can occur with having blood drawn, such as:

- fainting or feeling lightheaded
- hematoma (blood accumulating under the skin causing a lump or bruise)
- pain associated with multiple punctures to locate a vein

Helping Your Child

Having a blood test is relatively painless. Still, many kids are afraid of needles. Explaining the test in terms your child can understand might help ease some of the fear.

Allow your child to ask the technician any questions he or she might have. Tell your child to try to relax and stay still during the procedure, as tensing muscles and moving can make it harder and more painful to draw blood. It also may help for your child to look away when the needle is being inserted into the skin.

If You Have Questions

If you have questions about the allergen-specific IgE test, speak with your doctor.

Chapter 15

Laboratory Tests Used to Diagnose and Evaluate Lupus

What Is Lupus?

Lupus is one of many disorders of the immune system known as autoimmune diseases. In autoimmune diseases, the immune system turns against parts of the body it is designed to protect. This leads to inflammation and damage to various body tissues. Lupus can affect many parts of the body, including the joints, skin, kidneys, heart, lungs, blood vessels, and brain.

Typically, lupus is characterized by periods of illness, called flares, and periods of wellness, or remission. Understanding how to prevent flares and how to treat them when they do occur helps people with lupus maintain better health.

Who Gets Lupus?

We know that many more women than men have lupus. Lupus is more common in African American women than in Caucasian women and is also more common in women of Hispanic, Asian, and

This chapter includes text excerpted from "Lupus," National Institute of Arthritis and Musculoskeletal and Skin Diseases (NIAMS), February 2015.

Native American descent. African American and Hispanic women are also more likely to have active disease and serious organ system involvement. In addition, lupus can run in families, but the risk that a child or a brother or sister of a patient will also have lupus is still quite low.

It is difficult to estimate how many people in the United States have the disease, because its symptoms vary widely and its onset is often hard to pinpoint. Although systemic lupus erythematosus (SLE) usually first affects people between the ages of 15 and 45 years, it can occur in childhood or later in life as well.

Understanding What Causes Lupus

Lupus is a complex disease, and its cause is not fully understood. Research suggests that genetics plays an important role, but it also shows that genes alone do not determine who gets lupus, and that other factors play a role. Some of the factors scientists are studying include sunlight, stress, hormones, cigarette smoke, certain drugs, and infectious agents such as viruses. Studies have confirmed that one virus, Epstein-Barr virus (EBV), which causes mononucleosis, is a cause of lupus in genetically susceptible people.

Scientists believe there is no single gene that predisposes people to lupus. Rather, studies suggest that a number of different genes may be involved in determining a person's likelihood of developing the disease, which tissues and organs are affected, and the severity of disease.

In lupus, the body's immune system does not work as it should. A healthy immune system produces proteins called antibodies and specific cells called lymphocytes that help fight and destroy viruses, bacteria, and other foreign substances that invade the body. In lupus, the immune system produces antibodies against the body's healthy cells and tissues. These antibodies, called autoantibodies, contribute to the inflammation of various parts of the body and can cause damage to organs and tissues. The most common type of autoantibody that develops in people with lupus is called an antinuclear antibody (ANA) because it reacts with parts of the cell's nucleus (command center). Doctors and scientists do not yet understand all of the factors that cause inflammation and tissue damage in lupus, and researchers are actively exploring them.

Common Symptoms of Lupus

- Painful or swollen joints and muscle pain
- Unexplained fever

- Red rashes, most commonly on the face

- Chest pain upon deep breathing

- Unusual loss of hair

- Pale or purple fingers or toes from cold or stress (Raynaud phenomenon)

- Sensitivity to the sun

- Swelling (edema) in legs or around eyes

- Mouth ulcers

- Swollen glands

- Extreme fatigue

Diagnosing Lupus

Diagnosing lupus can be difficult. It may take months or even years for doctors to piece together the symptoms to diagnose this complex disease accurately. Making a correct diagnosis of lupus requires knowledge and awareness on the part of the doctor and good communication on the part of the patient. Giving the doctor a complete, accurate medical history (for example, what health problems you have had and for how long) is critical to the process of diagnosis. This information, along with a physical examination and the results of laboratory tests, helps the doctor consider other diseases that may mimic lupus, or determine if you truly have the disease. Reaching a diagnosis may take time as new symptoms appear.

No single test can determine whether a person has lupus, but several laboratory tests may help the doctor to confirm a diagnosis of lupus or rule out other causes for a person's symptoms. The most useful tests identify certain autoantibodies often present in the blood of people with lupus. For example, the antinuclear antibody (ANA) test is commonly used to look for autoantibodies that react against components of the nucleus, or "command center," of the body's cells. Most people with lupus test positive for ANA; however, there are a number of other causes of a positive ANA besides lupus, including infections and other autoimmune diseases. Occasionally, it is also found in healthy people. The ANA test simply provides another clue for the doctor to consider in making a diagnosis. In addition, there are blood tests for individual types of autoantibodies that are more specific to people with lupus, although not all people with lupus test positive for these and not all people with these antibodies have lupus. These antibodies include anti-DNA, anti-Sm, anti-RNP, anti-Ro (SSA), and anti-La (SSB). The doctor may use these antibody tests to help make a diagnosis of lupus.

Some tests are used less frequently but may be helpful if the cause of a person's symptoms remains unclear. The doctor may order a biopsy of the skin or kidneys if those body systems are affected. Some doctors may order a test for anticardiolipin (or antiphospholipid) antibody. The presence of this antibody may indicate increased risk for blood clotting and increased risk for miscarriage in pregnant women with lupus. Again, all these tests merely serve as tools to give the doctor clues and information in making a diagnosis. The doctor will look at the entire picture—medical history, symptoms, and test results—to determine if a person has lupus.

Diagnostic Tools for Lupus

- Medical history
- Complete physical examination
- Laboratory tests:
- Complete blood count (CBC)
- Erythrocyte sedimentation rate (ESR)
- Urinalysis
- Blood chemistries
- Complement levels
- Antinuclear antibody test (ANA)
- Other autoantibody tests (anti-DNA, anti-Sm, anti-RNP, anti-Ro [SSA], antiLa [SSB])
- Anticardiolipin antibody test
- Skin biopsy
- Kidney biopsy

Other laboratory tests are used to monitor the progress of the disease once it has been diagnosed. A complete blood count, urinalysis, blood chemistries, and the erythrocyte sedimentation rate test (a test to measure inflammation) can provide valuable information. Another common test measures the blood level of a group of substances called complement, which help antibodies fight invaders. A low level of complement could mean the substance is being used up because of an immune response in the body, such as that which occurs during a flare of lupus.

X-rays and other imaging tests can help doctors see the organs affected by SLE.

Part Three

Inherited Immune
Deficiency Diseases

Chapter 16

Primary Immune Deficiency Diseases (PIDDs)

Chapter Contents

Section 16.1

Primary Immune Deficiency Diseases (PIDDs) Explained

This section includes text excerpted from "Primary Immune Deficiency Diseases (PIDDs)," National Institute of Allergy and Infectious Diseases (NIAID), June 12, 2015.

Primary immune deficiency diseases (PIDDs) are rare, genetic disorders that impair the immune system. Without a functional immune response, people with PIDDs may be subject to chronic, debilitating infections, such as Epstein-Barr virus (EBV), which can increase the risk of developing cancer. Some PIDDs can be fatal. PIDDs may be diagnosed in infancy, childhood, or adulthood, depending on disease severity.

Genetics and Inheritance

PIDDs are caused by genetic abnormalities that prevent the body from developing normal immune responses.

All of the body's cells contain instructions on how to do their jobs. These instructions are packaged into 23 pairs of chromosomes—22 pairs of numbered chromosomes, called autosomes, and one pair of sex chromosomes (XX for girls and XY for boys). One chromosome in each pair is inherited from the person's mother and the other from the father. Each chromosome contains many genes, which are made up of DNA, the carrier of genetic information. Errors, or mutations, in genes can cause diseases such as PIDDs.

Genetic mutations sometimes appear randomly. For example, *de novo*, or "new," mutations occur as a result of a mutation in the egg or sperm of one of the parents or in the fertilized egg itself. In these cases, the affected person does not have a family history of disease.

Most often, genetic mutations run in families. Several types of inherited mutations can cause PIDDs.

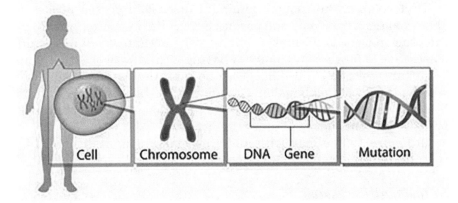

Figure 16.1. *Mutation on a Gene on a Chromosome in a Cell within the Human Body*

Autosomal Dominant

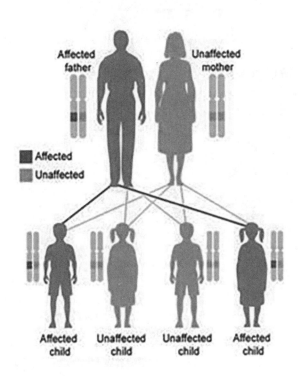

Figure 16.2. *Inheritance of Autosomal Dominant Disorder*

To develop an autosomal dominant disease, a person needs an abnormal gene from only one parent, even if the matching gene from the other parent is normal. A parent with an autosomal dominant disease has a 50 percent chance of having a child with the condition. The chance of one child inheriting the mutation is independent of whether his or her siblings have the mutation. In other words, if the first two children in a family have the mutation, the third child still has a 50 percent chance of inheriting it.

In Figure 16.2, a man with an autosomal dominant disorder has two affected children and two unaffected children.

Autosomal Recessive

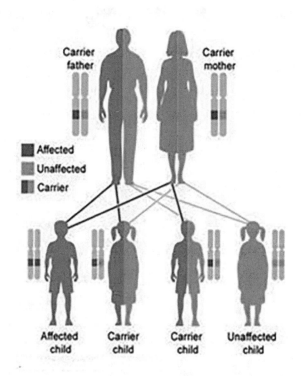

Figure 16.3. *Inheritance of Autosomal Recessive Disorder*

Two copies of an abnormal gene—one from each parent—must be present for an autosomal recessive disease to develop. Typically, both parents of an affected child carry one abnormal gene and are unaffected by the disease because the normal gene on the other chromosome continues to function. In this case, each child has a 25 percent, or one in four, chance of being affected by the disease. Each child also has a 50 percent chance of inheriting one copy of the mutated gene. People who inherit one abnormal gene copy will not develop the disease, but they can pass the mutation on to their children.

In Figure 16.3, two unaffected parents each carry one copy of a gene mutation for an autosomal recessive disorder. They have one affected child and three unaffected children, two of which carry one copy of the gene mutation.

X-Linked Recessive

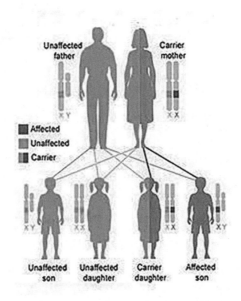

Figure 16.4. *Inheritance of X-Linked Recessive Disorder*

X-linked recessive diseases are caused by genes located on the X chromosome. Boys have only one copy of X-linked genes because they have one X chromosome. If a boy inherits a disease-causing mutation in a gene located on the X chromosome, he will develop the disease.

Girls usually do not develop X-linked recessive diseases because they have two X chromosomes and would need to inherit two abnormal copies of the gene—one from each parent—to be affected by the disease. Even if a girl carries the mutated gene on one X chromosome, the normal gene on the other X chromosome continues to function and she remains unaffected by the disease. Women who inherit one abnormal gene copy can pass the mutated gene on to their children.

In Figure 16.4, an unaffected woman carries one copy of a gene mutation for an X-linked recessive disorder. She has an affected son, an unaffected daughter who carries one copy of the mutation, and two unaffected children who do not have the mutation.

Talking to Your Doctor

We rely on our immune system to fight harmful bacteria or viruses—either on its own or with the help of antibiotics or antivirals—every day. Most of us recover quickly from infectious illnesses, and our immune system helps protect us from repeat infections in the future.

People with PIDDs, however, have defects in one or more parts of their immune system. They often cannot overcome infections, even with the aid of medicine.

Are You or Your Child at Risk for a PIDD?

- Do you get multiple, serious infections that are difficult to treat within a year?

- Have you had bacterial infections that don't get better, even after you've taken antibiotics?

- When you are sick, do you need to go to the hospital and/or receive intravenous antibiotics to get well?

- Do you have a family history of primary immune deficiency?

If you answered "yes" to any of these questions, you may be at risk for a PIDD. Consult with your doctor to get tested for an immune deficiency.

What to Ask Your Doctor

- Based on my medical and family history, am I at risk for an immune deficiency?

- What tests will be performed to determine my diagnosis, and how long will it take to get the results back?

- What precautions should I take to reduce my risk of infection?

- Should I see a specialist?

To diagnose a potential immune deficiency, your doctor will need to take a blood sample and send it to a lab for an initial screening test. If that test shows that you may be at risk for a PIDD, you'll need additional testing.

What to Bring to Your Doctor's Appointment

- A current list of medicines you have taken in the past and their effects

- Specific questions you want to have answered

- A journal to write down answers to your questions or to take notes

Section 16.2

Congenital Neutropenia Syndromes

This section includes text excerpted from "Congenital Neutropenia Syndromes," National Institute of Allergy and Infectious Diseases (NIAID), June 21, 2016.

Congenital neutropenia syndromes are a group of disorders characterized by low levels of neutrophils—white blood cells necessary for combating infections—present from birth. Congenital neutropenia syndromes also may be called congenital agranulocytosis, severe congenital neutropenia, severe infantile genetic neutropenia, infantile genetic agranulocytosis or Kostmann disease.

Causes

Researchers have identified a number of genetic mutations that cause congenital neutropenia syndromes. These disorders are inherited in several ways, including autosomal recessive, autosomal dominant, and X-linked.

Genes linked to these syndromes include the following:

- *ELANE*

- *HAX1*

- *G6PC3*
- *GFI1*
- *CSF3R*
- X-linked *WAS*
- *CXCR4*
- *VPS45A*
- *JAGN1*

Generally, mutations that result in congenital neutropenia affect the development, lifespan, or function of neutrophils. In some people, however, the disease-causing mutation of their congenital neutropenia syndrome is unknown.

Symptoms and Diagnosis

Signs and Symptoms

People with congenital neutropenia will experience bacterial infections early on in life. These may cause inflammation of the umbilical cord stump, abscesses (or boils) on the skin, oral infections, and pneumonia.

Congenital neutropenia also increases one's risk for developing myelodysplastic syndromes (MDS), blood disorders that are distinguished by low levels of various blood cells. Additionally, MDS may progress to a type of blood cell cancer called acute myeloid leukemia (AML).

Diagnosis

Bone marrow and blood tests can measure the levels of various white blood cells to test for deficiencies. A person suspected of having the disorder may undergo genetic testing for one of the known genetic mutations.

Treatment

Standard therapy includes being injected with granulocyte colony-stimulating factor (G-CSF), an immune-cell-growth molecule that can help restore the function of the immune system. People on G-CSF therapy may have a lower incidence and severity of infections, improving their quality of life, but effects vary between individuals. For some individuals, a bone marrow transplantation may be recommended to replace defective immune cells with those of a healthy donor.

Section 16.3

Glycosylation Disorders with Immunodeficiency

This section includes text excerpted from "Glycosylation Disorders with Immunodeficiency," National Institute of Allergy and Infectious Diseases (NIAID), June 24, 2016.

Glycosylation refers to the attachment of sugars to proteins, a normal process required for the healthy function of cells. Defects in glycosylation can impair the growth or function of cells and tissues in the body, and in some cases, the immune system is disrupted, resulting in immunodeficiency.

Causes

Researchers have not discovered the cause of many forms of glycosylation disorders with immunodeficiency. However, in 2014, researchers at the National Institutes of Health (NIH) discovered a new immunodeficiency caused by glycosylation defects. People with this disorder have mutations in the *PGM3* gene, resulting in defective sugar metabolism that leads to problems with glycosylation, especially in immune cells. These findings suggest that glycosylation defects may be involved in other common immune disorders, like allergy or autoimmunity.

Symptoms and Diagnosis

Signs and Symptoms

Glycosylation can impact how cells communicate, respond to their environment, grow, and function. Because it regulates a wide range of activities in cells found throughout the body, defects in glycosylation can cause extensive and severe symptoms.

People with *PGM3* gene mutations that cause some cases of glycosylation disorders may experience the following symptoms:

- susceptibility to bacterial and viral infections

- allergies, including food allergy

- asthma

- eczema

- autoimmunity

- developmental delays, including motor and cognitive impairments

Interestingly, glycosylation defects may protect people against microbes that rely on glycosylation for growth and infection. In 2014, NIH researchers identified two cases where defective glycosylation protected against specific viral infections.

Diagnosis

Glycosylation disorders with immunodeficiency cover a range of symptoms and are not limited to *PGM3* gene mutations. If a clinician suspects a patient may have a glycosylation defect, protein samples may be analyzed to measure sugars and look for deficiencies or abnormalities.

Treatment

People with these disorders may receive therapies commonly used to treat infections, allergies, and skin problems. For people with PGM3 defects, NIH researchers are evaluating ways to boost the production of the missing sugars by supplementing with other types of sugar. Based on insights gleaned from the study of glycosylation disorders, investigators at NIH are also exploring the use of glycosylation inhibitors to prevent and control viral infections.

Chapter 17

Ataxia-Telangiectasia

Ataxia-telangiectasia is a rare inherited disorder that affects the nervous system, immune system, and other body systems. This disorder is characterized by progressive difficulty with coordinating movements (ataxia) beginning in early childhood, usually before age 5. Affected children typically develop difficulty walking, problems with balance and hand coordination, involuntary jerking movements (chorea), muscle twitches (myoclonus), and disturbances in nerve function (neuropathy). The movement problems typically cause people to require wheelchair assistance by adolescence. People with this disorder also have slurred speech and trouble moving their eyes to look side-to-side (oculomotor apraxia). Small clusters of enlarged blood vessels called telangiectases, which occur in the eyes and on the surface of the skin, are also characteristic of this condition.

Affected individuals tend to have high amounts of a protein called alpha-fetoprotein (AFP) in their blood. The level of this protein is normally increased in the bloodstream of pregnant women, but it is unknown why individuals with ataxia-telangiectasia have elevated AFP or what effects it has in these individuals.

People with ataxia-telangiectasia often have a weakened immune system, and many develop chronic lung infections. They also have an increased risk of developing cancer, particularly cancer of blood-forming cells (leukemia) and cancer of immune system cells (lymphoma).

This chapter includes text excerpted from "Ataxia-Telangiectasia," Genetics Home Reference (GHR), National Institutes of Health (NIH), January 2013.

Affected individuals are very sensitive to the effects of radiation exposure, including medical X-rays. The life expectancy of people with ataxia-telangiectasia varies greatly, but affected individuals typically live into early adulthood.

Frequency

Ataxia-telangiectasia occurs in 1 in 40,000 to 100,000 people worldwide.

Genetic Changes

Mutations in the *ATM* gene cause ataxia-telangiectasia. The *ATM* gene provides instructions for making a protein that helps control cell division and is involved in DNA repair. This protein plays an important role in the normal development and activity of several body systems, including the nervous system and immune system. The ATM protein assists cells in recognizing damaged or broken DNA strands and coordinates DNA repair by activating enzymes that fix the broken strands. Efficient repair of damaged DNA strands helps maintain the stability of the cell's genetic information.

Mutations in the ATM gene reduce or eliminate the function of the ATM protein. Without this protein, cells become unstable and die. Cells in the part of the brain involved in coordinating movements (the cerebellum) are particularly affected by loss of the ATM protein. The loss of these brain cells causes some of the movement problems characteristic of ataxia-telangiectasia. Mutations in the *ATM* gene also prevent cells from responding correctly to DNA damage, which allows breaks in DNA strands to accumulate and can lead to the formation of cancerous tumors.

Inheritance Pattern

Ataxia-telangiectasia is inherited in an autosomal recessive pattern, which means both copies of the *ATM* gene in each cell have mutations. Most often, the parents of an individual with an autosomal recessive condition each carry one copy of the mutated gene, but do not show signs and symptoms of the condition.

About 1 percent of the United States population carries one mutated copy and one normal copy of the *ATM* gene in each cell. These individuals are called carriers. Although ATM mutation carriers do not have ataxia-telangiectasia, they are more likely than people without an ATM mutation to develop cancer; female carriers are particularly at risk for developing breast cancer. Carriers of a mutation in the ATM gene also may have an increased risk of heart disease.

Other Names for This Condition

- A-T
- Ataxia Telangiectasia Syndrome
- ATM
- Louis-Bar Syndrome
- Telangiectasia, Cerebello-Oculocutaneous

Chapter 18

Chediak-Higashi Syndrome

What Is Chediak-Higashi Syndrome?

Chediak-Higashi syndrome is a condition that affects many parts of the body, particularly the immune system. This disease damages immune system cells, leaving them less able to fight off invaders such as viruses and bacteria. As a result, most people with Chediak-Higashi syndrome have repeated and persistent infections starting in infancy or early childhood. These infections tend to be very serious or life-threatening.

Chediak-Higashi syndrome is also characterized by a condition called oculocutaneous albinism, which causes abnormally light coloring (pigmentation) of the skin, hair, and eyes. Affected individuals typically have fair skin and light-colored hair, often with a metallic sheen. Oculocutaneous albinism also causes vision problems such as reduced sharpness; rapid, involuntary eye movements (nystagmus); and increased sensitivity to light (photophobia).

Many people with Chediak-Higashi syndrome have problems with blood clotting (coagulation) that lead to easy bruising and abnormal bleeding. In adulthood, Chediak-Higashi syndrome can also affect the nervous system, causing weakness, clumsiness, difficulty with walking, and seizures.

If the disease is not successfully treated, most children with Chediak-Higashi syndrome reach a stage of the disorder known as the

This chapter includes text excerpted from "Chediak-Higashi Syndrome," Genetics Home Reference (GHR), National Institutes of Health (NIH), January, 2014.

accelerated phase. This severe phase of the disease is thought to be triggered by a viral infection. In the accelerated phase, white blood cells (which normally help fight infection) divide uncontrollably and invade many of the body's organs. The accelerated phase is associated with fever, episodes of abnormal bleeding, overwhelming infections, and organ failure. These medical problems are usually life-threatening in childhood.

A small percentage of people with Chediak-Higashi syndrome have a milder form of the condition that appears later in life. People with the adult form of the disorder have less noticeable changes in pigmentation and are less likely to have recurrent, severe infections. They do, however, have a significant risk of progressive neurological problems such as tremors, difficulty with movement and balance (ataxia), reduced sensation and weakness in the arms and legs (peripheral neuropathy), and a decline in intellectual functioning.

Frequency

Chediak-Higashi syndrome is a rare disorder. About 200 cases of the condition have been reported worldwide.

Genetic Changes

Chediak-Higashi syndrome is caused by mutations in the *LYST* gene. This gene provides instructions for making a protein known as the lysosomal trafficking regulator. Researchers believe that this protein plays a role in the transport (trafficking) of materials into structures called lysosomes and similar cell structures. Lysosomes act as recycling centers within cells. They use digestive enzymes to break down toxic substances, digest bacteria that invade the cell, and recycle worn-out cell components.

Mutations in the *LYST* gene impair the normal function of the lysosomal trafficking regulator protein, which disrupts the size, structure, and function of lysosomes and related structures in cells throughout the body. In many cells, the lysosomes are abnormally large and interfere with normal cell functions. For example, enlarged lysosomes in certain immune system cells prevent these cells from responding appropriately to bacteria and other foreign invaders. As a result, the malfunctioning immune system cannot protect the body from infections.

In pigment cells called melanocytes, cellular structures called melanosomes (which are related to lysosomes) are abnormally large.

116

Melanosomes produce and distribute a pigment called melanin, which is the substance that gives skin, hair, and eyes their color. People with Chediak-Higashi syndrome have oculocutaneous albinism because melanin is trapped within the giant melanosomes and is unable to contribute to skin, hair, and eye pigmentation.

Researchers believe that abnormal lysosome-like structures inside blood cells called platelets underlie the abnormal bruising and bleeding seen in people with Chediak-Higashi syndrome. Similarly, abnormal lysosomes in nerve cells probably cause the neurological problems associated with this disease.

Inheritance Pattern

This condition is inherited in an autosomal recessive pattern, which means both copies of the gene in each cell have mutations. The parents of an individual with an autosomal recessive condition each carry one copy of the mutated gene, but they typically do not show signs and symptoms of the condition.

Other Names for This Condition

- Chediak-Steinbrinck-Higashi syndrome
- CHS
- Oculocutaneous albinism with leukocyte defect

Chapter 19

Chronic Granulomatous Disease (CGD)

Chronic granulomatous disease (CGD) is a genetic disorder in which white blood cells called phagocytes are unable to kill certain bacteria and fungi. People with CGD have increased susceptibility to infections caused by certain types of bacteria and fungi, such as *Staphylococcus aureus, Serratia marcescens, Burkholderia cepacia, Nocardia* species, and *Aspergillus* species.

Causes

CGD is caused by defects in an enzyme called NAPDH oxidase that phagocytes need to kill bacteria and fungi. Mutations in one of five different genes can cause this defect, which leads to frequent and sometimes life-threatening infections of the skin, lungs, liver, and bones, with accumulations of inflammatory cells called abscesses (boils) or granulomas (inflamed masses of tissue).

Symptoms and Diagnosis

CGD may be suspected in children or adults with the abscesses that involve the lungs, liver, spleen, bones, or skin; infections caused

This chapter includes text excerpted from "Chronic Granulomatous Disease (CGD)," National Institute of Allergy and Infectious Diseases (NIAID), July 26, 2016.

by germs that are not usually harmful, such as fungi or *Nocardia*; and granulomas (tissue masses that can obstruct the bowel or urinary tract and complicate wounds). In some people, granulomas can cause an inflammatory bowel disease similar to Crohn's disease.

Furthermore, heart or kidney problems, diabetes, and autoimmune disease may occur in people with CGD. However, the incidence of these issues varies depending on which gene is mutated. CGD is diagnosed by special blood tests that show how well phagocytes produce hydrogen peroxide, an indicator that they are functioning properly.

Treatment

The key to managing CGD is early diagnosis and treatment with appropriate medications. The goal is to prevent infections and complications. Antibiotics are taken throughout life help prevent bacterial infections, and antifungals are taken throughout life help prevent fungal infections. Injections with interferon gamma, a protein that improves the activity of phagocytes, may also be helpful. Abscesses need aggressive care, which may include surgery. Granulomas may require steroid therapy. Some people have been treated successfully with bone marrow transplantation.

Chapter 20

CTLA4 Deficiency

CTLA4 deficiency impairs normal regulation of the immune system, resulting in excessive numbers of immune cells called lymphocytes, autoimmunity, low levels of antibodies, and recurrent infections.

Causes

CTLA4 deficiency is caused by mutations in the gene *CTLA4*, which provides cellular instructions for the production of the CTLA-4 protein. This protein functions as a "brake" to slow down and control the action of the immune system. Each person has two copies of the *CTLA4* gene—one from each parent. In 2014, NIAID scientists found that people with only one functional copy of *CTLA4* experience severe symptoms, including abnormal T cell activity and the disruption of organs by infiltrating immune cells. The researchers determined that having a single working copy of *CTLA4* is not sufficient to produce enough CTLA-4 protein for a normal immune system, hence the term haploinsufficiency (the prefix haplo- means "single").

Symptoms and Diagnosis

Signs and Symptoms

CTLA4 deficiency is characterized by infiltration of immune cells into the gut, lungs, bone marrow, central nervous system, kidneys,

---

This chapter includes text excerpted from "CTLA4 Deficiency," National Institute of Allergy and Infectious Diseases (NIAID), July 25, 2016.

and possibly other organs. Most people with CTLA4 deficiency experience diarrhea or intestinal disease. Enlarged lymph nodes, liver, and spleen also are common, as are respiratory infections. People with CTLA4 deficiency often experience autoimmune problems that can affect various organs and tissues, including the blood, thyroid, skin, and joints. It also may slightly increase the risk of lymphoma, a type of immune cell cancer.

Diagnosis

CTLA4 deficiency is diagnosed based on clinical symptoms, laboratory findings, and genetic testing. Most people with CTLA4 deficiency develop reduced levels of at least one type of immunoglobulin, or antibody. People with CTLA4 deficiency also may have low levels of healthy antibody-producing B cells, high levels of autoimmune B cells, and overactivation of T cells.

Treatment

Treatment may include standard therapies for autoimmune problems and immunoglobulin deficiencies. A drug called CTLA-4-Ig mimics the action of CTLA-4 and reduces immune activity. This drug is a potential therapy for people with CTLA4 deficiency and requires further exploration.

Chapter 21

DiGeorge Syndrome (22q11.2 Deletion Syndrome)

What Is 22q11.2 Deletion Syndrome?

22q11.2 deletion syndrome is a disorder caused by the deletion of a small piece of chromosome 22. The deletion occurs near the middle of the chromosome at a location designated q11.2.

22q11.2 deletion syndrome has many possible signs and symptoms that can affect almost any part of the body. The features of this syndrome vary widely, even among affected members of the same family. Common signs and symptoms include heart abnormalities that are often present from birth, an opening in the roof of the mouth (a cleft palate), and distinctive facial features. People with 22q11.2 deletion syndrome often experience recurrent infections caused by problems with the immune system, and some develop autoimmune disorders such as rheumatoid arthritis and Graves disease in which the immune system attacks the body's own tissues and organs. Affected individuals may also have breathing problems, kidney abnormalities, low levels of calcium in the blood (which can result in seizures), a decrease in

This chapter includes text excerpted from "22q11.2 Deletion Syndrome," Genetics Home Reference (GHR), National Institutes of Health (NIH), September 8, 2016.

blood platelets (thrombocytopenia), significant feeding difficulties, gastrointestinal problems, and hearing loss. Skeletal differences are possible, including mild short stature and, less frequently, abnormalities of the spinal bones.

Many children with 22q11.2 deletion syndrome have developmental delays, including delayed growth and speech development, and learning disabilities. Later in life, they are at an increased risk of developing mental illnesses such as schizophrenia, depression, anxiety, and bipolar disorder. Additionally, affected children are more likely than children without 22q11.2 deletion syndrome to have attention deficit hyperactivity disorder (ADHD) and developmental conditions such as autism spectrum disorders that affect communication and social interaction.

Because the signs and symptoms of 22q11.2 deletion syndrome are so varied, different groupings of features were once described as separate conditions. Doctors named these conditions DiGeorge syndrome, velocardiofacial syndrome (also called Shprintzen syndrome), and conotruncal anomaly face syndrome. In addition, some children with the 22q11.2 deletion were diagnosed with the autosomal dominant form of Opitz G/BBB syndrome and Cayler cardiofacial syndrome. Once the genetic basis for these disorders was identified, doctors determined that they were all part of a single syndrome with many possible signs and symptoms. To avoid confusion, this condition is usually called 22q11.2 deletion syndrome, a description based on its underlying genetic cause.

Frequency

22q11.2 deletion syndrome affects an estimated 1 in 4,000 people. However, the condition may actually be more common than this estimate because doctors and researchers suspect it is underdiagnosed due to its variable features. The condition may not be identified in people with mild signs and symptoms, or it may be mistaken for other disorders with overlapping features.

Genetic Changes

Most people with 22q11.2 deletion syndrome are missing a sequence of about 3 million DNA building blocks (base pairs) on one copy of chromosome 22 in each cell. This region contains 30 to 40 genes, many of which have not been well characterized. A small percentage of affected individuals have shorter deletions in the same region. This condition is described as a contiguous gene deletion syndrome because it results from the loss of many genes that are close together.

Researchers are working to identify all of the genes that contribute to the features of 22q11.2 deletion syndrome. They have determined that the loss of a particular gene on chromosome 22, *TBX1*, is probably responsible for many of the syndrome's characteristic signs (such as heart defects, a cleft palate, distinctive facial features, hearing loss, and low calcium levels). Some studies suggest that a deletion of this gene may contribute to behavioral problems as well. The loss of another gene, *COMT*, in the same region of chromosome 22 may also help explain the increased risk of behavioral problems and mental illness. The loss of additional genes in the deleted region likely contributes to the varied features of 22q11.2 deletion syndrome.

Inheritance Pattern

The inheritance of 22q11.2 deletion syndrome is considered autosomal dominant because a deletion in one copy of chromosome 22 in each cell is sufficient to cause the condition. Most cases of 22q11.2 deletion syndrome are not inherited, however. The deletion occurs most often as a random event during the formation of reproductive cells (eggs or sperm) or in early fetal development. Affected people typically have no history of the disorder in their family, though they can pass the condition to their children. In about 10 percent of cases, a person with this condition inherits the deletion in chromosome 22 from a parent. In inherited cases, other family members may be affected as well.

Other Names for This Condition

- 22q11.2DS
- Autosomal dominant opitz G/BBB syndrome
- CATCH22
- Cayler cardiofacial syndrome
- Conotruncal anomaly face syndrome (CTAF)
- Deletion 22q11.2 syndrome
- DiGeorge syndrome

- Sedlackova syndrome
- Shprintzen syndrome
- VCFS
- Velo-cardio-facial syndrome
- Velocardiofacial syndrome

Chapter 22

DOCK8 Deficiency

DOCK8 deficiency is a rare immune disorder named after the mutated gene responsible for the disease. The disorder causes decreased numbers and dysfunction of immune cells, as well as poor ability of immune cells to move across dense tissues like the skin. The abnormalities resulting from DOCK8 defects lead to recurrent infections.

Causes

DOCK8 deficiency is caused by mutations in the *DOCK8* gene. Initially, the disease was called autosomal recessive hyper IgE syndrome (AR-HIES) and considered a rare form of HIES, a primary immune deficiency disorder that National Institute of Allergy and Infectious Diseases (NIAID) also studies. In 2009 however, NIAID researchers discovered that many cases of AR-HIES are caused by a separate disease that results from mutations in the DOCK8 gene. As a result, the disease was renamed DOCK8 deficiency.

Symptoms and Diagnosis

Signs and Symptoms

DOCK8 deficiency causes persistent skin infections from viruses, such as herpes simplex virus that causes cold sores, human

This chapter includes text excerpted from "DOCK8 Deficiency," National Institute of Allergy and Infectious Diseases (NIAID), July 25 2016.

papillomavirus that causes warts, molluscum contagiosum that causes pox-like lesions, and varicella-zoster virus that causes shingles. People with DOCK8 deficiency commonly also have eczema, allergies, asthma, and a higher risk of developing certain cancers, such as squamous cell carcinoma and lymphoma.

People with DOCK8 deficiency do not typically have the joint, bone, and facial changes that are seen in patients with AD-HIES or Job syndrome.

Diagnosis

Genetic testing for mutations in the *DOCK8* gene can confirm the diagnosis of DOCK8 deficiency in people suspected of having the disease.

Treatment

Individuals with DOCK8 deficiency are given prolonged antibiotics and sometimes antibody replacement therapy to prevent infections. Bone marrow transplantation is frequently recommended for patients with DOCK8 deficiency.

Chapter 23

Hyper-Immunoglobulin M (Hyper-IgM) Syndromes

Hyper-Immunoglobulin M (Hyper-IgM) syndromes are conditions in which the immune system fails to produce normal levels of immunoglobulin A (IgA), IgG, and IgE antibodies but can produce normal or elevated levels of IgM. Various gene defects can cause hyper-IgM syndromes.

Causes

Hyper-IgM syndromes are caused by problems in communication between T cells and antibody-producing B cells. This leads to B cells that do not mature properly and only produce IgM antibodies because production of other antibody types, such as IgA, IgG, and IgE, requires normal T and B cell interaction. Scientists have identified mutations in six genes that can result in hyper-IgM syndromes. Four forms of hyper-IgM syndrome are autosomal recessive, and two are X-linked.

Symptoms and Diagnosis

Infants with a hyper-IgM syndrome usually develop severe respiratory infections within the first year of life. Some people with a

This chapter includes text excerpted from "Hyper-Immunoglobulin M (Hyper-IgM) Syndromes," National Institute of Allergy and Infectious Diseases (NIAID), July 15, 2012. Reviewed October 2016.

hyper-IgM syndrome may have low levels of white blood cells called neutrophils (a condition called neutropenia) and an increased risk of unusual infections, such as *Pneumocystis jiroveci* pneumonia or chronic diarrhea caused by infection with the parasite *Cryptosporidium*. People with X-linked hyper-IgM syndrome also may experience bone loss. Unusual infections and low antibody levels may indicate hyper-IgM syndrome. Normal numbers of T and B cells but elevated levels of IgM are very suggestive of this condition.

Treatment

People with a hyper-IgM syndrome must receive regular intravenous or subcutaneous antibody replacement therapy. Hyper-IgM patients with neutropenia also may take a drug called granulocyte-colony stimulating factor (G-CSF) to stimulate the body to produce more white blood cells. Some patients also may take anti-fungal medications to prevent pneumonia caused by the fungus *Pneumocystis jiroveci*.

Depending on the genetic defect that causes their particular form of hyper-IgM syndrome, some people can be treated with a bone marrow transplant from a healthy donor, which can reset and replenish the immune system.

Chapter 24

PI3 Kinase Disease

Discovered by National Institutes of Health (NIH) scientists in 2013, PI3 Kinase (P13K) disease is named after the genetic mutations that cause the disorder and its symptoms. People with PI3K disease have a weakened immune system and experience frequent bacterial and viral infections. PI3K disease also increases a person's risk of lymphoma, a type of immune cell cancer.

The disease also is called PI3K-p110δ activating mutation causing senescent T cells, lymphadenopathy, and immunodeficiency (PASLI) or activating PI3K delta syndrome (APDS)

Cause

PI3K disease is caused by mutations in the gene *PIK3CD*, which provides instructions for production of a protein called PI3K-p110δ. Mutations in *PIK3CD* affect the immune system by over-activating an important immune system signaling pathway. This launches a chain reaction leading to disruptions in the normal development of B and T cells and an increase in a person's susceptibility to infection. Mutations in other, related genes can cause similar versions of this disorder.

PI3K disease is inherited in an autosomal dominant manner, meaning a person only needs to inherit one copy of a mutated gene from one parent. However, not all people who inherit a mutation have severe disease, and some may have no symptoms at all. This variation, called

This chapter includes text excerpted from "PI3 Kinase Disease," National Institute of Allergy and Infectious Diseases (NIAID), July 25, 2016.

variable penetrance expressivity, can be striking, even within the same family.

Symptoms and Diagnosis

Signs and Symptoms

PI3K disease is characterized by recurrent respiratory infections, which can lead to progressive airway damage. People with PI3K disease also may experience:

- Lymphoproliferation, or the buildup of immune cells called lymphocytes. This can lead to enlarged lymph nodes and spleen.

- Chronic high levels of viruses such as Epstein-Barr virus (EBV) or cytomegalovirus in the blood.

- Cytopenias, or reductions in the number of blood cells. Cytopenias can cause fatigue, infections, increased risk of bleeding, or slow wound healing.

- EBV-driven B-cell lymphoma, a type of immune cell cancer associated with EBV infection.

Diagnosis

PI3K disease is diagnosed based on symptoms, genetic testing, and laboratory findings. People with PI3K disease have too few of some immune cell types and too many of other types, which can be determined with blood tests. Many also have abnormal levels of certain types of immunoglobulins, or antibodies.

Treatment

Researchers have had some success treating PI3K disease with medications that inhibit the immune system pathway that is over-activated in people with the disease. In early studies, this strategy reduced swelling of the lymph nodes, most likely by restoring the normal balance of immune cells. More research is needed to determine the most effective timing and dosage of this medication and to investigate other treatment options, such as PI3K-specific drugs.

Chapter 25

PLCG2-associated Antibody Deficiency and Immune Dysregulation (PLAID)

PLAID and PLAID-like diseases are rare immune disorders with overlapping features, and an allergic response to cold, called cold urticaria, is the most distinct symptom.

Cause

PLAID is a genetic disorder caused by mutations in the phospholipase C-gamma2 (*PLCG2*) gene, which is involved in the activity of specific immune cells, including B cells, NK cells, and myeloid cells. PLAID was discovered by NIAID scientists in 2012.

PLAID-like disease refers to a disorder that resembles PLAID, but mutations in *PLCG2* have not been identified. Mutations in other genes that regulate immune activity along with *PLCG2* are likely responsible, and research on PLAID-like disease is ongoing.

This chapter includes text excerpted from "PLCG2-Associated Antibody Deficiency and Immune Dysregulation (PLAID)," National Institute of Allergy and Infectious Diseases (NIAID), July 25, 2016.

Symptoms and Diagnosis

Signs and Symptoms

People with PLAID experience cold urticaria from infancy. This allergic response to cold tends to result from evaporative cooling, like exposure to cool air while sweating, and less so from touching cold objects. Additionally, some can develop a burn-like rash at birth in areas more likely to get cold, such as the nose. Other symptoms include recurrent bacterial infections and skin granulomas, which are accumulations of inflammatory immune cells. Eating cold foods may cause a burning sensation in the throat or chest but does not progress to anaphylaxis.

People with PLAID tend to have high levels of anti-nuclear antibodies, which react against their own cells and tissues and increase the likelihood of developing an autoimmune disease. They also may be more susceptible to bacterial infections. However, some people experience cold urticaria and no other symptoms.

Diagnosis

Low levels of IgA and IgM antibodies, low levels of NK cells, and a poor response to vaccination also may occur. Notably, people with PLAID lack abnormal proteins—cold agglutinins and cryoglobulins—observed in other cold-induced disorders.

Treatment

Currently, people with PLAID are advised to avoid triggers by warming rapidly after showers, avoiding drafts, and toweling off sweat. Antihistamines are used to treat allergic reactions. The allergic response to cold likely results from abnormal activation of immune cells at low temperatures. NIAID researchers have shown that immune cells from PLAID patients, including mast cells, which release histamine; B cells; neutrophils; and monocytes, are abnormally activated by cold temperature. In the future, it may be possible to develop therapies that target the *PLCG2* defect in order to restore normal immune function.

Chapter 26

Severe Combined Immunodeficiency (SCID)

Severe combined immunodeficiency (SCID) is a group of rare disorders caused by mutations in different genes involved in the development and function of infection-fighting T, B, and natural killer cells. Infants with SCID appear healthy at birth but are highly susceptible to severe infections. The condition is fatal, usually within the first year or two of life, unless infants receive immune-restoring treatments, such as transplants of blood-forming stem cells, gene therapy, or enzyme therapy. More than 80 percent of SCID infants do not have a family history of the condition. However, development of a newborn screening test has made it possible to detect SCID before symptoms appear, helping ensure that affected infants receive life-saving treatments.

Causes

SCID is caused by defects in different genes involved in the development and function of infection-fighting immune cells. More than a dozen genes have been implicated in SCID, but gene defects are unknown in approximately 15 percent of newborn-screened SCID infants, according to an study funded by National Institutes of Health (NIH).

This chapter includes text excerpted from "Severe Combined Immunodeficiency (SCID)," National Institute of Allergy and Infectious Diseases (NIAID), July 26, 2016.

Most often, SCID is inherited in an autosomal recessive pattern, in which both copies of a particular gene—one inherited from the mother and one from the father—contain defects. The best-known form of autosomal recessive SCID is caused by adenosine deaminase (ADA) deficiency, in which infants lack the ADA enzyme necessary for T-cell survival.

X-linked SCID, which is caused by mutations in a gene on the X chromosome, primarily affects male infants. Boys with this type of SCID have lymphocytes that grow and develop abnormally. As a consequence, they have low numbers of T cells and natural killer cells, and their B cells do not function.

Symptoms and Diagnosis

Typically, symptoms of SCID occur in infancy and include serious or life-threatening infections, especially viral infections, which result in pneumonia and chronic diarrhea. *Candida* (yeast) infections of the mouth and diaper area and pneumonia caused by the fungus *Pneumocystis jirovecii* also are common in affected infants.

The SCID newborn screening test, originally developed at NIH, measures T cell receptor excision circles (TRECs), a byproduct of T-cell development. Because SCID infants have few or no T cells, the absence of TRECs may indicate SCID. To confirm a SCID diagnosis, a doctor will evaluate the numbers and types of T and B cells present and their ability to function.

Research supported by NIAID and other organizations has shown that early diagnosis of SCID through newborn screening leads to prompt treatment and high survival rates. SCID was added in 2010 to the U.S. Department of Health and Human Services' (HHS') Recommended Uniform Screening Panel for newborns, and today, the majority of states screen newborns for SCID.

Treatment

Hematopoietic (blood-forming) stem cell transplantation is the standard treatment for infants with SCID. Ideally, SCID infants receive stem cells from a sibling who is a close tissue match. Transplants from matched siblings lead to the best restoration of immune function, but if a matched sibling is not available, infants may receive stem cells from a parent or an unrelated donor.

NIAID-supported research has shown that early transplantation is critical to achieving the best outcomes for SCID infants. Investigators analyzed data from 240 SCID infants at 25 transplant centers across North America, finding that infants who received transplants before the age of 3.5 months were most likely to survive, regardless of the type of stem cell donor used. Babies of any age who did not have infections at the time of transplant also had high survival rates.

Studies have shown that gene therapy can be an effective treatment for some types of SCID, including X-linked SCID. In gene therapy, doctors remove stem cells from the patient's bone marrow, insert one or more copies of the normal gene into the stem cells using a carrier known as a vector, and return the corrected cells to the patient. Initial efforts to treat X-linked SCID with gene therapy successfully restored children's T-cell function. However, approximately one-quarter of the children developed leukemia two to five years after treatment. Scientists suspect that the vectors used in these studies activated genes that control cell growth, contributing to leukemia. In 2014, NIAID-funded researchers reported development of a modified vector that appears effective and safe.

Children who have SCID with ADA deficiency have been treated somewhat successfully with enzyme replacement therapy called PEG-ADA.

Chapter 27

Warts, Hypogammaglobulinemia, Infections, and Myelokathexis Syndrome (WHIMS)

Warts, hypogammaglobulinemia, infections, and myelokathexis syndrome (WHIMS) is a rare immune disorder named after its symptoms: warts, hypogammaglobulinemia, infections, and myelokathexis. People with WHIMS have low levels of infection-fighting white blood cells, especially neutrophils, in their bloodstream. This deficiency predisposes them to frequent infections and persistent warts.

Causes

WHIMS is caused by mutations in the CXC chemokine receptor 4 (*CXCR4*) gene. One of the many functions of *CXCR4* is to tether white blood cells to the bone marrow, where the cells originate. WHIMS

This chapter includes text excerpted from "Warts, Hypogammaglobulinemia, Infections, and Myelokathexis Syndrome (WHIMS)," National Institute of Allergy and Infectious Diseases (NIAID), July 26, 2016.

mutations result in excessive *CXCR4* activity, which traps the cells inside the bone marrow and prevents their movement into the bloodstream and the rest of the body.

Symptoms and Diagnosis

People with WHIMS experience the following symptoms:

- warts of the skin, mouth, and genitals caused by human papillomavirus (HPV)

- hypogammaglobulinemia, a deficiency in specific infection-fighting antibodies in the blood

- infections that recur frequently

- myelokathexis, the failure of neutrophils, a type of white blood cell, to move from the bone marrow into the bloodstream

WHIMS patients also have trouble distributing most other types of immune cells to the blood. Such defects in the immune system predispose WHIMS patients to frequent infections and an increased risk of developing cancer caused by HPV.

Almost all WHIMS patients have mutations in the *CXCR4* gene.

Treatment

Standard therapy for WHIMS, which is aimed at restoring deficient components of the blood, includes intravenous immunoglobulin, a blood product containing antibodies, or granulocyte colony-stimulating factor (G-CSF), an immune-cell-growth molecule. However, these treatments do not specifically target the *CXCR4* genetic defect and evidence of their efficacy from direct tests in clinical trials is lacking.

In 2011, NIAID investigators tested the drug plerixafor (Genzyme/Sanofi) in WHIMS patients over the course of 1 week to investigate safety and to establish the minimally effective dose for raising the neutrophil count to a level at which infections would be unlikely to occur. Plerixafor, which blocks the activity of *CXCR4*, is approved by the U.S. Food and Drug Administration (FDA) to mobilize blood-forming stem cells from the bone marrow for collection and eventual transplantation after cancer therapy. Because it can mobilize immune cells to the blood in healthy people and targets *CXCR4* specifically, it was considered an ideal drug candidate for treating patients with WHIMS. In this study, the drug was safe and could elevate neutrophils to a safe level using approximately 5 percent of the FDA-approved dose for stem cell mobilization.

In 2014, a study by NIAID researchers revealed that low-dose plerixafor, designed to reduce but not eliminate *CXCR4* activity, was safe and effective at raising the neutrophil count in the blood over the course of 6 months. The study also provided preliminary evidence of efficacy at reducing wart burden and the incidence of infection. Currently, NIAID scientists are comparing the safety and efficacy of plerixafor to that of G-CSF, a standard treatment, in clinical trials for the treatment of WHIMS.

Interestingly in 2015, NIAID researchers reported the spontaneous cure of a person with WHIMS that likely was the result of a genetic phenomenon called chromothripsis, or "chromosome shattering," which caused a random and fortuitous deletion of the mutant *CXCR4* gene. Presumably, a stem cell lacking mutant *CXCR4* survived and repopulated all of the person's neutrophils. The NIAID team is exploring how to apply the study findings to improve bone marrow transplantation, which relies on the ability of donor stem cells to repopulate in a recipient.

Chapter 28

Wiskott-Aldrich Syndrome (WAS)

People with Wiskott-Aldrich Syndrome (WAS) have problems with their B cells, T cells, and platelets (blood components that aid in clotting). This can result in prolonged episodes of bleeding, recurrent bacterial and fungal infections, and increased risk of cancers and autoimmune diseases.

Cause

WAS is an X-linked recessive disease caused by mutations in the WAS gene, which provides instructions for production of Wiskott-Aldrich Syndrome Protein (WASP).

Symptoms and Diagnosis

Mutations in the *WAS* gene differ from person to person, and some mutations result in more severe disease than others. Classic symptoms of WAS include the following:

- reduced platelet counts that lead to small bruises or bleeding in the skin, bowels, and gums or prolonged nose bleeds

- upper respiratory tract infections such as sinusitis

This chapter includes text excerpted from "Wiskott-Aldrich Syndrome (WAS)," National Institute of Allergy and Infectious Diseases (NIAID), June 27, 2016.

- lower respiratory infections and pneumonia

- eczema

More severe forms of WAS can lead to the following:

- bloodstream infections, meningitis, and severe viral infections

- autoimmune-like symptoms, including blood vessel inflammation, anemia, and production of antibodies against the body's own platelets

- lymphoma or leukemia

Blood tests will indicate low platelet counts in boys who show unusual bleeding or bruises; low platelet counts also can be determined using blood samples. Children with WAS fail to produce effective antibodies to bacteria and vaccines; skin tests can reveal abnormal T-cell function that leads to this failure.

Treatment

Intravenous (through the vein) immunglobulin replacement therapy and iron supplements are given to children with WAS. Bone marrow transplant, which re-sets and replenishes the immune system, has been shown to be effective.

Chapter 29

X-Linked Agammaglobulinemia (XLA)

X-Linked Agammaglobulinemia (XLA) is an inherited immune disorder caused by an inability to produce B cells or the immunoglobulins (antibodies) that the B cells make. The mutated gene responsible for XLA (Bruton tyrosine kinase or *BTK*) is located on the X chromosome. XLA is also called by Bruton type agammaglobulinemia, X-linked infantile agammaglobulinemia, and congenital agammaglobulinemia.

Causes

XLA is caused by mutations in the *BTK* gene found on the X chromosome. This gene normally produces a protein that is required for the development of B cells. XLA is an X-linked recessive disease. Because males only have one X chromosome, they are affected if they inherit an X chromosome containing mutated *BTK*.

Symptoms and Diagnosis

Infants with XLA develop frequent infections of the ears, throat, lungs, and sinuses. Serious infections also can develop in the bloodstream, central nervous system, skin, and internal organs. These

---

This chapter includes text excerpted from "X-Linked Agammaglobulinemia (XLA)," National Institute of Allergy and Infectious Diseases (NIAID), July 26, 2016.

children tend to cope well with most short-term viral infections but are very susceptible to chronic viral infections such as hepatitis and polio. They usually lack or have very small tonsils.

People with XLA have extremely low numbers of B cells, and blood tests will show extremely low levels of all types of immunoglobulins (antibodies). People with XLA fail to develop antibodies to specific germs and will not produce protective antibodies after immunizations. Most laboratories can examine B cell numbers in blood samples, while specialized labs can test for the *BTK* mutation.

Treatment

People with XLA receive intravenous (through the vein) or subcutaneous (just under the skin) immunoglobulin regularly and antibiotics to treat infections. National Institutes of Health (NIH) researchers have improved methods to identify the specific microbes responsible for infections in people with XLA. By identifying hard-to-detect bacteria, physicians can prescribe the correct treatments.

Chapter 30

X-Linked Immunodeficiency with Magnesium Defect, Epstein-Barr Virus Infection, and Neoplasia (XMEN)

X-linked immunodeficiency with magnesium defect, Epstein-Barr virus infection, and neoplasia (typically known by the acronym XMEN) is a disorder that affects the immune system in males. In XMEN, certain types of immune system cells called T cells are reduced in number or do not function properly. Normally these cells recognize foreign invaders, such as viruses, bacteria, and fungi, and are then turned on (activated) to attack these invaders in order to prevent infection and illness. Because males with XMEN do not have enough functional T cells, they have frequent infections, such as ear infections, sinus infections, and pneumonia.

In particular, affected individuals are vulnerable to the Epstein-Barr virus (EBV). EBV is a very common virus that infects more than 90 percent of the general population and in most cases goes unnoticed. Normally, after initial infection, EBV remains in the body for the rest of a person's life. However, the virus is generally inactive (latent)

This chapter includes text excerpted from "X-Linked Immunodeficiency with Magnesium Defect, Epstein-Barr Virus Infection, and Neoplasia," Genetics Home Reference (GHR), National Institutes of Health (NIH), June 2014.

because it is controlled by T cells. In males with XMEN, however, the T cells cannot control the virus, and EBV infection can lead to cancers of immune system cells (lymphomas). The word "neoplasia" in the condition name refers to these lymphomas; neoplasia is a general term meaning abnormal growths of tissue. The EBV infection itself usually does not cause any other symptoms in males with XMEN, and affected individuals may not come to medical attention until they develop lymphoma.

Frequency

The prevalence of XMEN is unknown. Only a few affected individuals have been described in the medical literature.

Genetic Changes

XMEN is caused by mutations in the *MAGT1* gene. This gene provides instructions for making a protein called a magnesium transporter, which moves charged atoms (ions) of magnesium ($Mg2+$) into certain T cells. Specifically, the magnesium transporter produced from the *MAGT1* gene is active in CD8+ T cells, which are especially important in controlling viral infections such as the EBV. These cells normally take in magnesium when they detect a foreign invader, and the magnesium is involved in activating the T cell's response.

Researchers suggest that magnesium transport may also be involved in the production of another type of T cell called helper T cells (CD4+ T cells) in a gland called the thymus. CD4+ T cells direct and assist the functions of the immune system by influencing the activities of other immune system cells.

Mutations in the *MAGT1* gene impair the magnesium transporter's function, reducing the amount of magnesium that gets into T cells. This magnesium deficiency prevents the efficient activation of the T cells to target EBV and other infections. Uncontrolled EBV infection increases the likelihood of developing lymphoma. Impaired production of CD4+ T cells resulting from abnormal magnesium transport likely accounts for the deficiency of this type of T cell in people with XMEN, contributing to the decreased ability to prevent infection and illness.

Inheritance Pattern

This condition is inherited in an X-linked recessive pattern. The gene associated with this condition is located on the X chromosome, which is one of the two sex chromosomes. In males (who have only one X chromosome), one altered copy of the gene in each cell is sufficient to cause the condition. In females (who have two X chromosomes), a mutation would have to occur in both copies of the gene to cause the disorder. Because it is unlikely that females will have two altered copies of this gene, males are affected by X-linked recessive disorders much more frequently than females. A characteristic of X-linked inheritance is that fathers cannot pass X-linked traits to their sons.

Other Names for This Condition

- Immunodeficiency, X-linked, with magnesium defect, Epstein-Barr virus infection, and neoplasia

Chapter 31

X-Linked Lymphoproliferative Disease (XLP)

X-linked lymphoproliferative disease (XLP) primarily affects boys and is characterized by a life-long vulnerability to Epstein-Barr virus (EBV), a common type of herpesvirus that usually does not cause symptoms other than a brief infection or mononucleosis. Boys with XLP, however, can have severe reactions to EBV infections.

Causes

XLP is associated with mutations in a gene called *SH2D1A*, which is located on the X chromosome and provides instructions for making SAP protein. These mutations can alter the structure and function of SAP or the amount of SAP produced. Lack of functional SAP causes defects in T- and B-cell interactions, which leads to abnormal immune responses to EBV.

Symptoms and Diagnosis

Boys with XLP are healthy until they are exposed to Epstein-Barr virus (EBV). Then, they can become seriously ill and experience

This chapter includes text excerpted from "X-Linked Lymphoproliferative Disease (XLP)," National Institute of Allergy and Infectious Diseases (NIAID), July 26, 2016.

swollen lymph nodes, an enlarged liver and spleen, hepatitis, and lymphoma. Some boys with XLP have developed lymphoma in the absence of EBV infection.

XLP may be suspected based on an overactive immune response to viral infection, such as development of severe mononucleosis in response to EBV infection. A blood test showing low antibody, or immunoglobulin, levels also may suggest XLP. Diagnosis of XLP requires a demonstrated lack of functional SAP or identification of a loss-of-function mutation in the *SH2D1A* gene.

Treatment

Evidence suggests that rituximab, a drug that targets B cells, can be life-saving in boys with XLP and severe mononucleosis caused by EBV. Doctors may use immunoglobulin replacement therapy to treat the low level of immunoglobulin that occurs in some patients with XLP, but this will not necessarily protect a child against EBV infection. Bone marrow or umbilical cord blood transplantation, which re-set and replenish the immune system, can effectively cure XLP.

Chapter 32

Rare Primary Immunodeficiency Diseases

Chapter Contents

Section 32.1

Interferon Gamma, Interleukin 12, Interleukin 23 Deficiencies

This section includes text excerpted from "Interferon Gamma, Interleukin 12, and Interleukin 23 Deficiencies," National Institute of Allergy and Infectious Diseases (NIAID), July 15, 2012. Reviewed October 2016.

The immune system is a network of cells, tissues, and organs that work together to protect the body from infection. Immune cells communicate using a series of signals that can be secreted into the cell's environment or expressed on the surface of the cell. Interferon gamma (IFN-γ), interleukin 12 (IL-12), and interleukin 23 (IL-23) are key signal molecules that raise an alert against bacteria and other infectious microbes. People with deficiencies in one or more of these signal molecules are susceptible to infections caused by certain bacteria, such as *Mycobacteria*, S*almonella*, and *Listeria*, and viruses, such as herpes.

Causes

Disease-causing mutations that interfere with IFN-γ, IL-12, and IL-23 signaling have been identified in the following genes: *IFNGR1, IFNGR2, STAT1, IL12B, IL12RB1, NEMO*. Generally, mutations in these genes will render immune cells unresponsive to IFN-γ, IL-12, or IL-23 signals in the surrounding tissue or prevent immune cells from producing IL-12 and IL-23 altogether. These mutations can be inherited in an autosomal dominant or recessive pattern.

Symptoms and Diagnosis

People with deficiencies in IFN-γ, IL-12, or IL-23 experience severe, recurring infections, especially those caused by *Mycobacteria*. As a result of these infections, patients with these signal molecule deficiencies may develop granulomas, inflammatory lesions that form in tissues and organs. Depending on which mutation is causing the disease, symptoms may appear early, during infancy and childhood, or later on in life. Genetic testing can determine if a person has a mutation in one of the genes involved in IFN-γ, IL-12, or IL-23 signaling.

Treatment

A physician may prescribe antibiotic therapy to prevent infections. Bone marrow transplantation, which replaces defective immune cells with those from a healthy donor, has been used in patients with these deficiencies successfully.

Section 32.2

Common Variable Immunodeficiency (CVID)

This section includes text excerpted from "Common Variable Immunodeficiency (CVID)," National Institute of Allergy and Infectious Diseases (NIAID), June 21, 2016.

Common variable immunodeficiency (CVID) is characterized by low levels of antibodies and an increased risk of infections. Although the disease usually is diagnosed in adults, it also can occur in children. CVID also is known as hypogammaglobulinemia, adult-onset agammaglobulinemia, late-onset hypogammaglobulinemia, and acquired agammaglobulinemia.

Causes

CVID is caused by a variety of different genetic abnormalities that result in a defect in the capability of immune cells to produce normal amounts of all types of antibodies, also called immunoglobulins. Only a few of these defects have been identified, and therefore the cause of most cases of CVID is unknown. Many people with CVID carry a DNA variation called a polymorphism in a gene known as *TACI*. However, while this genetic abnormality confers increased risk of developing CVID, it is not capable of causing CVID alone.

IgA deficiency is a related condition in which only the level of the antibody immunoglobulin A (IgA) is definitely low, while levels of other immunoglobulin types such as IgG and IgM are usually normal or near normal. IgA deficiency typically occurs alone, but in some cases it may precede the development of CVID or occur in family members of CVID patients.

Symptoms and Diagnosis

Signs and Symptoms

People with CVID can experience frequent bacterial and viral infections of the upper airway, sinuses, and lungs. Acute lung infections can cause pneumonia, and long-term lung infections may cause a chronic form of bronchitis known as bronchiectasis, which is characterized by thickened airway walls colonized by bacteria.

Respiratory infection may be associated with

- Diarrhea and problems absorbing food nutrients
- Reduced liver function and impaired blood flow to the liver
- Painful swollen joints in the knee, ankle, elbow, or wrist
- Enlarged spleen and swollen glands or lymph nodes
- Autoimmune problems that cause reduced levels of blood cells or platelets
- Increased risk of developing some cancers

Diagnosis

Doctors can diagnose CVID by weighing several factors:

- History of recurrent infections, especially of the lungs
- Occurrence of digestive system problems
- Lab tests showing very low immunoglobulin levels
- Low antibody responses to immunization

Treatment

CVID is treated with intravenous immunoglobulin infusion every three to four weeks or subcutaneous (under the skin) immunoglobulin injection weekly to partially restore immunoglobulin levels. The immunoglobulin given by either method provides antibodies from the blood of healthy donors. The frequent bacterial infections experienced by people with CVID are treated with antibiotics. Other problems caused by CVID may require additional, tailored treatments.

Section 32.3

Hyper-Immunoglobulin E Syndrome (Job Syndrome)

This section includes text excerpted from "Hyper-Immunoglobulin E Syndrome (HIES) or Job's Syndrome," National Institute of Allergy and Infectious Diseases (NIAID), July 25, 2016.

People with hyper-immunoglobulin E syndrome, or HIES, have recurrent infections of the skin and lungs caused by bacteria. Patients with HIES typically also have eczema, very high levels of a type of antibody called immunoglobulin E (IgE), distinct facial features, and a tendency to experience bone fractures. HIES is also called Job syndrome.

Causes

Typical cases of HIES are considered autosomal dominant HIES (AD-HIES) and result from mutations in the gene that encodes a signaling molecule called *STAT3*. This molecule is involved in many different activities of the body, explaining why HIES affects facial appearance, bones, lungs, skin, and arteries.

A distinct disease called DOCK8 deficiency is sometimes referred to as autosomal recessive HIES (AR-HIES). In 2009, National Institute of Allergy and Infectious Diseases (NIAID) researchers discovered that the cause of many cases of AR-HIES are explained by a separate disease caused by mutations in the *DOCK8* gene.

Symptoms and Diagnosis

Signs and Symptoms

People with HIES may have recurrent infections of the skin and lungs. These infections are often caused by the bacteria *Staphylococcus aureus* but also may be caused by other bacteria and fungi. Furthermore, people with HIES tend to have recurrent bone fractures, unusually flexible joints, and inflamed skin. Baby teeth in people with

157

HIES often do not fall out on their own. In 2008, NIAID scientists discovered that important immune cells called Th17 cells are missing in people with HIES. In 2011, NIAID researchers also identified that an unusually low number of immune memory cells may cause people with HIES to be more susceptible to some viral infections.

People with HIES often have distinctive facial characteristics, such as the following:

- uneven facial features
- prominent forehead
- deep-set eyes
- broad nasal bridge
- wide, fleshy nose tip
- protruding lower jaw

Diagnosis

A doctor will suspect HIES in a person with eczema, recurrent boils, and pneumonias.

Blood tests diagnosing HIES will show normal levels of IgG, IgA, and IgM antibodies but very high levels of IgE antibodies. Patients with HIES also may show a high number of white blood cells called eosinophils and a poor response to immunizations.

Treatment

The most effective treatments for HIES are continuous antibiotics and antifungals as needed. Some patients receive antibody replacement therapy. Antiseptic approaches, such as dilute bleach baths, are often helpful to prevent skin infections and improve eczema.

Section 32.4

Leukocyte Adhesion Deficiency (LAD)

This section includes text excerpted from "Leukocyte Adhesion Deficiency (LAD)," National Institute of Allergy and Infectious Diseases (NIAID), July 25, 2016.

Leukocyte adhesion deficiency (LAD) is an immune deficiency in which immune cells called phagocytes are unable to move to the site of an infection to fight off invading germs. This inability to fight germs results in recurrent, life-threatening infections and poor wound healing.

Cause

LAD is caused by the absence of a molecule called CD18. These molecules are normally found on the outer surface of phagocytes. Without them, phagocytes cannot attach to blood vessel walls and enter infected tissues, where they help fight infection. *ITGB2* is the gene that instructs, or codes for, the production of CD18. Mutations in this gene cause LAD. LAD is an autosomal recessive disease, meaning an affected person receives a copy of an abnormal gene from both parents.

Symptoms and Diagnosis

Signs and Symptoms

- Children with LAD cannot fight off infection and may have any of the following:
- severe infections of the soft tissue, including skin, muscles, ligaments, and tendons
- eroding skin sores without pus
- severe infections of the gums with tooth loss
- infections of the digestive system
- or wounds that heal slowly or not at all

The more severe form of LAD, known as type 1 LAD, may lead to death in infancy or early childhood. Children with a more moderate form of the disease may survive into young adulthood.

Diagnosis

Blood tests can diagnose children with LAD, who have a very high number of white blood cells and very low levels of CD18. A doctor may suspect LAD if wounds do not heal properly and children develop severe infections caused by bacteria.

Treatment

Doctors prescribe antibiotics to prevent and treat infections. Some children with LAD have been treated successfully with bone marrow transplants, which replace defective immune cells with those of a healthy donor.

Part Four

Acquired Immune
Deficiency Diseases

Chapter 33

Acquired Immunodeficiency Syndrome (AIDS) and Human Immunodeficiency Virus (HIV)

What Is HIV/AIDS?

Human Immunodeficiency Virus (HIV)

HIV stands for human immunodeficiency virus. If left untreated, HIV can lead to the disease AIDS (acquired immunodeficiency syndrome).

Unlike some other viruses, the human body can't get rid of HIV completely. So once you have HIV, you have it for life.

HIV attacks the body's immune system, specifically the CD4 cells (T cells), which help the immune system fight off infections. If left untreated, HIV reduces the number of CD4 cells (T cells) in the body, making the person more likely to get infections or infection-related cancers. Over time, HIV can destroy so many of these cells that the body can't fight off infections and disease. These opportunistic infections

This chapter includes text excerpted from "HIV/AIDS 101," AIDS.gov, U.S. Department of Health and Human Services (HHS), December 31, 2015.

or cancers take advantage of a very weak immune system and signal that the person has AIDS, the last state of HIV infection.

No effective cure for HIV currently exists, but with proper treatment and medical care, HIV can be controlled. The medicine used to treat HIV is called antiretroviral therapy or ART. If taken the right way, every day, this medicine can dramatically prolong the lives of many people with HIV, keep them healthy, and greatly lower their chance of transmitting the virus to others. Today, a person who is diagnosed with HIV, treated before the disease is far advanced, and stays on treatment can live a nearly as long as someone who does not have HIV.

The only way to know for sure if you have HIV is to get tested. Testing is relatively simple. You can ask your healthcare provider for an HIV test. Many medical clinics, substance abuse programs, community health centers, and hospitals offer them too. You can also buy a home testing kit at a pharmacy or online.

Acquired Immunodeficiency Syndrome (AIDS)

AIDS stands for acquired immunodeficiency syndrome. AIDS is the final stage of HIV infection, and not everyone who has HIV advances to this stage.

AIDS is the stage of infection that occurs when your immune system is badly damaged and you become vulnerable to opportunistic infections. When the number of your CD4 cells falls below 200 cells per cubic millimeter of blood (200 cells/mm^3), you are considered to have progressed to AIDS. (The CD4 count of an uninfected adult/adolescent who is generally in good health ranges from 500 cells/mm^3 to 1,600 cells/mm^3.) You can also be diagnosed with AIDS if you develop one or more opportunistic infections, regardless of your CD4 count.

Without treatment, people who are diagnosed with AIDS typically survive about 3 years. Once someone has a dangerous opportunistic illness, life expectancy without treatment falls to about 1 year. People with AIDS need medical treatment to prevent death.

Where Did HIV Come from?

Scientists identified a type of chimpanzee in Central Africa as the source of HIV infection in humans. They believe that the chimpanzee version of the immunodeficiency virus (called simian immunodeficiency virus, or SIV) most likely was transmitted to humans and mutated into HIV when humans hunted these chimpanzees for meat and came into contact with their infected blood. Studies show that HIV may have jumped from apes to humans as far back as the late 1800s. Over decades, the virus slowly spread across Africa and later into other parts of the world. We know that the virus has existed in the United States since at least the mid- to late-1970s.

How Do You Get HIV or AIDS?

How Is HIV Spread?

You can get or transmit HIV only through specific activities. Most commonly, people get or transmit HIV through sexual behaviors and needle or syringe use.

HIV is not spread easily. Only certain body fluids from a person who has HIV can transmit HIV:

- blood

- semen (cum)

- pre-seminal fluid (pre-cum)

- rectal fluids

- vaginal fluids

- breast milk

These body fluids must come into contact with a mucous membrane or damaged tissue or be directly injected into your bloodstream (by a needle or syringe) for transmission to occur. Mucous membranes are found inside the rectum, vagina, penis, and mouth.

Ways HIV Is Transmitted

In the United States, HIV is spread mainly by:

- Having anal or vaginal sex with someone who has HIV without using a condom or taking medicines to prevent or treat HIV.

  - Anal sex is the highest-risk sexual behavior. For the HIV-negative partner, receptive anal sex ("bottoming") is riskier than insertive anal sex ("topping").

  - Vaginal sex is the second highest-risk sexual behavior.

- Sharing needles or syringes, rinse water, or other equipment ("works") used to prepare injection drugs with someone who has

HIV. HIV can live in a used needle up to 42 days depending on temperature and other factors.

Less commonly, HIV may be spread:

- From mother to child during pregnancy, birth, or breastfeeding. Although the risk can be high if a mother is living with HIV and not taking medicine, recommendations to test all pregnant women for HIV and start HIV treatment immediately have lowered the number of babies who are born with HIV.

- By being stuck with an HIV-contaminated needle or other sharp object. This is a risk mainly for healthcare workers.

In extremely rare cases, HIV has been transmitted by:

- Oral sex—putting the mouth on the penis (fellatio), vagina (cunnilingus), or anus (rimming). In general, there is little to no risk of getting HIV from oral sex. But transmission of HIV, though extremely rare, is theoretically possible if an HIV-positive man ejaculates in his partner's mouth during oral sex.

- Receiving blood transfusions, blood products, or organ/tissue transplants that are contaminated with HIV. This was more common in the early years of HIV, but now the risk is extremely small because of rigorous testing of the U.S. blood supply and donated organs and tissues.

- Eating food that has been pre-chewed by an HIV-infected person. The contamination occurs when infected blood from a caregiver's mouth mixes with food while chewing. The only known cases are among infants.

- Being bitten by a person with HIV. Each of the very small number of documented cases has involved severe trauma with extensive tissue damage and the presence of blood. There is no risk of transmission if the skin is not broken.

- Contact between broken skin, wounds, or mucous membranes and HIV-infected blood or blood-contaminated body fluids.

- Deep, open-mouth kissing if the person with HIV has sores or bleeding gums and blood from the HIV-positive partner gets into the bloodstream of the HIV-negative partner. HIV is not spread through saliva.

HIV Is Not Spread By...

HIV does not survive long outside the human body (such as on surfaces) and it cannot reproduce outside a human host. It is **not** spread by:

- air or water
- mosquitoes, ticks or other insects
- saliva, tears, or sweat that is not mixed with the blood of an HIV-positive person
- shaking hands, hugging, sharing toilets, sharing dishes/drinking glasses, or closed-mouth or "social" kissing with someone who is HIV-positive
- drinking fountains
- other sexual activities that don't involve the exchange of body fluids (for example, touching)

HIV Treatment Reduces Transmission Risk

People with HIV who are using antiretroviral therapy (ART) consistently and who have achieved viral suppression (having the virus reduced to an undetectable level in the body) are very unlikely to transmit the virus to their uninfected partners. However, there is still some risk of transmission, so even with an undetectable viral load, people with HIV and their partners should continue to take steps to reduce the risk of HIV transmission.

I Have HIV, Does That Mean I Have AIDS?

No. The terms "HIV" and "AIDS" can be confusing because both terms refer to the same disease. However, "HIV" refers to the virus itself, and "AIDS" refers to the late stage of HIV infection, when an HIV-infected person's immune system is severely damaged and has difficulty fighting diseases and certain cancers. Before the development of certain medications, people with HIV could progress to AIDS in just a few years. But today, most people who are HIV-positive do not progress to AIDS. That's because if you have HIV and you take ART consistently, you can keep the level of HIV in your body low. This will help keep your body strong and healthy and reduce the likelihood that you will ever progress to AIDS. It will also help lower your risk of transmitting HIV to others.

Symptoms of HIV

How Can I Tell If I Have HIV?

You cannot rely on symptoms to tell whether you have HIV. **The only way to know for sure if you have HIV is to get tested.** Knowing your status is important because it helps you make healthy decisions to prevent getting or transmitting HIV.

The symptoms of HIV vary, depending on the individual and what stage of the disease you are in: the early stage, the clinical latency stage, or AIDS (the late stage of HIV infection). Below are the symptoms that some individuals may experience in these three stages. Not all individuals will experience these symptoms.

Early Stage of HIV

Some people may experience a flu-like illness within 2–4 weeks after HIV infection. But some people may not feel sick during this stage.

Flu-like symptoms can include:

- fever

- chills

- rash

- night sweats

- muscle aches

- sore throat

- fatigue

- swollen lymph nodes

- mouth ulcers

These symptoms can last anywhere from a few days to several weeks. During this time, HIV infection may not show up on an HIV test, but people who have it are highly infectious and can spread the infection to others.

You should not assume you have HIV just because you have any of these symptoms. Each of these symptoms can be caused by other illnesses. And some people who have HIV do not show any symptoms at all for 10 years or more.

If you think you may have been exposed to HIV, get an HIV test. Most HIV tests detect antibodies (proteins your body makes as a reaction against the presence of HIV), not HIV itself. But it takes a few weeks for your body to produce these antibodies, so if you test too early, you might not get an accurate test result. A new HIV test is available that can detect HIV directly during this early stage of infection. So be sure to let your testing site know if you think you may have been recently infected with HIV.

After you get tested, it's important to find out the result of your test so you can talk to your healthcare provider about treatment options if you're HIV-positive or learn ways to prevent getting HIV if you're HIV-negative.

You are at high risk of transmitting HIV to others during the early stage of HIV infection, even if you have no symptoms. For this reason, it is very important to take steps to reduce your risk of transmission.

Clinical Latency Stage

After the early stage of HIV infection, the disease moves into a stage called the clinical latency stage (also called "chronic HIV infection"). During this stage, HIV is still active but reproduces at very low levels. People with chronic HIV infection may not have any HIV-related symptoms, or only mild ones.

For people who aren't taking medicine to treat HIV (called antiretroviral therapy or ART), this period can last a decade or longer, but some may progress through this phase faster. People who are taking medicine to treat HIV the right way, every day may be in this stage for several decades because treatment helps keep the virus in check.

It's important to remember that people can still transmit HIV to others during this phase even if they have no symptoms, although people who are on ART and stay virally suppressed (having a very low level of virus in their blood) are much less likely to transmit HIV than those who are not virally suppressed.

Progression to AIDS

If you have HIV and you are not on ART, eventually the virus will weaken your body's immune system and you will progress to AIDS, the late stage of HIV infection.

Symptoms can include:

- rapid weight loss

- recurring fever or profuse night sweats

- extreme and unexplained tiredness

- prolonged swelling of the lymph glands in the armpits, groin, or neck
- diarrhea that lasts for more than a week
- sores of the mouth, anus, or genitals
- pneumonia
- red, brown, pink, or purplish blotches on or under the skin or inside the mouth, nose, or eyelids
- memory loss, depression, and other neurologic disorders

Each of these symptoms can also be related to other illnesses. So the only way to know for sure if you have HIV is to get tested.

Many of the severe symptoms and illnesses of HIV disease come from the opportunistic infections that occur because your body's immune system has been damaged.

Chapter 34

Opportunistic Infections

Opportunistic infections (OIs) are infections that occur more frequently and are more severe in individuals with weakened immune systems, including people with HIV. OIs are less common now than they were in the early days of HIV and AIDS because better treatments reduce the amount of HIV in a person's body and keep a person's immune system stronger. However, many people with HIV still develop OIs because they may not know of their HIV infection, they may not be on treatment, or their treatment may not be keeping their HIV levels low enough for their immune system to fight off infections.

For those reasons, it is important for individuals with HIV to be familiar with the most common OIs so that they can work with their healthcare provider to prevent them or to obtain treatment for them as early as possible.

Most Common Opportunistic Infections

When a person living with HIV gets certain infections (called opportunistic infections, or OIs), he or she will get a diagnosis of AIDS, the most serious stage of HIV infection. AIDS is also diagnosed if a type of blood cell that fights infection (known as CD4 cells) falls below a certain level in persons with HIV. These blood cells are a critical part of a person's immune system.

This chapter includes text excerpted from "Opportunistic Infections," Centers for Disease Control and Prevention (CDC), August 25, 2016.

Centers for Disease Control and Prevention (CDC) has developed a list of OIs that indicate a person has AIDS. It does not matter how many CD4 cells a person has, receiving a diagnosis with any of these OIs means HIV infection has progressed to AIDS. HIV treatment can help restore the person's immune system.

Candidiasis

This illness is caused by infection with a common (and usually harmless) type of fungus called *Candida*. Candidiasis, or infection with *Candida*, can affect the skin, nails, and mucous membranes throughout the body. Persons with HIV infection often have trouble with *Candida*, especially in the mouth and vagina. However, candidiasis is only considered an OI when it infects the esophagus (swallowing tube) or lower respiratory tract, such as the trachea and bronchi (breathing tube), or deeper lung tissue.

Invasive Cervical Cancer

This is a cancer that starts within the cervix, which is the lower part of the uterus at the top of the vagina, and then spreads (becomes invasive) to other parts of the body. This cancer can be prevented by having your care provider perform regular examinations of the cervix.

Coccidioidomycosis

This illness is caused by the fungus *Coccidioides immitis*. It most commonly acquired by inhaling fungal spores, which can lead to a pneumonia that is sometimes called desert fever, San Joaquin Valley fever, or valley fever. The disease is especially common in hot, dry regions of the southwestern United States, Central America, and South America.

Cryptococcosis

This illness is caused by infection with the fungus *Cryptococcus neoformans*. The fungus typically enters the body through the lungs and can cause pneumonia. It can also spread to the brain, causing swelling of the brain. It can infect any part of the body, but (after the brain and lungs) infections of skin, bones, or urinary tract are most common.

Cryptosporidiosis

This diarrheal disease is caused by the protozoan parasite *Cryptosporidium*. Symptoms include abdominal cramps and severe, chronic, watery diarrhea.

Cytomegalovirus Diseases (CMV)

This virus can infect multiple parts of the body and cause pneumonia, gastroenteritis (especially abdominal pain caused by infection of the colon), encephalitis (infection) of the brain, and sight-threatening retinitis (infection of the retina at the back of eye). People with CMV retinitis have difficulty with vision that worsens ever time. CMV retinitis is a medical emergency because it can cause blindness if not treated promptly.

Encephalopathy

This brain disorder is a result of HIV infection. It can occur as part of acute HIV infection or can result from chronic HIV infection. Its exact cause is unknown but it is thought to be related to infection of the brain with HIV and the resulting inflammation.

Herpes Simplex Virus (HSV)

Herpes simplex virus (HSV) is a very common virus that for most people never causes any major problems. HSV is usually acquired sexually or from an infected mother during birth. In most people with healthy immune systems, HSV is usually latent (inactive). However, stress, trauma, other infections, or suppression of the immune system, (such as by HIV), can reactivate the latent virus and symptoms can return. HSV can cause painful cold sores (sometime called fever blisters) in or around the mouth, or painful ulcers on or around the genitals or anus. In people with severely damaged immune systems, HSV can also cause infection of the bronchus (breathing tube), pneumonia (infection of the lungs) and esophagitis (infection of the esophagus, or swallowing tube).

Histoplasmosis

This illness is caused by the fungus *Histoplasma capsulatum*. *Histoplasma* most often infects the lungs and produces symptoms that are similar to those of influenza or pneumonia. People with severely damaged immune systems can get a very serious form of the disease called progressive disseminated histoplasmosis. This form of histoplasmosis can last a long time and involves organs other than the lungs.

Isosporiasis

This infection is caused by the parasite *Isospora belli*, which can enter the body through contaminated food or water. Symptoms include diarrhea, fever, headache, abdominal pain, vomiting, and weight loss.

Kaposi Sarcoma (KS)

This cancer, also known as KS, is caused by a virus called Kaposi sarcoma herpesvirus (KSHV) or human herpesvirus 8 (HHV-8). KS causes small blood vessels, called capillaries, to grow abnormally. Because capillaries are located throughout the body, KS can occur anywhere. KS appears as firm pink or purple spots on the skin that can be raised or flat. KS can be life-threatening when it affects organs inside the body, such the lung, lymph nodes or intestines.

Lymphoma

Lymphoma refers to cancer of the lymph nodes and other lymphoid tissues in the body. There are many different kinds of lymphomas. Some types, such as non-Hodgkin lymphoma and Hodgkin lymphoma, are associated with HIV infection.

Tuberculosis (TB)

Tuberculosis (TB) infection is caused by the bacteria *Mycobacterium tuberculosis*. TB can be spread through the air when a person with active TB coughs, sneezes, or speaks. Breathing in the bacteria can lead to infection in the lungs. Symptoms of TB in the lungs include cough, tiredness, weight loss, fever, and night sweats. Although the disease usually occurs in the lungs, it may also affect other parts of the body, most often the larynx, lymph nodes, brain, kidneys, or bones.

Mycobacterium Avium Complex (MAC) or Mycobacterium Kansasii

MAC is caused by infection with different types of mycobacterium: *Mycobacterium avium*, *Mycobacterium intracellulare*, or *Mycobacterium kansasii*. These mycobacteria live in our environment, including in soil and dust particles. They rarely cause problems for persons with healthy immune systems. In people with severely damaged immune systems, infections with these bacteria spread throughout the body and can be life-threatening.

Pneumocystis Carinii Pneumonia (PCP)

This lung infection, also called PCP, is caused by a fungus, which used to be called *Pneumocystis carinii*, but now is named *Pneumocystis jirovecii*. PCP occurs in people with weakened immune systems, including people with HIV. The first signs of infection are difficulty breathing, high fever, and dry cough.

Pneumonia

Pneumonia is an infection in one or both of the lungs. Many germs, including bacteria, viruses, and fungi can cause pneumonia, with symptoms such as a cough (with mucous), fever, chills, and trouble breathing. In people with immune systems severely damaged by HIV, one of the most common and life-threatening causes of pneumonia is infection with the bacteria *Streptococcus pneumoniae*, also called *Pneumococcus*. There are now effective vaccines that can prevent infection with *Streptococcus pneumoniae* and all persons with HIV infection should be vaccinated.

Progressive Multifocal Leukoencephalopathy

This rare brain and spinal cord disease is caused by the John Cunningham (JC) virus. It is seen almost exclusively in persons whose immune systems have been severely damaged by HIV. Symptoms may include loss of muscle control, paralysis, blindness, speech problems, and an altered mental state. This disease often progresses rapidly and may be fatal.

Salmonella *Septicemia*

Salmonella are a kind of bacteria that typically enter the body through ingestion of contaminated food or water. Infection with salmonella (called salmonellosis) can affect anyone and usually causes a self-limited illness with nausea, vomiting, and diarrhea. *Salmonella* septicemia is a severe form of infection in which the bacteria circulate through the whole body and exceeds the immune system's ability to control it.

Toxoplasmosis

This infection, often called toxo, is caused by the parasite *Toxoplasma gondii*. The parasite is carried by warm-blooded animals including cats, rodents, and birds and is excreted by these animals in their feces. Humans can become infected with it by inhaling dust or eating food contaminated with the parasite. *Toxoplasma* can also occur in commercial meats, especially red meats and pork, but rarely poultry. Infection with toxo can occur in the lungs, retina of the eye, heart, pancreas, liver, colon, testes, and brain. Although cats can transmit toxoplasmosis, litter boxes can be changed safely by wearing gloves and washing hands thoroughly with soap and water afterwards. All raw red meats that have not been frozen for at least 24 hours should be cooked through to an internal temperature of at least 150°F.

Wasting Syndrome Due to HIV

Wasting is defined as the involuntary loss of more than 10 percent of one's body weight while having experienced diarrhea or weakness and fever for more than 30 days. Wasting refers to the loss of muscle mass, although part of the weight loss may also be due to loss of fat.

Preventing Opportunistic Infections

The best ways to prevent getting an OI are to get into and stay on medical care and to take HIV medications as prescribed. Sometimes, your healthcare provider will also prescribe medications specifically to prevent certain OIs. By staying on HIV medications, you can keep the amount of HIV in your body as low as possible and keep your immune system healthy. It is especially important that you get regular check-ups and take all of your medications as prescribed by your care giver. Taking HIV medications is a life-long commitment.

In addition to taking HIV medications to keep your immune system strong, there are other steps you can take to prevent getting an OI.

- Use condoms consistently and correctly to prevent exposure to sexually transmitted infections.

- Don't share drug injection equipment. Blood with hepatitis C in it can remain in syringes and needles after use and the infection can be transmitted to the next user.

- Get vaccinated—your doctor can tell you what vaccines you need. If he or she doesn't, you should ask.

- Understand what germs you are exposed to (such as tuberculosis or germs found in the stools, saliva, or on the skin of animals) and limit your exposure to them.

- Don't consume certain foods, including undercooked eggs, unpasteurized (raw) milk and cheeses, unpasteurized fruit juices, or raw seed sprouts.

- Don't drink untreated water such as water directly from lakes or rivers. Tap water in foreign countries is also often not safe. Use bottled water or water filters.

- Ask your doctor to review with you the other things you do at work, at home, and on vacation to make sure you aren't exposed to an OI.

Treating Opportunistic Infections

If you do develop an OI, there are treatments available, such as antibiotics or antifungal drugs. Having an OI may be a very serious medical situation and its treatment can be challenging. The development of an OI likely means that your immune system is weakened and that your HIV is not under control. That is why it is so important to be on medication, take it as prescribed, see your care provider regularly, and undergo the routine monitoring he or she recommends to ensure your viral load is reduced and your immune system is healthy.

Chapter 35

Graft Versus Host Disease

The immune system is the body's tool that fights infection and disease. It works by seeing harmful cells as "foreign" and attacking them. When you receive a donor's stem cells (the "graft"), the stem cells recreate the donor's immune system in your body (the "host"). Graft versus host disease (GVHD) is the term used when this new immune system from the donor attacks your body. Your donor's cells see your body as "foreign" and attack it, which causes damage. GVHD can range from mild to moderate to severe. Acute GVHD usually occurs within the first 100 days after your transplant or infusion of T-cells (in a donor lymphocyte infusion, or DLI). Acute GVHD commonly affects your skin, liver, and gastrointestinal (GI) tract. Chronic GVHD can happen 60–100 days after transplant and can reoccur for several years after transplant.

What Are the Signs and Symptoms of GVHD?

Skin GVHD

- Red rash
- Itching
- Darkening of skin

This chapter includes text excerpted from "NIH Clinical Center Patient Education Materials—GVHD (Graft-Versus-Host Disease): A Guide for Patients and Families after Stem Cell Transplant," Clinical Center, U.S. Department of Health and Human Services (HHS), May 2015.

Liver GVHD

- Elevated liver enzymes determined through blood tests
- Yellowing of the skin and whites of the eyes
- Abdominal pain

Gastrointestinal (GI) GVHD

- Watery diarrhea
- Stomach cramps (especially before and during bowel movements and after eating)
- Persistent nausea

Can I Prevent GVHD?

The medical team cannot predict if you will get GVHD. Depending on the type of stem cell transplant that you have, your doctor may give you medications to lessen the chance of getting GVHD. These medications suppress your new immune system so that it will not attack your body's cells.

You play an important role in helping the medical team prevent GVHD by taking your medications and protecting yourself from the sun.

- Take the medications prescribed for you after your transplant. Medications such as cyclosporine, tacrolimus, and sirolimus, suppress your immune system to make GVHD less severe. You may need to take these medications for several months after your transplant. It is important to take these medications as prescribed and to report any side effects. If you are unable to take your medications for any reason, or if you have any changes in your skin or in your bowel movements, report that information to your medical team as soon as possible. You will be at greater risk for infection while you take these medications.

- Protect yourself from the sun. Sun exposure can trigger GVHD or make it worse. When you go outside, wear a hat, long sleeves, long pants, and sunscreen. The best protection is to avoid being out in the sun.

How Is GVHD Diagnosed?

Your doctor can diagnose GVHD from your symptoms, as well as from results of laboratory tests and tissue samples. The early symptoms of GVHD are often the same as some side effects and complications after a transplant, so diagnosing GVHD can be hard. Before your doctor can make a diagnosis, your medical team will first make sure that there are not other reasons for the symptoms. You can help your medical team by immediately reporting changes in your symptoms or about the onset of new symptoms.

How Is GVHD Treated?

The goal of GVHD treatment is to lower the graft's immune response against your body, so you will be given medication to do this. Steroids, such as prednisone and methylprednisolone, are medications commonly used. Other medications that lower the immune response, like tacrolimus and sirolimus, are also used. Your treatment may be medications that you take by mouth or put on your skin or an infusion through a vascular access device. Also, treatment may either be outpatient or inpatient. All of these are determined by the severity of your symptoms and concern for complications.

You will be at greater risk for infection while you take steroids. Medications can also cause high blood pressure and other issues. So, along with medication for GVHD, your doctor may admit you to the hospital if you cannot manage your symptoms at home.

How Can I Manage GVHD Symptoms?

Along with your treatment plan, there are also things that you can do to help manage GVHD.

Skin care

- Avoid scratching.
- Use moisturizing lotion. Avoid perfumed lotions.
- Use sunscreen with SPF 30 or greater, and reapply every 1–2 hours while outside.
- Avoid prolonged sun exposure.
- Wear a hat.
- Wear long sleeves and pants.

Diarrhea

- Follow the diet prescribed by your doctor and dietitian to prevent worsening diarrhea.

- Avoid spicy foods.

- Avoid skin problems (such as irritation) around your rectal area. It is very important to keep this area clean. Cleanse this area well after each time that you have diarrhea. Tell your nurse if this area gets red, cracked, painful, or infected.

Preventing infection

- Wash your hands often.

- Stay away from sick family members and friends.

- If your medical team suggests that you wear a mask that covers your nose and mouth, then wear one.

Part Five

Autoimmune Diseases

Chapter 36

Understanding Autoimmune Diseases

When an intruder invades your body—like a cold virus or bacteria on a thorn that pricks your skin—your immune system protects you. It tries to identify, kill and eliminate the invaders that might hurt you. But sometimes problems with your immune system cause it to mistake your body's own healthy cells as invaders and then repeatedly attacks them. This is called an autoimmune disease. ("Autoimmune" means immunity against the self.)

The Immune System

Your immune system is the network of cells and tissues throughout your body that work together to defend you from invasion and infection. You can think of it as having two parts: the acquired and the innate immune systems.

The acquired (or adaptive) immune system develops as a person grows. It "remembers" invaders so that it can fight them if they come back. When the immune system is working properly, foreign invaders provoke the body to activate immune cells against the invaders and to produce proteins called antibodies that attach to the invaders so that they can be recognized and destroyed. The more primitive innate (or

This chapter includes text excerpted from "Understanding Autoimmune Diseases," National Institute of Arthritis and Musculoskeletal and Skin Diseases (NIAMS), March 2016.

185

inborn) immune system activates white blood cells to destroy invaders, without using antibodies.

Autoimmune diseases refer to problems with the acquired immune system's reactions. In an autoimmune reaction, antibodies and immune cells target the body's own healthy tissues by mistake, signaling the body to attack them.

Autoimmune Diseases

Autoimmune diseases can affect almost any part of the body, including the heart, brain, nerves, muscles, skin, eyes, joints, lungs, kidneys, glands, the digestive tract, and blood vessels.

The classic sign of an autoimmune disease is inflammation, which can cause redness, heat, pain, and swelling. How an autoimmune disease affects you depends on what part of the body is targeted. If the disease affects the joints, as in rheumatoid arthritis, you might have joint pain, stiffness, and loss of function. If it affects the thyroid, as in Graves disease and thyroiditis, it might cause tiredness, weight gain, and muscle aches. If it attacks the skin, as it does in scleroderma/ systemic sclerosis, vitiligo, and systemic lupus erythematosus (SLE), it can cause rashes, blisters, and color changes.

Many autoimmune diseases don't restrict themselves to one part of the body. For example, SLE can affect the skin, joints, kidneys, heart, nerves, blood vessels, and more. Type 1 diabetes can affect your glands, eyes, kidneys, muscles, and more.

No one is sure what causes autoimmune diseases. In most cases, a combination of factors is probably at work. For example, you might have a genetic tendency to develop a disease and then, under the right conditions, an outside invader like a virus might trigger it.

The list of diseases that fall into the autoimmune category includes

- alopecia areata

- autoimmune hemolytic anemia

- autoimmune hepatitis

- dermatomyositis

- diabetes (type 1)

- some forms of juvenile idiopathic arthritis

- glomerulonephritis

- Graves disease

- Guillain-Barré syndrome
- idiopathic thrombocytopenic purpura
- myasthenia gravis
- some forms of myocarditis
- multiple sclerosis
- pemphigus/pemphigoid
- pernicious anemia
- polyarteritis nodosa
- polymyositis
- primary biliary cirrhosis
- psoriasis
- rheumatoid arthritis
- scleroderma/systemic sclerosis
- Sjögren syndrome
- systemic lupus erythematosus
- some forms of thyroiditis
- some forms of uveitis
- vitiligo
- granulomatosis with polyangiitis (Wegener's)

The treatment depends on the disease, but in most cases one important goal is to reduce inflammation. Sometimes doctors prescribe corticosteroids or immunosuppressive drugs.

Chapter 37

Autoimmune Disease in Women

What Are Autoimmune Diseases?

Our bodies have an immune system, which is a complex network of special cells and organs that defends the body from germs and other foreign invaders. At the core of the immune system is the ability to tell the difference between self and nonself: what's you and what's foreign. A flaw can make the body unable to tell the difference between self and nonself. When this happens, the body makes autoantibodies that attack normal cells by mistake. At the same time special cells called regulatory T cells fail to do their job of keeping the immune system in line. The result is a misguided attack on your own body. This causes the damage we know as autoimmune disease. The body parts that are affected depend on the type of autoimmune disease. There are more than 80 known types.

How Common Are Autoimmune Diseases?

Overall, autoimmune diseases are common, affecting more than 23.5 million Americans. They are a leading cause of death and

This chapter includes text excerpted from "Autoimmune Diseases Fact Sheet," Office on Women's Health (OWH), U.S. Department of Health and Human Services (HHS), July 16, 2012. Reviewed October 2016.

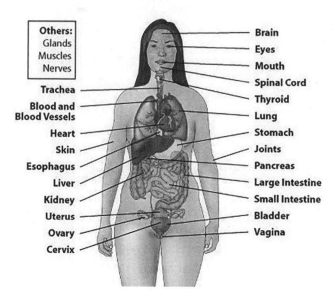

Others:
Glands
Muscles
Nerves
Trachea
Blood and
Blood Vessels
Heart
Skin
Esophagus
Liver
Kidney
Uterus
Ovary
Cervix

Brain
Eyes
Mouth
Spinal Cord
Thyroid
Lung
Stomach
Joints
Pancreas
Large Intestine
Small Intestine
Bladder
Vagina

Figure 37.1. *Body Parts That Can Be Affected by Autoimmune Diseases*

disability. Yet some autoimmune diseases are rare, while others, such as Hashimoto disease, affect many people.

Who Gets Autoimmune Diseases?

Autoimmune diseases can affect anyone. Yet certain people are at greater risk, including:

- **Women of childbearing age**—More women than men have autoimmune diseases, which often start during their childbearing years.

- **People with a family history**—Some autoimmune diseases run in families, such as lupus and multiple sclerosis. It is also common for different types of autoimmune diseases to affect different members of a single family. Inheriting certain genes can make it more likely to get an autoimmune disease. But a combination of genes and other factors may trigger the disease to start.

- **People who are around certain things in the environment**—Certain events or environmental exposures may cause some autoimmune diseases, or make them worse. Sunlight, chemicals called solvents, and viral and bacterial infections are linked to many autoimmune diseases.

- **People of certain races or ethnic backgrounds**—Some autoimmune diseases are more common or more severely affect certain groups of people more than others. For instance, type 1 diabetes is more common in white people. Lupus is most severe for African-American and Hispanic people.

What Autoimmune Diseases Affect Women, and What Are Their Symptoms?

The diseases listed here either are more common in women than men or affect many women and men. They are listed in A-to-Z order.

Although each disease is unique, many share hallmark symptoms, such as fatigue, dizziness, and low-grade fever. For many autoimmune diseases, symptoms come and go, or can be mild sometimes and severe at others. When symptoms go away for a while, it's called remission. Flares are the sudden and severe onset of symptoms.

Table 37.1. Types of Autoimmune Diseases and Their Symptoms

Disease	Symptoms
Alopecia areata The immune system attacks hair follicles (the structures from which hair grows). It usually does not threaten health, but it can greatly affect the way a person looks.	• Patchy hair loss on the scalp, face, or other areas of your body
Antiphospholipid antibody syndrome (aPL) A disease that causes problems in the inner lining of blood vessels resulting in blood clots in arteries or veins.	• Blood clots in veins or arteries • Multiple miscarriages • Lacy, net-like red rash on the wrists and knees
Autoimmune hepatitis The immune system attacks and destroys the liver cells. This can lead to scarring and hardening of the liver, and possibly liver failure.	• Fatigue • Enlarged liver • Yellowing of the skin or whites of eyes • Itchy skin • Joint pain • Stomach pain or upset

Table 37.1. Continued

Disease	Symptoms
Celiac disease A disease in which people can't tolerate gluten, a substance found in wheat, rye, and barley, and also some medicines. When people with celiac disease eat foods or use products that have gluten, the immune system responds by damaging the lining of the small intestines.	• Abdominal bloating and pain • Diarrhea or constipation • Weight loss or weight gain • Fatigue • Missed menstrual periods • Itchy skin rash • Infertility or miscarriages
Diabetes type 1 A disease in which your immune system attacks the cells that make insulin, a hormone needed to control blood sugar levels. As a result, your body cannot make insulin. Without insulin, too much sugar stays in your blood. Too high blood sugar can hurt the eyes, kidneys, nerves, and gums and teeth. But the most serious problem caused by diabetes is heart disease.	• Being very thirsty • Urinating often • Feeling very hungry or tired • Losing weight without trying • Having sores that heal slowly • Dry, itchy skin • Losing the feeling in your feet or having tingling in your feet • Having blurry eyesight
Graves disease (overactive thyroid) A disease that causes the thyroid to make too much thyroid hormone.	• Insomnia • Irritability • Weight loss • Heat sensitivity • Sweating • Fine brittle hair • Muscle weakness • Light menstrual periods • Bulging eyes • Shaky hands Sometimes there are no symptoms
Guillain-Barre syndrome The immune system attacks the nerves that connect your brain and spinal cord with the rest of your body. Damage to the nerves makes it hard for them to transmit signals. As a result, the muscles have trouble responding to the brain.	• Weakness or tingling feeling in the legs that might spread to the upper body • Paralysis in severe cases • Symptoms often progress relatively quickly, over a period of days or weeks, and often occur on both sides of the body.

Table 37.1. Continued

Disease	Symptoms
Hashimoto disease (underactive thyroid) A disease that causes the thyroid to not make enough thyroid hormone.	• Fatigue • Weakness • Weight gain • Sensitivity to cold • Muscle aches and stiff joints • Facial swelling • Constipation
Hemolytic anemia The immune system destroys the red blood cells. Yet the body can't make new red blood cells fast enough to meet the body's needs. As a result, your body does not get the oxygen it needs to function well, and your heart must work harder to move oxygen-rich blood throughout the body.	• Fatigue • Shortness of breath • Dizziness • Headache • Cold hands or feet • Paleness • Yellowish skin or whites of eyes • Heart problems, including heart failure
Idiopathic thrombocytopenic purpura (ITP) A disease in which the immune system destroys blood platelets, which are needed for blood to clot.	• Very heavy menstrual period • Tiny purple or red dots on the skin that might look like a rash. • Easy bruising • Nosebleed or bleeding in the mouth

Inflammatory bowel disease (IBD) A disease that causes chronic inflammation of the digestive tract. Crohn's disease and ulcerative colitis are the most common forms of IBD.	• Abdominal pain
	• Diarrhea, which may be bloody
	• Some people also have:
	  • Rectal bleeding
	  • Fever
	  • Weight loss
	  • Fatigue
	  • Mouth ulcers (in Crohn's disease)
	  • Painful or difficult bowel movements (in ulcerative colitis)

Table 37.1. Continued

Disease	Symptoms

Inflammatory myopathies A group of diseases that involve muscle inflammation and muscle weakness. **Polymyositis** and **dermatomyositis** are 2 types more common in women than men.	• Slow but progressive muscle weakness beginning in the muscles closest to the trunk of the body. Polymyositis affects muscles involved with making movement on both sides of the body. With dermatomyositis, a skin rash comes before or at the same time as muscle weakness.
	• May also have:
	  • Fatigue after walking or standing
	  • Tripping or falling
	  • Difficulty swallowing or breathing

Multiple sclerosis (MS) A disease in which the immune system attacks the protective coating around the nerves. The damage affects the brain and spinal cord.	• Weakness and trouble with coordination, balance, speaking, and walking • Paralysis • Tremors • Numbness and tingling feeling in arms, legs, hands, and feet Symptoms vary because the location and extent of each attack vary
Myasthenia gravis (MG) A disease in which the immune system attacks the nerves and muscles throughout the body.	• Double vision, trouble keeping a steady gaze, and drooping eyelids • Trouble swallowing, with frequent gagging or choking • Weakness or paralysis • Muscles that work better after rest • Drooping head • Trouble climbing stairs or lifting things • Trouble talking
Primary biliary cirrhosis The immune system slowly destroys the liver's bile ducts. Bile is a substance made in the liver. It travels through the bile ducts to help with digestion. When the ducts are destroyed, the bile builds up in the liver and hurts it. The damage causes the liver to harden and scar, and eventually stop working.	• Fatigue • Itchy skin • Dry eyes and mouth • Yellowing of skin and whites of eyes

Table 37.1. Continued

Disease	Symptoms
Psoriasis A disease that causes new skin cells that grow deep in your skin to rise too fast and pile up on the skin surface.	• Thick red patches, covered with scales, usually appearing on the head, elbows, and knees • Itching and pain, which can make it hard to sleep, walk, and care for yourself • May have: • A form of arthritis that often affects the joints and the ends of the fingers and toes. Back pain can occur if the spine is involved.
Rheumatoid arthritis A disease in which the immune system attacks the lining of the joints throughout the body.	• Painful, stiff, swollen, and deformed joints • Reduced movement and function • May have: • Fatigue • Fever • Weight loss • Eye inflammation • Lung disease • Lumps of tissue under the skin, often the elbows • Anemia
Scleroderma A disease causing abnormal growth of connective tissue in the skin and blood vessels.	• Fingers and toes that turn white, red, or blue in response to heat and cold • Pain, stiffness, and swelling of fingers and joints • Thickening of the skin • Skin that looks shiny on the hands and forearm • Tight and mask-like facial skin • Sores on the fingers or toes • Trouble swallowing • Weight loss • Diarrhea or constipation • Shortness of breath
Sjögren syndrome A disease in which the immune system targets the glands that make moisture, such as tears and saliva.	• Dry eyes or eyes that itch • Dryness of the mouth, which can cause sores • Trouble swallowing • Loss of sense of taste • Severe dental cavities • Hoarse voice • Fatigue • Joint swelling or pain • Swollen glands • Cloudy eyes

195

Table 37.1. Continued

Disease	Symptoms
Systemic lupus erythematosus A disease that can damage the joints, skin, kidneys, heart, lungs, and other parts of the body. Also called SLE or lupus.	• Fever • Weight loss • Hair loss • Mouth sores • Fatigue • "Butterfly" rash across the nose and cheeks • Rashes on other parts of the body • Painful or swollen joints and muscle pain • Sensitivity to the sun • Chest pain • Headache, dizziness, seizure, memory problems, or change in behavior
Vitiligo The immune system destroys the cells that give your skin its color. It also can affect the tissue inside your mouth and nose.	• White patches on areas exposed to the sun, or on armpits, genitals, and rectum • Hair turns gray early • Loss of color inside your mouth

FAQs on Autoimmune Disease in Women

Are There Alternative Treatments That Can Help?

Many people try some form of complimentary and alternative medicine (CAM) at some point in their lives. Some examples of CAM are herbal products, chiropractic, acupuncture, and hypnosis. If you have an autoimmune disease, you might wonder if CAM therapies can help some of your symptoms. This is hard to know. Studies on CAM therapies are limited. Also, some CAM products can cause health problems or interfere with how the medicines you might need work. If you want to try a CAM treatment, be sure to discuss it with your doctor. Your doctor can tell you about the possible benefits and risks of trying CAM.

I Want to Have a Baby. Does Having an Autoimmune Disease Affect Pregnancy?

Women with autoimmune diseases can safely have children. But there could be some risks for the mother or baby, depending on the disease and how severe it is. For instance, pregnant women with lupus have a higher risk of preterm birth and stillbirth. Pregnant women with myasthenia gravis (MG) might have symptoms that lead to trouble breathing during pregnancy. For some women, symptoms tend to improve during pregnancy, while others find their symptoms tend to flare up. Also, some medicines used to treat autoimmune diseases might not be safe to use during pregnancy.

If you want to have a baby, talk to your doctor before you start trying to get pregnant. Your doctor might suggest that you wait until your disease is in remission or suggest a change in medicines before you start trying. You also might need to see a doctor who cares for women with high-risk pregnancies.

Some women with autoimmune diseases may have problems getting pregnant. This can happen for many reasons. Tests can tell if fertility problems are caused by an autoimmune disease or an unrelated reason. Fertility treatments are able to help some women with autoimmune disease become pregnant.

How Can I Manage My Life Now That I Have an Autoimmune Disease?

Although most autoimmune diseases don't go away, you can treat your symptoms and learn to manage your disease, so you can enjoy life! Women with autoimmune diseases lead full, active lives. Your life goals should not have to change. It is important, though, to see a doctor who specializes in these types of diseases, follow your treatment plan, and adopt a healthy lifestyle.

How Can I Deal with Flares?

Flares are the sudden and severe onset of symptoms. You might notice that certain triggers, such as stress or being out in the sun, cause your symptoms to flare. Knowing your triggers, following your treatment plan, and seeing your doctor regularly can help you to prevent flares or keep them from becoming severe. If you suspect a flare is coming, call your doctor. Don't try a "cure" you heard about from a friend or relative.

What Are Some Things I Can Do to Feel Better?

If you are living with an autoimmune disease, there are things you can do each day to feel better:

- **Eat healthy, well-balanced meals.** Make sure to include fruits and vegetables, whole grains, fat-free or low-fat milk products, and lean sources of protein. Limit saturated fat, *trans* fat, cholesterol, salt, and added sugars. If you follow a healthy eating plan, you will get the nutrients you need from food.

- **Get regular physical activity. But be careful not to overdo it.** Talk with your doctor about what types of physical activity you can do. A gradual and gentle exercise program often works well for people with long-lasting muscle and joint pain. Some types of yoga or tai chi exercises may be helpful.

- **Get enough rest.** Rest allows your body tissues and joints the time they need to repair. Sleeping is a great way you can help both your body and mind. If you don't get enough sleep, your stress level and your symptoms could get worse. You also can't fight off sickness as well when you sleep poorly. When you are well-rested, you can tackle your problems better and lower your risk for illness. Most people need at least 7 to 9 hours of sleep each day to feel well-rested.

- **Reduce stress.** Stress and anxiety can trigger symptoms to flare up with some autoimmune diseases. So finding ways to simplify your life and cope with daily stressors will help you to feel your best. Meditation, self-hypnosis, and guided imagery, are simple relaxation techniques that might help you to reduce stress, lessen your pain, and deal with other aspects of living with your disease. You can learn to do these through self-help books, tapes, or with the help of an instructor. Joining a support group or talking with a counselor might also help you to manage your stress and cope with your disease.

You have some power to lessen your pain! Try using imagery for 15 minutes, two or three times each day.

1. Put on your favorite calming music.

2. Lie back on your favorite chair or sofa. Or if you are at work, sit back and relax in your chair.

3. Close your eyes.

4. Imagine your pain or discomfort.

5. Imagine something that confronts this pain and watch it "destroy" the pain.

Chapter 38

Addison Disease

What Is Autoimmune Addison Disease?

Autoimmune Addison disease affects the function of the adrenal glands, which are small hormone-producing glands located on top of each kidney. It is classified as an autoimmune disorder because it results from a malfunctioning immune system that attacks the adrenal glands. As a result, the production of several hormones is disrupted, which affects many body systems.

The signs and symptoms of autoimmune Addison disease can begin at any time, although they most commonly begin between ages 30 and 50. Common features of this condition include extreme tiredness (fatigue), nausea, decreased appetite, and weight loss. In addition, many affected individuals have low blood pressure (hypotension), which can lead to dizziness when standing up quickly; muscle cramps; and a craving for salty foods. A characteristic feature of autoimmune Addison disease is abnormally dark areas of skin (hyperpigmentation), especially in regions that experience a lot of friction, such as the armpits, elbows, knuckles, and palm creases. The lips and the inside lining of the mouth can also be unusually dark. Because of an imbalance of hormones involved in development of sexual characteristics, women with this condition may lose their underarm and pubic hair.

Other signs and symptoms of autoimmune Addison disease include low levels of sugar (hypoglycemia) and sodium (hyponatremia) and

This chapter includes text excerpted from "Autoimmune Addison Disease," Genetics Home Reference (GHR), National Institutes of Health (NIH), June 2014.

high levels of potassium (hyperkalemia) in the blood. Affected individuals may also have a shortage of red blood cells (anemia) and an increase in the number of white blood cells (lymphocytosis), particularly those known as eosinophils (eosinophilia).

Autoimmune Addison disease can lead to a life-threatening adrenal crisis, characterized by vomiting, abdominal pain, back or leg cramps, and severe hypotension leading to shock. The adrenal crisis is often triggered by a stressor, such as surgery, trauma, or infection.

Individuals with autoimmune Addison disease or their family members often have another autoimmune disorder, most commonly autoimmune thyroid disease or type 1 diabetes.

Frequency

Addison disease affects approximately 11 to 14 in 100,000 people of European descent. The autoimmune form of the disorder is the most common form in developed countries, accounting for up to 90 percent of cases.

Genetic Changes

The cause of autoimmune Addison disease is complex and not completely understood. A combination of environmental and genetic factors plays a role in the disorder, and changes in multiple genes are thought to affect the risk of developing the condition.

The genes that have been associated with autoimmune Addison disease participate in the body's immune response. The most commonly associated genes belong to a family of genes called the human leukocyte antigen (HLA) complex. The HLA complex helps the immune system distinguish the body's own proteins from proteins made by foreign invaders (such as viruses and bacteria). Each HLA gene has many different normal variations, allowing each person's immune system to react to a wide range of foreign proteins. The most well-known risk factor for autoimmune Addison disease is a variant of the *HLA-DRB1* gene called *HLA-DRB1*04:04*. This and other disease-associated HLA gene variants likely contribute to an inappropriate immune response that leads to autoimmune Addison disease, although the mechanism is unknown.

Normally, the immune system responds only to proteins made by foreign invaders, not to the body's own proteins. In autoimmune Addison disease, however, an immune response is triggered by a normal adrenal gland protein, typically a protein called 21-hydroxylase. This protein plays a key role in producing certain hormones in the adrenal glands. The prolonged immune attack triggered by 21-hydroxylase damages the adrenal glands (specifically the outer layers of the glands known, collectively, as the adrenal cortex), preventing hormone production. A shortage of adrenal hormones (adrenal insufficiency) disrupts several normal functions in the body, leading to hypoglycemia, hyponatremia, hypotension, muscle cramps, skin hyperpigmentation and other features of autoimmune Addison disease.

Rarely, Addison disease is not caused by an autoimmune reaction. Other causes include infections that damage the adrenal glands, such as tuberculosis, or tumors in the adrenal glands. Addison disease can also be one of several features of other genetic conditions, including X-linked adrenoleukodystrophy and autoimmune polyglandular syndrome, type 1, which are caused by mutations in other genes.

Inheritance Pattern

A predisposition to develop autoimmune Addison disease is passed through generations in families, but the inheritance pattern is unknown.

Other Names for This Conditon

- Autoimmune Addison disease
- Autoimmune adrenalitis
- Classic Addison disease
- Primary Addison disease

Chapter 39

Alopecia Areata

What Is Alopecia Areata?

Alopecia areata is considered an autoimmune disease, in which the immune system, which is designed to protect the body from foreign invaders such as viruses and bacteria, mistakenly attacks the hair follicles, the structures from which hairs grow. This can lead to hair loss on the scalp and elsewhere.

In most cases, hair falls out in small, round patches about the size of a quarter. In many cases, the disease does not extend beyond a few bare patches. In some people, hair loss is more extensive. Although uncommon, the disease can progress to cause total loss of hair on the scalp (referred to as alopecia areata totalis) or complete loss of hair on the scalp, face, and body (alopecia areata universalis).

In alopecia areata, immune system cells called white blood cells attack the rapidly growing cells in the hair follicles. The affected hair follicles become small and drastically slow down hair production. Fortunately, the stem cells that continuously supply the follicle with new cells do not seem to be targeted. So the follicle always has the potential to regrow hair.

Scientists do not know exactly why the hair follicles undergo these changes, but they suspect that a combination of genes may predispose some people to the disease. In those who are genetically predisposed,

This chapter includes text excerpted from "Alopecia Areata," National Institute of Arthritis and Musculoskeletal and Skin Diseases (NIAMS), May 2016.

some type of trigger—perhaps a virus or something in the person's environment—brings on the attack against the hair follicles.

Who Is Most Likely to Get It?

Alopecia areata affects nearly 2 percent of Americans of both sexes and of all ages and ethnic backgrounds. It often begins in childhood.

If you have a close family member with the disease, your risk of developing it is slightly increased. If your family member lost his or her first patch of hair before age 30, the risk to other family members is greater.

Is My Hair Loss a Symptom of a Serious Disease?

Alopecia areata is not a life-threatening disease. It does not cause any physical pain, and people with the condition are generally healthy otherwise. But for most people, a disease that unpredictably affects their appearance the way alopecia areata does is a serious matter.

The effects of alopecia areata are primarily socially and emotionally disturbing. In alopecia universalis, however, loss of eyelashes and eyebrows and hair in the nose and ears can make the person more vulnerable to dust, germs, and foreign particles entering the eyes, nose, and ears.

Alopecia areata often occurs in people whose family members have other autoimmune diseases, such as type 1 diabetes, rheumatoid arthritis, thyroid disease, systemic lupus erythematosus, pernicious anemia, or Addison disease. People who have alopecia areata do not usually have other autoimmune diseases, but they do have a higher occurrence of thyroid disease, atopic eczema, nasal allergies, and asthma.

Can I Pass It On to My Children?

It is possible for alopecia areata to be inherited. However, most children with alopecia areata do not have a parent with the disease, and the vast majority of parents with alopecia areata do not pass it along to their children.

What Causes It?

Alopecia areata is not like some genetic diseases in which a child has a 50-50 chance of developing the disease if one parent has it.

Scientists believe that there may be a number of genes that predispose certain people to the disease. It is highly unlikely that a child would inherit all of the genes needed to predispose him or her to the disease.

Even with the right (or wrong) combination of genes, alopecia areata is not a certainty. Studies suggest that in identical twins, who share all of the same genes, the concordance rate is only 55 percent. In other words, if one twin has the disease, there is only a 55 percent chance that the other twin will have it as well. This shows that other factors besides genetics are required to trigger the disease.

Will My Hair Ever Grow Back?

There is every chance that your hair will regrow with or without treatment, but it may also fall out again. No one can predict when it might regrow or fall out. The course of the disease varies from person to person. Some people lose just a few patches of hair, then the hair regrows, and the condition never recurs. Other people continue to lose and regrow hair for many years. A few lose all the hair on the scalp; some lose all the hair on the scalp, face, and body. Even in those who lose all their hair, the possibility for full regrowth remains. The course of alopecia areata is highly unpredictable, and the uncertainty of what will happen next is probably the most difficult and frustrating aspect of the disease.

In some, the initial hair regrowth is white, with a gradual return of the original hair color. In most, the regrown hair is ultimately the same color and texture as the original hair.

How Is It Treated?

Although there is neither a cure for alopecia areata nor drugs approved for its treatment, some people find that medications approved for other purposes can help hair grow back, at least temporarily. Keep in mind that although these treatments may promote hair growth, none of them prevent new patches or actually cure the underlying disease. Consult your healthcare professional about the best option for you. A combination of treatments may work best. Ask how long the treatment may last, how long it will take before you see results, and about the possible side effects.

In addition to treatments to help hair grow, there are measures that can be taken to minimize the effects of excessive sun exposure or discomforts of lost hair.

- Sunscreens are important for the scalp, face, and all exposed areas.

- Eyeglasses (or sunglasses) protect the eyes from excessive sun and from dust and debris when eyebrows or eyelashes are missing.

- Wigs, caps, or scarves protect the scalp from the sun and keep the head warm.

- An ointment applied inside the nostrils keeps them moisturized and helps to protect against organisms invading the nose when nostril hair is missing.

How Will Alopecia Areata Affect My Life?

This is a common question, particularly for children, teens, and young adults who are beginning to form lifelong goals and who may live with the effects of alopecia areata for many years. The comforting news is that alopecia areata is not a painful disease and does not make people feel physically sick. It is not contagious, and people who have the disease are generally healthy otherwise. It does not reduce life expectancy, and it should not interfere with going to school, playing sports and exercising, pursuing any career, working, marrying, and raising a family.

The emotional aspects of living with hair loss, however, can be challenging. Many people cope by learning as much as they can about the disease, speaking with others who are facing the same problem, and, if necessary, seeking counseling to help build a positive self-image.

Chapter 40

Autoimmune-Related Anemias

Chapter Contents

Section 40.1

Autoimmune Hemolytic Anemia

This section includes text excerpted from "Hemolytic Anemia,"
National Heart, Lung, and Blood Institute (NHLBI), March 21, 2014.

What Is Hemolytic Anemia?

Hemolytic anemia is a condition in which red blood cells are destroyed and removed from the bloodstream before their normal lifespan is over.

Red blood cells are disc-shaped and look like doughnuts without holes in the center. These cells carry oxygen to your body. They also remove carbon dioxide (a waste product) from your body.

Red blood cells are made in the bone marrow—a sponge-like tissue inside the bones. They live for about 120 days in the bloodstream and then die.

White blood cells and platelets also are made in the bone marrow. White blood cells help fight infections. Platelets stick together to seal small cuts or breaks on blood vessel walls and stop bleeding.

When blood cells die, the body's bone marrow makes more blood cells to replace them. However, in hemolytic anemia, the bone marrow can't make red blood cells fast enough to meet the body's needs.

Hemolytic anemia can lead to many health problems, such as fatigue (tiredness), pain, irregular heartbeats called arrhythmias, an enlarged heart, and heart failure.

Types of Hemolytic Anemia

There are many types of hemolytic anemia. The condition can be inherited or acquired. "Inherited" means your parents passed the gene for the condition on to you. "Acquired" means you aren't born with the condition, but you develop it.

The following are various types of hemolytic anemias:

- Inherited Hemolytic Anemias
  - Sickle cell anemia

- Thalassemias
- Hereditary spherocytosis
- Hereditary elliptocytosis (ovalocytosis)
- Glucose-6-phosphate dehydrogenase (G6PD) Deficiency
- Pyruvate kinase deficiency
- Acquired Hemolytic Anemias
  - Immune hemolytic anemia
  - Autoimmune hemolytic anemia (AIHA)
  - Alloimmune hemolytic anemia
  - Mechanical hemolytic anemias
  - Paroxysmal nocturnal hemoglobinuria

Other Names for Hemolytic Anemia

- Alloimmune hemolytic anemia
- Drug-induced hemolytic anemia
- Glucose-6-phosphate dehydrogenase (G6PD) deficiency
- Hereditary elliptocytosis
- Hereditary ovalocytosis
- Hereditary spherocytosis
- Immune hemolytic anemia
- Microangiopathic hemolytic anemia
- Paroxysmal nocturnal hemoglobinuria (PNH)
- Pyruvate kinase deficiency
- Sickle cell anemia
- Thalassemias

What Causes Hemolytic Anemia?

The immediate cause of hemolytic anemia is the early destruction of red blood cells. This means that red blood cells are destroyed and removed from the bloodstream before their normal lifespan is over.

Many diseases, conditions, and factors can cause the body to destroy its red blood cells. These causes can be inherited or acquired. "Inherited" means your parents passed the gene for the condition on to you. "Acquired" means you aren't born with the condition, but you develop it.

Who Is at Risk for Hemolytic Anemia?

Hemolytic anemia can affect people of all ages and races and both sexes. Some types of hemolytic anemia are more likely to occur in certain populations than others.

For example, glucose-6-phosphate dehydrogenase (G6PD) deficiency mostly affects males of African or Mediterranean descent. In the United States, the condition is more common among African Americans than Caucasians.

In the United States, sickle cell anemia mainly affects African Americans.

What Are the Signs and Symptoms of Hemolytic Anemia?

The signs and symptoms of hemolytic anemia will depend on the type and severity of the disease.

People who have mild hemolytic anemia often have no signs or symptoms. More severe hemolytic anemia may cause many signs and symptoms, and they may be serious.

Many of the signs and symptoms of hemolytic anemia apply to all types of anemia:

- jaundice
- pain in the upper abdomen
- leg ulcers and pain
- a severe reaction to a blood transfusion

How Is Hemolytic Anemia Diagnosed?

Your doctor will diagnose hemolytic anemia based on your medical and family histories, a physical exam, and test results.

Specialists Involved

Primary care doctors, such as a family doctor or pediatrician, may help diagnose and treat hemolytic anemia. Your primary care doctor also may refer you to a hematologist. This is a doctor who specializes in diagnosing and treating blood diseases and disorders.

Doctors and clinics that specialize in treating inherited blood disorders, such as sickle cell anemia and thalassemias, also may be involved.

If your hemolytic anemia is inherited, you may want to consult a genetic counselor. A counselor can help you understand your risk of having a child who has the condition. He or she also can explain the choices that are available to you.

How Is Hemolytic Anemia Treated?

Treatments for hemolytic anemia include blood transfusions, medicines, plasmapheresis, surgery, blood and marrow stem cell transplants, and lifestyle changes.

People who have mild hemolytic anemia may not need treatment, as long as the condition doesn't worsen. People who have severe hemolytic anemia usually need ongoing treatment. Severe hemolytic anemia can be fatal if it's not properly treated.

How Can Hemolytic Anemia Be Prevented?

You can't prevent inherited types of hemolytic anemia. One exception is glucose-6-phosphate dehydrogenase (G6PD) deficiency.

If you're born with G6PD deficiency, you can avoid substances that may trigger the condition. For example, avoid fava beans, naphthalene (a substance found in some moth balls), and certain medicines (as your doctor advises).

Some types of acquired hemolytic anemia can be prevented. For example, reactions to blood transfusions, which can cause hemolytic anemia, can be prevented. This requires careful matching of blood types between the blood donor and the recipient.

Prompt and proper prenatal care can help you avoid the problems of Rh incompatibility. This condition can occur during pregnancy if a woman has Rh-negative blood and her baby has Rh-positive blood. "Rh-negative" and "Rh-positive" refer to whether your blood has Rh factor. Rh factor is a protein on red blood cells.

Rh incompatibility can lead to hemolytic anemia in a fetus or newborn.

Section 40.2

Pernicious Anemia

This section includes text excerpted from "Pernicious Anemia,"
National Heart, Lung, and Blood Institute (NHLBI), April 1, 2011.
Reviewed October 2016.

What Is Pernicious Anemia?

Pernicious anemia is a condition in which the body can't make enough healthy red blood cells because it doesn't have enough vitamin B12.

Vitamin B12 is a nutrient found in some foods. The body needs this nutrient to make healthy red blood cells and to keep its nervous system working properly.

People who have pernicious anemia can't absorb enough vitamin B12 from food. This is because they lack intrinsic factor, a protein made in the stomach. A lack of this protein leads to vitamin B12 deficiency.

Other conditions and factors also can cause vitamin B12 deficiency. Examples include infections, surgery, medicines, and diet. Technically, the term "pernicious anemia" refers to vitamin B12 deficiency due to a lack of intrinsic factor. Often though, vitamin B12 deficiency due to other causes also is called pernicious anemia.

This section discusses pernicious anemia due to a lack of intrinsic factor and other causes.

Other Names for Pernicious Anemia

Pernicious anemia is one of two major types of "macrocystic" or "megaloblastic" anemia. These terms refer to anemia in which the red blood cells are larger than normal. (The other major type of macrocystic anemia is caused by folic acid deficiency.)

Rarely, children are born with an inherited disorder that prevents their bodies from making intrinsic factor. This disorder is called congenital pernicious anemia.

Vitamin B12 deficiency also is called cobalamin deficiency and combined systems disease.

What Causes Pernicious Anemia?

Pernicious anemia is caused by a lack of intrinsic factor (a protein made in the stomach) or other causes, such as infections, surgery, medicines, or diet.

Who Is at Risk for Pernicious Anemia?

Pernicious anemia is more common in people of Northern European and African descent than in other ethnic groups.

Older people also are at higher risk for the condition. This is mainly due to a lack of stomach acid and intrinsic factor, which prevents the small intestine from absorbing vitamin B12. As people grow older, they tend to make less stomach acid.

Pernicious anemia also can occur in younger people and other populations. You're at higher risk for pernicious anemia if you:

- Have a family history of the condition.

- Have had part or all of your stomach surgically removed. The stomach makes intrinsic factor. This protein helps your body absorb vitamin B12.

- Have an autoimmune disorder that involves the endocrine glands, such as Addison disease, type 1 diabetes, Grave disease, or vitiligo. Research suggests a link may exist between these autoimmune disorders and pernicious anemia that's caused by an autoimmune response.

- Have had part or all of your small intestine surgically removed. The small intestine is where vitamin B12 is absorbed.

- Have certain intestinal diseases or other disorders that may prevent your body from properly absorbing vitamin B12. Examples include Crohn's disease, intestinal infections, and HIV.

- Take medicines that prevent your body from properly absorbing vitamin B12. Examples of such medicines include antibiotics and certain seizure medicines.

- Are a strict vegetarian who doesn't eat any animal or dairy products and doesn't take a vitamin B12 supplement, or if you eat poorly overall.

What Are the Signs and Symptoms of Pernicious Anemia?

A lack of vitamin B12 (vitamin B12 deficiency) causes the signs and symptoms of pernicious anemia. Without enough vitamin B12, your body can't make enough healthy red blood cells, which causes anemia.

Some of the signs and symptoms of pernicious anemia apply to all types of anemia. Other signs and symptoms are specific to a lack of vitamin B12.

How Is Pernicious Anemia Diagnosed?

Your doctor will diagnose pernicious anemia based on your medical and family histories, a physical exam, and test results.

Your doctor will want to find out whether the condition is due to a lack of intrinsic factor or another cause. He or she also will want to find out the severity of the condition, so it can be properly treated.

Specialists Involved

Primary care doctors—such as family doctors, internists, and pediatricians (doctors who treat children)—often diagnose and treat pernicious anemia. Other kinds of doctors also may be involved, including:

- a neurologist (nervous system specialist)

- a cardiologist (heart specialist)

- a hematologist (blood disease specialist)

- a gastroenterologist (digestive tract specialist)

How Is Pernicious Anemia Treated?

Doctors treat pernicious anemia by replacing the missing vitamin B12 in the body. People who have pernicious anemia may need lifelong treatment.

The goals of treating pernicious anemia include:

- Preventing or treating the anemia and its signs and symptoms

- Preventing or managing complications, such as heart and nerve damage

- Treating the cause of the pernicious anemia (if a cause can be found)

How Can Pernicious Anemia Be Prevented?

You can't prevent pernicious anemia caused by a lack of intrinsic factor. Without intrinsic factor, you won't be able to absorb vitamin B12 and will develop pernicious anemia.

Although uncommon, some people develop pernicious anemia because they don't get enough vitamin B12 in their diets. You can take steps to prevent pernicious anemia caused by dietary factors.

Eating foods high in vitamin B12 can help prevent low vitamin B12 levels. Good food sources of vitamin B12 include:

- breakfast cereals with added vitamin B12

- meats such as beef, liver, poultry, and fish

- eggs and dairy products (such as milk, yogurt, and cheese)

- foods fortified with vitamin B12, such as soy-based beverages and vegetarian burgers

If you're a strict vegetarian, talk with your doctor about having your vitamin B12 level checked regularly.

Vitamin B12 also is found in multivitamins and B-complex vitamin supplements. Doctors may recommend supplements for people at risk for vitamin B12 deficiency, such as strict vegetarians or people who have had stomach surgery.

Older adults may have trouble absorbing vitamin B12. Thus, doctors may recommend that older adults eat foods fortified with vitamin B12 or take vitamin B12 supplements.

Chapter 41

Antiphospholipid Antibody Syndrome

What Is Antiphospholipid Antibody Syndrome?

Antiphospholipid antibody syndrome (APS) is an autoimmune disorder. Autoimmune disorders occur if the body's immune system makes antibodies that attack and damage tissues or cells.

Antibodies are a type of protein. They usually help defend the body against infections. In APS, however, the body makes antibodies that mistakenly attack phospholipids—a type of fat.

Phospholipids are found in all living cells and cell membranes, including blood cells and the lining of blood vessels.

When antibodies attack phospholipids, cells are damaged. This damage causes blood clots to form in the body's arteries and veins. (These are the vessels that carry blood to your heart and body.)

Usually, blood clotting is a normal bodily process. Blood clots help seal small cuts or breaks on blood vessel walls. This prevents you from losing too much blood. In APS, however, too much blood clotting can block blood flow and damage the body's organs.

This chapter includes text excerpted from "Antiphospholipid Antibody Syndrome," National Heart, Lung, and Blood Institute (NHLBI), May 17, 2012. Reviewed October 2016.

Other Names for Antiphospholipid Antibody Syndrome

- Anticardiolipin antibody syndrome, or aCL syndrome

- Antiphospholipid syndrome

- aPL syndrome

- Hughes syndrome

- Lupus anticoagulant syndrome

What Causes Antiphospholipid Antibody Syndrome?

Antiphospholipid antibody syndrome (APS) occurs if the body's immune system makes antibodies (proteins) that attack phospholipids.

Phospholipids are a type of fat found in all living cells and cell membranes, including blood cells and the lining of blood vessels. What causes the immune system to make antibodies against phospholipids isn't known.

APS causes unwanted blood clots to form in the body's arteries and veins. Usually, blood clotting is a normal bodily process. It helps seal small cuts or breaks on blood vessel walls. This prevents you from losing too much blood. In APS, however, too much blood clotting can block blood flow and damage the body's organs.

Researchers don't know why APS antibodies cause blood clots to form. Some believe that the antibodies damage or affect the inner lining of the blood vessels, which causes blood clots to form. Others believe that the immune system makes antibodies in response to blood clots damaging the blood vessels.

Who Is at Risk for Antiphospholipid Antibody Syndrome?

Antiphospholipid antibody syndrome (APS) can affect people of any age. The disorder is more common in women than men, but it affects both sexes.

APS also is more common in people who have other autoimmune or rheumatic disorders, such as lupus. ("Rheumatic" refers to disorders that affect the joints, bones, or muscles.)

About 10 percent of all people who have lupus also have APS. About half of all people who have APS also have another autoimmune or rheumatic disorder.

Some people have APS antibodies, but don't ever have signs or symptoms of the disorder. The mere presence of APS antibodies doesn't mean that you have APS. To be diagnosed with APS, you must have APS antibodies and a history of health problems related to the disorder.

However, people who have APS antibodies but no signs or symptoms are at risk of developing APS. Health problems, other than autoimmune disorders, that can trigger blood clots include:

- smoking

- prolonged bed rest

- pregnancy and the postpartum period

- birth control pills and hormone therapy

- cancer and kidney disease

What Are the Signs and Symptoms of Antiphospholipid Antibody Syndrome?

The signs and symptoms of antiphospholipid antibody syndrome (APS) are related to abnormal blood clotting. The outcome of a blood clot depends on its size and location.

Blood clots can form in, or travel to, the arteries or veins in the brain, heart, kidneys, lungs, and limbs. Clots can reduce or block blood flow. This can damage the body's organs and may cause death.

Major Signs and Symptoms

Major signs and symptoms of blood clots include:

- chest pain and shortness of breath

- pain, redness, warmth, and swelling in the limbs

- ongoing headaches

- speech changes

- upper body discomfort in the arms, back, neck, and jaw

- nausea (feeling sick to your stomach)

Other Signs and Symptoms

Other signs and symptoms of APS include chronic (ongoing) headaches, memory loss, and heart valve problems. Some people who have APS also get a lacy-looking red rash on their wrists and knees.

How Is Antiphospholipid Antibody Syndrome Diagnosed?

Your doctor will diagnose antiphospholipid antibody syndrome (APS) based on your medical history and the results from blood tests.

Specialists Involved

A hematologist often is involved in the care of people who have APS. This is a doctor who specializes in diagnosing and treating blood diseases and disorders.

You may have APS and another autoimmune disorder, such as lupus. If so, a doctor who specializes in that disorder also may provide treatment.

Many autoimmune disorders that occur with APS also affect the joints, bones, or muscles. Rheumatologists specialize in treating these types of disorders.

Medical History

Some people have APS antibodies but no signs or symptoms of the disorder. Having APS antibodies doesn't mean that you have APS. To be diagnosed with APS, you must have APS antibodies and a history of health problems related to the disorder.

Blood Tests

Your doctor can use blood tests to confirm a diagnosis of APS. These tests check your blood for any of the three APS antibodies: anticardiolipin, beta-2 glycoprotein I (β2GPI), and lupus anticoagulant.

How Is Antiphospholipid Antibody Syndrome Treated?

Antiphospholipid antibody syndrome (APS) has no cure. However, medicines can help prevent complications. The goals of treatment are to prevent blood clots from forming and keep existing clots from getting larger.

You may have APS and another autoimmune disorder, such as lupus. If so, it's important to control that condition as well. When the other condition is controlled, APS may cause fewer problems.

Research is ongoing for new ways to treat APS.

Chapter 42

Arthritis

Chapter Contents

Section 42.1

Ankylosing Spondylitis

This section includes text excerpted from "Ankylosing
Spondylitis," National Institute of Arthritis and
Musculoskeletal and Skin Diseases (NIAMS), June 2016.

What Is Ankylosing Spondylitis?

Ankylosing spondylitis is a form of progressive arthritis due to
chronic inflammation of the joints in the spine. Its name comes from
the Greek words *"ankylos,"* meaning stiffening of a joint, and *"spon-
dylo,"* meaning vertebra. Spondylitis refers to inflammation of the
spine or one or more of the adjacent structures of the vertebrae.

Ankylosing spondylitis belongs to a group of disorders called seronegative spondyloarthropathies. Seronegative means an individual
has tested negative for an autoantibody called rheumatoid factor. The
spondyloarthropathies are a family of similar diseases that usually
cause joint and spine inflammation. Other well-established syndromes
in this group include psoriatic arthritis, the arthritis of inflammatory
bowel disease, chronic reactive arthritis, and enthesitis-related idiopathic juvenile arthritis.

Although these disorders have similarities, they also have features
that distinguish them from one another. The hallmark of ankylosing
spondylitis is "sacroiliitis," or inflammation of the sacroiliac (SI) joints,
where the spine joins the pelvis.

In some people, ankylosing spondylitis can affect joints outside
of the spine, like the shoulders, ribs, hips, knees, and feet. It can
also affect entheses, which are sites where the tendons and ligaments
attach to the bones. It is possible that it can affect other organs, such
as the eyes, bowel, and—more rarely—the heart and lungs.

Although many people with ankylosing spondylitis have mild episodes of back pain that come and go, others have severe, ongoing pain
accompanied by loss of flexibility of the spine. In the most severe cases,
long-term inflammation leads to calcification that causes two or more
bones of the spine to fuse. Fusion can also stiffen the rib cage, resulting
in restricted lung capacity and function.

Who Has Ankylosing Spondylitis?

Ankylosing spondylitis typically begins in adolescents and young adults, but it affects people for the rest of their lives. Men are more likely to develop ankylosing spondylitis than are women.

What Causes Ankylosing Spondylitis?

The cause of ankylosing spondylitis is unknown, but it is likely that both genes and factors in the environment play a role. The main gene associated with susceptibility to ankylosing spondylitis is called *HLA-B27*. But while most people with ankylosing spondylitis have this genetic marker, only a small percentage of people with the gene develop the disease.

How Is Ankylosing Spondylitis Diagnosed?

A diagnosis of ankylosing spondylitis is based largely on the findings of a medical history and physical exam. Radiologic tests and lab tests may be used to help confirm a diagnosis, but both have some limitations.

What Type of Doctor Diagnoses and Treats Ankylosing Spondylitis?

The diagnosis of ankylosing spondylitis is often made by a rheumatologist, a doctor specially trained to diagnose and treat arthritis and related conditions of the musculoskeletal system. However, because ankylosing spondylitis can affect different parts of the body, a person with the disorder may need to see several different types of doctors for treatment. In addition to a rheumatologist, there are many different specialists who treat ankylosing spondylitis. These may include:

- An **ophthalmologist**, who treats eye disease.
- A **gastroenterologist**, who treats bowel disease.
- A **physiatrist**, a medical doctor who specializes in physical medicine and rehabilitation.
- A **physical therapist** or **rehabilitation specialist**, who supervises stretching and exercise regimens.

Often, it is helpful to the doctors and the patient for one doctor to manage the complete treatment plan.

Can Ankylosing Spondylitis Be Cured?

There is no cure for ankylosing spondylitis, but some treatments relieve symptoms of the disorder and may possibly prevent its progression. In most cases, treatment involves a combination of medication, exercise, and self-help measures. In some cases, surgery may be used to repair some of the joint damage caused by the disease.

What Medications Are Used to Treat Ankylosing Spondylitis?

Several classes of medications are used to treat ankylosing spondylitis. Because there are many medication options, it's important to work with your doctor to find the safest and most effective treatment plan for you. A treatment plan for ankylosing spondylitis will likely include one or more of the following:

- nonsteroidal anti-inflammatory drugs (NSAIDs)

- corticosteroids

- disease-modifying antirheumatic drugs (DMARDs)

- biologic agents

When Might Surgery Be Necessary, and How Can It Help?

If ankylosing spondylitis causes severe joint damage that makes it difficult to do your daily activities, total joint replacement may be an option. This involves removing the damaged joint and replacing it with a prosthesis made of metals, plastics, and/or ceramic materials. The most commonly replaced joints are the knee and hip.

In very rare cases, a procedure called osteotomy may be used to straighten a spine that has fused into a curved-forward position. This surgery involves cutting through the spine so that it can be realigned to a more vertical position. After the bones are realigned, hardware may be implanted to hold them in their new position while the spine heals.

Surgery to straighten the spine can only be done by a surgeon with significant experience in the procedure. Many doctors and surgeons consider the procedure high risk.

What Are Some Things I Can Do to Help Myself?

Aside from seeing your doctor regularly and following your prescribed treatment plan, staying active is probably the best thing you can do for ankylosing spondylitis. Regular exercise can help relieve pain, improve posture, and maintain flexibility. Before beginning an exercise program, speak with your doctor or physical therapist about designing a program that's right for you.

Another important thing you can do for yourself is to practice good posture. A good test for posture is to check yourself in a mirror. First, stand with a full-length mirror to your side and, if possible, turn your head to look at your profile. Next, imagine you have dropped a weighted string from the top of your head to the soles of your feet. Where does the string fall? If your posture is good, it should pass through your earlobe, the front of your shoulder, the center of your hip, behind your kneecap, and in front of your anklebone. If you are not standing that way already, practice holding your body that way in front of a mirror until you know well how it feels. Practicing good posture can help you avoid some of the complications that can occur with ankylosing spondylitis.

What Is the Prognosis for People with Ankylosing Spondylitis?

The course of ankylosing spondylitis varies from person to person. Some people will have only mild episodes of back pain that come and go, while others will have chronic severe back pain. In almost all cases, the condition is characterized by acute, painful episodes and remissions, or periods of time where the pain lessens.

In the sacroiliac joints and spine, inflammation can cause pain and stiffness. Over time, bony outgrowths called syndesmophytes can develop that cause the vertebrae to grow together, or fuse. Fusion can also stiffen the rib cage, resulting in restricted lung capacity and restricted lung function.

A number of factors are associated with an ankylosing spondylitis prognosis. One study found that among people who had ankylosing spondylitis for at least 20 years, those who had physically demanding jobs, other health problems, or smoked had greater functional limitations from their disease. People with higher levels of education and a history of ankylosing spondylitis in the family tended to have less severe limitations from their disease.

A study supported by the NIAMS found that the likelihood of having severe joint damage increased with age at disease onset, and that men were twice as likely as women to be in that group. The study also found that current smokers were more than four times as likely to have severe damage as nonsmokers, and that having a genetic marker called DRB1*0801 seemed to protect against severe spine damage.

Will Diet and Exercise Help?

A healthy diet and exercise are good for everyone, but may be especially helpful if you have ankylosing spondylitis.

Exercise and stretching, when done carefully and increased gradually, may help painful, stiff joints.

- **Strengthening exercises**, performed with weights or done by tightening muscles without moving the joints, build the muscles around painful joints to better support them. Exercises that don't require joint movement can be done even when your joints are painful and inflamed.

- **Range-of-motion exercises** improve movement and flexibility and reduce stiffness in the affected joint. If the spine is painful and/or inflamed, exercises to stretch and extend the back can be helpful in preventing long-term disability.

Many people with ankylosing spondylitis find it helpful to exercise in water.

Before beginning an exercise program, it's important to speak with a health professional who can recommend appropriate exercises.

Section 42.2

Juvenile Arthritis

This section includes text excerpted from "Juvenile Arthritis,"
National Institute of Arthritis and Musculoskeletal and Skin
Diseases (NIAMS), June 2015.

What Is Juvenile Arthritis?

"Arthritis" means joint inflammation. This term refers to a group of
diseases that cause pain, swelling, stiffness, and loss of motion in the
joints. Arthritis is also used more generally to describe the more than
100 rheumatic diseases that may affect the joints but can also cause pain,
swelling, and stiffness in other supporting structures of the body such as
muscles, tendons, ligaments, and bones. Some rheumatic diseases can
affect other parts of the body, including various internal organs. **Juvenile arthritis (JA)** is a term often used to describe arthritis in children.
Children can develop almost all types of arthritis that affect adults, but
the most common type that affects children is juvenile idiopathic arthritis.

Both **juvenile idiopathic arthritis (JIA)** and **juvenile rheumatoid arthritis (JRA)** are classification systems for chronic arthritis in
children. The juvenile rheumatoid arthritis classification system was
developed decades ago and had three different subtypes: polyarticular,
pauciarticular, and systemic-onset. More recently, pediatric rheumatologists throughout the world developed the juvenile idiopathic arthritis
classification system, which includes more types of chronic arthritis
that affect children. This classification system also provides a more
accurate separation of the three juvenile rheumatoid arthritis subtypes.

Prevalence statistics for juvenile arthritis vary, but according to
a 2008 report from the National Arthritis Data Workgroup, about
294,000 children age 0 to 17 are affected with arthritis or other rheumatic conditions.

What Is Juvenile Idiopathic Arthritis?

Juvenile idiopathic arthritis is currently the most widely accepted
term to describe various types of chronic arthritis in children.

In general, the symptoms of juvenile idiopathic arthritis include joint pain, swelling, tenderness, warmth, and stiffness that last for more than 6 continuous weeks. It is divided into seven separate sub-types, each with characteristic symptoms:

1. **Systemic juvenile idiopathic arthritis (formerly known as systemic juvenile rheumatoid arthritis).** A patient has arthritis with, or that was preceded by, a fever that has lasted for at least 2 weeks. It must be documented as an intermittent fever, spiking for at least 3 days, and it must be accompanied by at least one or more of the following:

   • Generalized enlargement of the lymph nodes.

   • Enlargement of the liver or spleen.

   • Inflammation of the lining of the heart or the lungs (pericarditis or pleuritis).

   • The characteristic rheumatoid rash, which is flat, pale, pink, and generally not itchy. The individual spots of the rash are usually the size of a quarter or smaller. They are present for a few minutes to a few hours, and then disappear without any changes in the skin. The rash may move from one part of the body to another.

2. **Oligoarticular juvenile idiopathic arthritis (formerly known as pauciarticular juvenile rheumatoid arthritis).** A patient has arthritis affecting one to four joints during the first 6 months of disease. Two subcategories are recognized:

   • *Persistent oligoarthritis*, which means the child never has more than four joints involved throughout the disease course.

   • *Extended oligoarthritis*, which means that more than four joints are involved after the first 6 months of the disease.

3. **Polyarticular juvenile idiopathic arthritis—rheumatoid factor negative (formerly known as polyarticular juvenile rheumatoid arthritis—rheumatoid factor negative).** A patient has arthritis in five or more joints during the first 6 months of disease, and all tests for rheumatoid factor (proteins produced by the immune system that can attack healthy tissue, which are commonly found in rheumatoid arthritis and juvenile arthritis) are negative.

4. **Polyarticular juvenile idiopathic arthritis—rheumatoid factor positive (formerly known as polyarticular rheumatoid arthritis—rheumatoid factor positive).** A patient has arthritis in five or more joints during the first 6 months of the disease. Also, at least two tests for rheumatoid factor, at least 3 months apart, are positive.

5. **Psoriatic juvenile idiopathic arthritis.** Patients have both arthritis and psoriasis (a skin disease), or they have arthritis and at least two of the following:

   - inflammation and swelling of an entire finger or toe (this is called dactylitis)

   - nail pitting or splitting

   - a first-degree relative with psoriasis.

5. **Enthesitis-related juvenile idiopathic arthritis.** The enthesis is the point at which a ligament, tendon, or joint capsule attaches to the bone. If this point becomes inflamed, it can be tender, swollen, and painful with use. The most common locations are around the knee and at the Achilles tendon on the back of the ankle. Patients are diagnosed with this juvenile idiopathic arthritis subtype if they have both arthritis and inflammation of an enthesitis site, or if they have either arthritis or enthesitis with at least two of the following:

   - inflammation of the sacroiliac joints (at the bottom of the back) or pain and stiffness in the lumbosacral area (in the lower back)

   - a positive blood test for the human leukocyte antigen (HLA) *B27* gene

   - onset of arthritis in males after age 6 years

   - a first-degree relative diagnosed with ankylosing spondylitis, enthesitis-related arthritis, or inflammation of the sacroiliac joint in association with inflammatory bowel disease or acute inflammation of the eye.

7. **Undifferentiated arthritis.** A child is said to have this subtype of juvenile idiopathic arthritis if the arthritis manifestations do not fulfill the criteria for one of the other six categories or if they fulfill the criteria for more than one category.

What Causes Juvenile Arthritis?

Most forms of juvenile arthritis are autoimmune disorders, which means that the body's immune system—which normally helps to fight off bacteria or viruses—mistakenly attacks some of its own healthy cells and tissues. The result is inflammation, marked by redness, heat, pain, and swelling. Inflammation can cause joint damage. Doctors do not know why the immune system attacks healthy tissues in children who develop juvenile arthritis. Scientists suspect that it is a two-step process. First, something in a child's genetic makeup gives him or her a tendency to develop juvenile arthritis; then an environmental factor, such as a virus, triggers the development of the disease.

Not all cases of juvenile arthritis are autoimmune, however. Recent research has demonstrated that some people, such as many with systemic arthritis, have what is more accurately called an autoinflammatory condition. Although the two terms sound somewhat similar, the disease processes behind autoimmune and autoinflammatory disorders are different.

When the immune system is working properly, foreign invaders such as bacteria and viruses provoke the body to produce proteins called antibodies. Antibodies attach to these invaders so that they can be recognized and destroyed. In an autoimmune reaction, the antibodies attach to the body's own healthy tissues by mistake, signaling the body to attack them. Because they target the self, these proteins are called autoantibodies.

Like autoimmune disorders, autoinflammatory conditions also cause inflammation. And like autoimmune disorders, they also involve an overactive immune system. However, autoinflammation is not caused by autoantibodies. Instead, autoinflammation involves a more primitive part of the immune system that in healthy people causes white blood cells to destroy harmful substances. When this system goes awry, it causes inflammation for unknown reasons. In addition to inflammation, autoinflammatory diseases often cause fever and rashes.

What Are Its Symptoms and Signs?

The most common symptom of all types of juvenile arthritis is persistent joint swelling, pain, and stiffness that is typically worse in the morning or after a nap. The pain may limit movement of the affected joint, although many children, especially younger ones, will not complain of pain. Juvenile arthritis commonly affects the knees and the joints in the hands and feet. One of the earliest signs of juvenile arthritis may be limping in the morning because of an affected knee. Besides joint symptoms, children with systemic juvenile arthritis have a high fever and a skin rash. The rash and fever may appear and disappear very quickly. Systemic arthritis also may cause the lymph nodes located in the neck and other parts of the body to swell. In some cases (fewer than half), internal organs including the heart and (very rarely) the lungs, may be involved.

Eye inflammation is a potentially severe complication that commonly occurs in children with oligoarthritis but can also be seen in other types of juvenile arthritis. All children with juvenile arthritis need to have regular eye exams, including a special exam called a slit lamp exam. Eye diseases such as iritis or uveitis can be present at the beginning of arthritis but often develop some time after a child first develops juvenile arthritis. Very commonly, juvenile arthritis-associated eye inflammation does not cause any symptoms and is found only by performing eye exams.

Typically, there are periods when the symptoms of juvenile arthritis are better or disappear (remissions) and times when symptoms "flare," or get worse. Juvenile arthritis is different in each child; some may have just one or two flares and never have symptoms again, while others may experience many flares or even have symptoms that never go away.

Some children with juvenile arthritis have growth problems. Depending on the severity of the disease and the joints involved, bone growth at the affected joints may be too fast or too slow, causing one leg or arm to be longer than the other, for example, or resulting in a small or misshapen chin. Overall growth also may be slowed. Doctors are exploring the use of growth hormone to treat this problem. Juvenile arthritis may also cause joints to grow unevenly.

How Is It Diagnosed?

To be classified as juvenile arthritis, symptoms must have started before age 16. Doctors usually suspect juvenile arthritis, along with several other possible conditions, when they see children with persistent joint pain or swelling, unexplained skin rashes, and fever associated with swelling of lymph nodes or inflammation of internal organs. A diagnosis of juvenile arthritis also is considered in children with an unexplained limp or excessive clumsiness.

No single test can be used to diagnose juvenile arthritis. A doctor diagnoses juvenile arthritis by carefully examining the patient and considering his or her medical history and the results of tests that help confirm juvenile arthritis or rule out other conditions. Specific findings or problems that relate to the joints are the main factors that go into making a juvenile arthritis diagnosis.

Symptoms

When diagnosing juvenile arthritis, a doctor must consider not only the symptoms a child has but also the length of time these symptoms have been present. Joint swelling or other objective changes in the joint with arthritis must be present continuously for at least 6 weeks for the doctor to establish a diagnosis of juvenile arthritis. Because this factor is so important, it may be useful to keep a record of the symptoms and changes in the joints, noting when they first appeared and when they are worse or better.

Family History

It is very rare for more than one member of a family to have juvenile arthritis. But children with a family member who has juvenile arthritis are at a slightly increased risk of developing it. Research shows that juvenile arthritis is also more likely in families with a history of any autoimmune disease. One study showed that families of children with juvenile arthritis are more likely to have a member with an autoimmune disease such as rheumatoid arthritis, multiple sclerosis, or thyroid inflammation (Hashimoto's thyroiditis) than are families of children without juvenile arthritis. For that reason, having an autoimmune disease in the family may raise the doctor's suspicions that a child's joint symptoms are caused by juvenile arthritis or some other autoimmune disease.

Laboratory Tests

Laboratory tests, usually blood tests, cannot alone provide the doctor with a clear diagnosis. But these tests can be used to help rule out other conditions and classify the type of juvenile arthritis that a patient has. Blood samples may be taken to test for anti-CCP antibodies, rheumatoid factor, and antinuclear antibodies, and to determine the erythrocyte sedimentation rate (ESR), described below.

- **Anticyclic citrullinated peptide (anti-CCP) antibodies.**
  Anti-CCP antibodies may be detected in healthy individuals years before onset of clinical rheumatoid arthritis. They may predict the eventual development of undifferentiated arthritis into rheumatoid arthritis.

- **Rheumatoid factor (RF).** Rheumatoid factor, an autoantibody that is produced in large amounts in adults with rheumatoid arthritis, also may be detected in children with juvenile arthritis, although it is rare. The RF test helps the doctor differentiate among the different types of juvenile arthritis.

- **Antinuclear antibody (ANA).** An autoantibody directed against substances in the cells' nuclei, ANA is found in some juvenile arthritis patients. However, the presence of ANA in children generally points to some type of connective tissue disease, helping the doctor to narrow down the diagnosis. A positive test in a child with oligoarthritis markedly increases his or her risk of developing eye disease.

- **Erythrocyte sedimentation rate (ESR or sed rate).** This blood test, which measures how fast red blood cells fall to the bottom of a test tube, can tell the doctor if inflammation is present. Inflammation is a hallmark of juvenile arthritis and a number of other conditions.

X-rays

X-rays are needed if the doctor suspects injury to the bone or unusual bone development. Early in the disease, some X-rays can show changes in soft tissue. In general, X-rays are more useful later in the disease, when bones may be affected.

Other Tests

Because there are many causes of joint pain and swelling, the doctor must rule out other conditions before diagnosing juvenile arthritis. These include physical injury, bacterial or viral infection, Lyme disease, inflammatory bowel disease, lupus, dermatomyositis, and some forms of cancer. The doctor may use additional laboratory tests to help rule out these and other possible conditions.

How Is It Treated?

The main goals of treatment are to preserve a high level of physical and social functioning and maintain a good quality of life. To achieve these goals, doctors recommend treatments to reduce swelling, maintain full movement in the affected joints, relieve pain, and prevent, identify, and treat complications. Most children with juvenile arthritis need a combination of medication and nonmedication treatments to reach these goals.

Following are some of the most commonly used treatments.

Medication Treatments

- **Nonsteroidal anti-inflammatory drugs (NSAIDs).** Aspirin, ibuprofen, naproxen, and naproxen sodium are examples of NSAIDs. They are often the first type of medication used. All NSAIDs work similarly by blocking substances called prostaglandins that contribute to inflammation and pain. However, each NSAID is a different chemical, and each has a slightly different effect on the body.

- **Disease-modifying antirheumatic drugs (DMARDs).** If NSAIDs do not relieve symptoms of juvenile arthritis, the doctor may prescribe this type of medication. DMARDs slow the progression of juvenile arthritis, but because they may take weeks or months to relieve symptoms, they often are taken with an NSAID. Although many different types of DMARDs are available, doctors are most likely to use one particular DMARD, methotrexate, for children with juvenile arthritis.

  Researchers have learned that methotrexate is safe and effective for some children with juvenile arthritis whose symptoms are not relieved by other medications. Because only small doses of methotrexate are needed to relieve arthritis symptoms, potentially dangerous side effects rarely occur. The most serious complication is liver damage, but it can be avoided with regular blood screening tests and doctor follow-up. Careful monitoring for side effects is important for people taking methotrexate. When side effects are noticed early, the doctor can reduce the dose and eliminate the side effects.

- **Corticosteroids.** In children with very severe juvenile arthritis, stronger medicines may be needed to stop serious symptoms such as inflammation of the sac around the heart (pericarditis). Corticosteroids such as prednisone may be added to the treatment plan to control severe symptoms. This medication can be given either intravenously (directly into the vein) or by mouth. Corticosteroids can interfere with a child's normal growth and can cause other side effects, such as a round face, weakened bones, and increased susceptibility to infections. Once the medication controls severe symptoms, the doctor will reduce the dose gradually and eventually stop it completely. Because it can be dangerous to stop taking corticosteroids suddenly, it is important to carefully follow the doctor's instructions about how to take or reduce the dose. For inflammation in one or just a few joints, injecting a corticosteroid compound into the affected joint or joints can often bring quick relief without the systemic side effects of oral or intravenous medication.

- **Biologic agents.** Children with juvenile arthritis who have received little relief from other drugs may be given one of a newer class of drug treatments called biologic response modifiers, or biologic agents. Tumor necrosis factor (TNF) inhibitors work by blocking the actions of TNF, a naturally occurring protein in the body that helps cause inflammation. Other biologic agents block other inflammatory proteins such as interleukin-1 or immune cells called T cells. Different biologics tend to work better for different subtypes of the disease.

Treatments Without Medication

- **Physical therapy.** A regular, general exercise program is an important part of a child's treatment plan. It can help to maintain muscle tone and preserve and recover the range of motion of the joints. A physiatrist (rehabilitation specialist) or a physical therapist can design an appropriate exercise program for a person with juvenile arthritis. The specialist also may recommend using splints and other devices to help maintain normal bone and joint growth.

- **Complementary and alternative therapies.** Many adults seek alternative ways of treating arthritis, such as special diets, supplements, acupuncture, massage, or even magnetic jewelry or mattress pads. Research shows that increasing numbers of children are using alternative and complementary therapies as well.

Although there is little research to support many alternative treatments, some people seem to benefit from them. If a child's doctor feels the approach has value and is not harmful, it can be incorporated into the treatment plan. However, it is important not to neglect regular healthcare or treatment of serious symptoms.

How Can the Family Help a Child Live Well with Juvenile Arthritis?

Juvenile arthritis affects the entire family, all of whom must cope with the special challenges of this disease. Juvenile arthritis can strain a child's participation in social and after-school activities and make schoolwork more difficult. Family members can do several things to help the child physically and emotionally.

- **Get the best care possible.** Ensure that the child receives appropriate medical care and follows the doctor's instructions. If possible, have a pediatric rheumatologist manage your child's care. If such a specialist is not close by, consider having your child see one yearly or twice a year. A pediatric rheumatologist can devise a treatment plan and consult with your child's doctor, who will help you carry it out and monitor your child's progress.

- **Learn as much as you can about your child's disease and its treatment.** (The resources listed at the end of this publication can help.) Many treatment options are available, and because juvenile arthritis is different in each child, what works for one may not work for another. If the medications that the doctor prescribes do not relieve symptoms or if they cause unpleasant side effects, you and your child should discuss other choices with the doctor. A person with juvenile arthritis can be more active when symptoms are controlled.

- **Consider joining a support group.** Try to find other parents and kids who face similar experiences. It can help you—and your child—to know you're not alone. Some organizations have support groups for people with juvenile arthritis and their families.

- **Treat the child as normally as possible.** Try not to cut your child too much slack just because he or she has arthritis. Too much coddling can keep your child from being responsible and independent and can cause resentment in siblings.

- **Encourage exercise and physical therapy for the child.** For many young people, exercise and physical therapy play important roles in managing juvenile arthritis. Parents can arrange for children to participate in activities that the doctor recommends. During symptom-free periods, many doctors suggest playing team sports or doing other activities. The goal is to help keep the joints strong and flexible, to provide play time with other children, and to encourage appropriate social development.

- **Work closely with your child's school.** Help your child's school to develop a suitable lesson plan, and educate your child's teacher and classmates about juvenile arthritis. Some children with juvenile arthritis may be absent from school for prolonged periods and need to have the teacher send assignments home. Some minor changes—such as having an extra set of books or leaving class a few minutes early to get to the next class on time—can be a great help. With proper attention, most children progress normally through school.

- **Talk with your child.** Explain that getting juvenile arthritis is nobody's fault. Some children believe that juvenile arthritis is a punishment for something they did. Let your child know you are always available to listen, and help him or her in any way you can.

- **Work with therapists or social workers.** They can help you and your child adapt more easily to the lifestyle changes juvenile arthritis may bring.

Do These Children Have to Limit Activities?

Although pain sometimes limits physical activity, exercise is important for reducing the symptoms of juvenile arthritis and maintaining function and range of motion of the joints. Most children with juvenile arthritis can take part fully in physical activities and selected sports when their symptoms are under control. During a disease flare, however, the doctor may advise limiting certain activities, depending on the joints involved. Once the flare is over, the child can start regular activities again.

Swimming is particularly useful because it uses many joints and muscles without putting weight on the joints. A doctor or physical therapist can recommend exercises and activities.

Section 42.3

Rheumatoid Arthritis

This section includes text excerpted from "Rheumatoid Arthritis,"
National Institute of Arthritis and Musculoskeletal and Skin
Diseases (NIAMS), February 2016.

What Is Rheumatoid Arthritis?

Rheumatoid arthritis (RA) is an inflammatory disease that causes pain, swelling, stiffness, and loss of function in the joints. It occurs when the immune system, which normally defends the body from invading organisms, turns its attack against the membrane lining the joints.

Rheumatoid arthritis has several features that make it different from other kinds of arthritis. For example, rheumatoid arthritis generally occurs in a symmetrical pattern, meaning that if one knee or hand is involved, the other one also is. The disease often affects the wrist joints and the finger joints closest to the hand. It can also affect other parts of the body besides the joints. In addition, people with rheumatoid arthritis may have fatigue, occasional fevers, and a loss of energy.

The course of rheumatoid arthritis can range from mild to severe. In most cases it is chronic, meaning it lasts a long time—often a lifetime. For many people, periods of relatively mild disease activity are punctuated by flares, or times of heightened disease activity. In others, symptoms are constant.

Features of Rheumatoid Arthritis

- Tender, warm, swollen joints

- Symmetrical pattern of affected joints

- Joint inflammation *often* affecting the wrist and finger joints closest to the hand

- Joint inflammation *sometimes* affecting other joints, including the neck, shoulders, elbows, hips, knees, ankles, and feet

- Fatigue, occasional fevers, a loss of energy

- Pain and stiffness lasting for more than 30 minutes in the morning or after a long rest
- Symptoms that last for many years
- Variability of symptoms among people with the disease.

Who Has Rheumatoid Arthritis?

Scientists estimate that about 1.5 million people, or about 0.6 percent of the U.S. adult population, have rheumatoid arthritis. Interestingly, some recent studies have suggested that although the number of new cases of rheumatoid arthritis for older people is increasing, the overall number of new cases may actually be going down.

How Does Rheumatoid Arthritis Affect People's Lives?

Rheumatoid arthritis affects people differently. Some people have mild or moderate forms of the disease, with periods of worsening symptoms, called flares, and periods in which they feel better, called remissions. Others have a severe form of the disease that is active most of the time, lasts for many years or a lifetime, and leads to serious joint damage and disability.

Although rheumatoid arthritis is primarily a disease of the joints, its effects are not just physical. Many people with rheumatoid arthritis also experience issues related to:

- depression, anxiety
- feelings of helplessness
- low self-esteem.

Rheumatoid arthritis can affect virtually every area of a person's life from work life to family life. It can also interfere with the joys and responsibilities of family life and may affect the decision to have children.

Fortunately, current treatment strategies allow most people with the disease to lead active and productive lives. These strategies include pain-relieving drugs and medications that slow joint damage, a balance between rest and exercise, and patient education and support programs. In recent years, research has led to a new understanding of rheumatoid arthritis and has increased the likelihood that, in time, researchers will find even better ways to treat the disease.

What Causes Rheumatoid Arthritis?

Scientists still do not know exactly what causes the immune system to turn against the body's own tissues in rheumatoid arthritis, but research over the last few years has begun to piece together the factors involved.

Genetic (inherited) factors: Scientists have discovered that certain genes known to play a role in the immune system are associated with a tendency to develop rheumatoid arthritis. For the genes that have been linked to rheumatoid arthritis, the frequency of the risky gene is only modestly higher in those with rheumatoid arthritis compared with healthy controls. In other words, individual genes by themselves confer only a small relative risk of disease. Some people who have these particular genes never develop the disease. These observations suggest that although a person's genetic makeup plays an important role in determining if he or she will develop rheumatoid arthritis, it is not the only factor. What is clear, however, is that more than one gene is involved in determining whether a person develops rheumatoid arthritis and how severe the disease will become.

Environmental factors: Many scientists think that something must occur to trigger the disease process in people whose genetic makeup makes them susceptible to rheumatoid arthritis. A variety of factors have been suggested, but a specific agent has not been identified.

Other factors: Some scientists also think that a variety of hormonal factors may be involved. Women are more likely to develop rheumatoid arthritis than men. The disease may improve during pregnancy and flare after pregnancy. Breastfeeding may also aggravate the disease. Contraceptive use may increase a person's likelihood of developing rheumatoid arthritis. This suggests hormones, or possibly deficiencies or changes in certain hormones, may promote the development of rheumatoid arthritis in a genetically susceptible person who has been exposed to a triggering agent from the environment.

Even though all the answers are not known, one thing is certain: rheumatoid arthritis develops as a result of an interaction of many factors. Researchers are trying to understand these factors and how they work together.

How Is Rheumatoid Arthritis Diagnosed?

Rheumatoid arthritis can be difficult to diagnose in its early stages for several reasons. First, there is no single test for the disease. In addition, symptoms differ from person to person and can be more severe in some people than in others. Also, symptoms can be similar to those of other types of arthritis and joint conditions, and it may take some time for other conditions to be ruled out. Finally, the full range of symptoms develops over time, and only a few symptoms may be present in the early stages. As a result, doctors use a variety of the following tools to diagnose the disease and to rule out other conditions:

Medical history: The doctor begins by asking the patient to describe the symptoms, and when and how the condition started, as well as how the symptoms have changed over time. The doctor will also ask about any other medical problems the patient and close family members have and about any medications the patient is taking. Accurate answers to these questions can help the doctor make a diagnosis and understand the impact the disease has on the patient's life.

Physical examination: The doctor will check the patient's reflexes and general health, including muscle strength. The doctor will also examine bothersome joints and observe the patient's ability to walk, bend, and carry out activities of daily living. The doctor will also look at the skin for a rash and listen to the chest for signs of inflammation in the lungs.

Laboratory tests: A number of lab tests may be useful in confirming a diagnosis of rheumatoid arthritis. Following are some of the more common ones:

- **Rheumatoid factor (RF):** Rheumatoid factor is an antibody that is present eventually in the blood of most people with rheumatoid arthritis. (An antibody is a special protein made by the immune system that normally helps fight foreign substances in the body.) Not all people with rheumatoid arthritis test positive for rheumatoid factor, and some people test positive for rheumatoid factor, yet never develop the disease. Rheumatoid factor also can be positive in some other diseases; however, a positive RF in a person who has symptoms consistent with those of rheumatoid arthritis can be useful in confirming a diagnosis. Furthermore, high levels of rheumatoid factor are associated with more severe rheumatoid arthritis.

- **Anti-CCP antibodies:** This blood test detects antibodies to cyclic citrullinated peptide (anti-CCP). This test is positive in most people with rheumatoid arthritis and can even be positive years before rheumatoid arthritis symptoms develop. When used with the RF, this test's results are very useful in confirming a rheumatoid arthritis diagnosis.

241

- **Others:** Other common laboratory tests include a white blood cell count, a blood test for anemia, which is common in rheumatoid arthritis; the erythrocyte sedimentation rate (often called the sed rate), which measures inflammation in the body; and C-reactive protein, another common test for inflammation that is useful both in making a diagnosis and monitoring disease activity and response to anti-inflammatory therapy.

X-rays: X-rays are used to determine the degree of joint destruction. They are not useful in the early stages of rheumatoid arthritis before bone damage is evident; however, they may be used to rule out other causes of joint pain. They may also be used later to monitor the progression of the disease.

How Is Rheumatoid Arthritis Treated?

Doctors use a variety of approaches to treat rheumatoid arthritis. These are used in different combinations and at different times during the course of the disease and are chosen according to the patient's individual situation. No matter what treatment the doctor and patient choose, however, the goals are the same: to relieve pain, reduce inflammation, slow down or stop joint damage, and improve the person's sense of well-being and ability to function.

Good communication between the patient and doctor is necessary for effective treatment. Talking to the doctor can help ensure that exercise and pain management programs are provided as needed, and that drugs are prescribed appropriately. Talking to the doctor can also help people who are making decisions about surgery.

Goals of Treatment

- relieve pain.
- reduce inflammation.
- slow down or stop joint damage.
- improve a person's sense of well-being and ability to function.

Current Treatment Approaches

- lifestyle
- medications
- surgery
- routine monitoring and ongoing care.

Health behavior changes: Certain activities can help improve a person's ability to function independently and maintain a positive outlook.

- **Rest and exercise:** People with rheumatoid arthritis need a good balance between rest and exercise, with more rest when the disease is active and more exercise when it is not. Rest helps to reduce active joint inflammation and pain and to fight fatigue. The length of time for rest will vary from person to person, but in general, shorter rest breaks every now and then are more helpful than long times spent in bed.

  Exercise is important for maintaining healthy and strong muscles, preserving joint mobility, and maintaining flexibility. Exercise can also help people sleep well, reduce pain, maintain a positive attitude, and manage weight. Exercise programs should take into account the person's physical abilities, limitations, and changing needs.

- **Joint care:** Some people find using a splint for a short time around a painful joint reduces pain and swelling by supporting the joint and letting it rest. Splints are used mostly on wrists and hands, but also on ankles and feet. A doctor or a physical or occupational therapist can help a person choose a splint and make sure it fits properly. Other ways to reduce stress on joints include self-help devices (for example, zipper pullers, long-handled shoe horns); devices to help with getting on and off chairs, toilet seats, and beds; and changes in the ways that a person carries out daily activities.

- **Stress reduction:** People with rheumatoid arthritis face emotional challenges as well as physical ones. The emotions they feel because of the disease—fear, anger, and frustration—combined with any pain and physical limitations can increase their stress level. Although there is no evidence that stress plays a role in causing rheumatoid arthritis, it can make living with the disease difficult at times. Stress also may affect the amount of pain a person feels. There are a number of successful techniques for coping with stress. Regular rest periods can help, as can relaxation, distraction, or visualization exercises. Exercise programs, participation in support groups, and good communication with the healthcare team are other ways to reduce stress.

- **Healthful diet:** With the exception of several specific types of oils, there is no scientific evidence that any specific food or nutrient helps or harms people with rheumatoid arthritis. However, an overall nutritious diet with enough—but not an excess of—calories, protein, and calcium is important. Some people may need to be careful about drinking alcoholic beverages because of the medications they take for rheumatoid arthritis. Those taking methotrexate may need to avoid alcohol altogether because one of the most serious long-term side effects of methotrexate is liver damage.

- **Climate:** Some people notice that their arthritis gets worse when there is a sudden change in the weather. However, there is no evidence that a specific climate can prevent or reduce the effects of rheumatoid arthritis. Moving to a new place with a different climate usually does not make a long-term difference in a person's rheumatoid arthritis.

Medications: Most people who have rheumatoid arthritis take medications. Some medications (analgesics) are used only for pain relief; others, such as corticosteroids and nonsteroidal anti-inflammatory drugs (NSAIDs), are used to reduce inflammation. Still others, often called disease-modifying antirheumatic drugs (DMARDs), are used to try to slow the course of the disease. Common DMARDs include hydroxychloroquine, leflunomide, methotrexate, and sulfasalazine. Other DMARDs—called biologic response modifiers—may be used in people with more serious disease. These are genetically engineered medications that help reduce inflammation and structural damage to the joints by interrupting the cascade of events that drive inflammation. Currently, several biologic response modifiers are approved for rheumatoid arthritis, including abatacept, adalimumab, anakinra, certolizumab, etanercept, golimumab, infliximab, rituximab, and tocilizumab.

Another DMARD, tofacitinib, from a new class of drugs called Janus-associated kinase (JAK) inhibitors, fights inflammation from inside the cell to reduce inflammation in people with rheumatoid arthritis.

For many years, doctors initially prescribed aspirin or other pain-relieving drugs for rheumatoid arthritis, and they waited to prescribe more powerful drugs only if the disease worsened. In recent decades this approach to treatment has changed as studies have shown that early treatment with more powerful drugs—and the use of drug combinations instead of one medication alone—may be more effective in reducing or preventing joint damage. Someone with persistent rheumatoid arthritis symptoms should see a doctor familiar with the disease and its treatment to reduce the risk of damage.

Many of the drugs that help reduce disease in rheumatoid arthritis do so by reducing the inflammation that can cause pain and joint damage. However, in some instances, inflammation is one mechanism the body normally uses to maintain health, such as to fight infection and possibly to stop tumors from growing. The magnitude of the risk from the treatment is hard to judge because infections and cancer can occur in people with rheumatoid arthritis who are not on treatment, and probably more commonly than in healthy individuals. Nevertheless, appropriate caution and vigilance are justified.

Surgery: Several types of surgery are available to patients with severe joint damage. The primary purpose of these procedures is to reduce pain, improve the affected joint's function, and improve the patient's ability to perform daily activities. Surgery is not for everyone, however, and the decision should be made only after careful consideration by the patient and doctor. Together they should discuss the patient's overall health, the condition of the joint or tendon that will be operated on, and the reason for, as well as the risks and benefits of, the surgical procedure. Cost may be another factor.

Routine monitoring and ongoing care: Regular medical care is important to monitor the course of the disease, determine the effectiveness and any negative effects of medications, and change therapies as needed. Monitoring typically includes regular visits to the doctor. It also may include blood, urine, and other laboratory tests and X-rays.

People with rheumatoid arthritis may want to discuss preventing osteoporosis with their doctors as part of their long-term, ongoing care. Osteoporosis is a condition in which bones become weakened and fragile. Having rheumatoid arthritis increases the risk of developing osteoporosis for both men and women, particularly if a person takes corticosteroids. Such patients may want to discuss with their doctors the potential benefits of calcium and vitamin D supplements or other treatments for osteoporosis.

Alternative and complementary therapies: Special diets, vitamin supplements, and other alternative approaches have been suggested for treating rheumatoid arthritis. Research shows that some of these, for example, fish oil supplements, may help reduce arthritis inflammation. For most, however, controlled scientific studies either have not been conducted on them or have found no definite benefit to these therapies.

As with any therapy, patients should discuss the benefits and drawbacks with their doctors before beginning an alternative or new type of therapy. If the doctor feels the approach has value and will not be harmful, it can be incorporated into a person's treatment plan. However, it is important not to neglect regular healthcare.

Who Treats Rheumatoid Arthritis?

Diagnosing and treating rheumatoid arthritis requires a team effort involving the patient and several types of healthcare professionals.

The primary doctor to treat arthritis may be an **internist,** a doctor who specializes in the diagnosis and medical treatment of adults, or a **rheumatologist,** a doctor who specializes in arthritis and other diseases of the bones, joints, and muscles.

As treatment progresses, other professionals often help. These may include the following:

- **Orthopaedists:** Surgeons who specialize in the treatment of, and surgery for, bone and joint diseases.

- **Physical therapists:** Health professionals who work with patients to improve joint function.

- **Occupational therapists:** Health professionals who teach ways to protect joints, minimize pain, perform activities of daily living, and conserve energy.

- **Dietitians:** Health professionals who teach ways to use a good diet to improve health and maintain a healthy weight.

- **Nurse educators:** Nurses who specialize in helping patients understand their overall condition and implement their treatment plans.

- **Psychologists:** Health professionals who seek to help patients cope with difficulties in the home and workplace that may result from their medical conditions.

What You Can Do: The Importance of Self-Care

Although healthcare professionals can prescribe or recommend treatments to help patients manage their rheumatoid arthritis, the real key to living well with the disease lies with the patients themselves. Research shows that people who take part in their own care report less pain and make fewer doctor visits. They also enjoy a better quality of life.

Self-management programs teach about rheumatoid arthritis and its treatments, exercise and relaxation approaches, communication between patients and healthcare providers, and problem solving. Research on these programs has shown that they help people:

- understand the disease
- reduce their pain while remaining active
- cope physically, emotionally, and mentally
- feel greater control over the disease and build a sense of confidence in the ability to function and lead full, active, and independent lives.

Chapter 43

Autoimmune Hepatitis

What Is Autoimmune Hepatitis?

Autoimmune hepatitis is a chronic—or long lasting—disease in which the body's immune system attacks the normal components, or cells, of the liver and causes inflammation and liver damage. The immune system normally protects people from infection by identifying and destroying bacteria, viruses, and other potentially harmful foreign substances.

Autoimmune hepatitis is a serious condition that may worsen over time if not treated. Autoimmune hepatitis can lead to cirrhosis and liver failure. Cirrhosis occurs when scar tissue replaces healthy liver tissue and blocks the normal flow of blood through the liver. Liver failure occurs when the liver stops working properly.

What Are Autoimmune Diseases?

Autoimmune diseases are disorders in which the body's immune system attacks the body's own cells and organs with proteins called autoantibodies; this process is called autoimmunity.

The body's immune system normally makes large numbers of proteins called antibodies to help the body fight off infections. In some cases, however, the body makes autoantibodies. Certain environmental

This chapter includes text excerpted from "Autoimmune Hepatitis," National Institute of Diabetes and Digestive and Kidney Diseases (NIDDK), March 2014.

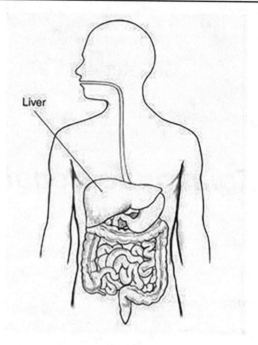

Figure 43.1. *Digestive System and Liver*

Autoimmune hepatitis is a chronic disease of the liver.

triggers can lead to autoimmunity. Environmental triggers are things originating outside the body, such as bacteria, viruses, toxins, and medications.

What Causes Autoimmune Hepatitis?

A combination of autoimmunity, environmental triggers, and a genetic predisposition can lead to autoimmune hepatitis.

Who Is More Likely to Develop Autoimmune Hepatitis?

Autoimmune hepatitis is more common in females. The disease can occur at any age and affects all ethnic groups.

What Are the Types of Autoimmune Hepatitis?

Autoimmune hepatitis is classified into several types. Type 1 autoimmune hepatitis is the most common form in North America. Type

1 can occur at any age; however, it most often starts in adolescence or young adulthood. About 70 percent of people with type 1 autoimmune hepatitis are female.

People with type 1 autoimmune hepatitis commonly have other autoimmune disorders, such as

- celiac disease, an autoimmune disease in which people cannot tolerate gluten because it damages the lining of their small intestine and prevents absorption of nutrients

- Crohn's disease, which causes inflammation and irritation of any part of the digestive tract

- Graves disease, the most common cause of hyperthyroidism in the United States

- Hashimoto disease, also called chronic lymphocytic thyroiditis or autoimmune thyroiditis, a form of chronic inflammation of the thyroid gland

- proliferative glomerulonephritis, or inflammation of the glomeruli, which are tiny clusters of looping blood vessels in the kidneys

- primary sclerosing cholangitis, which causes irritation, scarring, and narrowing of the bile ducts inside and outside the liver

- rheumatoid arthritis, which causes pain, swelling, stiffness, and loss of function in the joints

- Sjögren syndrome, which causes dryness in the mouth and eyes

- systemic lupus erythematosus, which causes kidney inflammation called lupus nephritis

- type 1 diabetes, a condition characterized by high blood glucose, also called blood sugar, levels caused by a total lack of insulin

- ulcerative colitis, a chronic disease that causes inflammation and sores, called ulcers, in the inner lining of the large intestine

Type 2 autoimmune hepatitis is less common and occurs more often in children than adults. People with type 2 can also have any of the above autoimmune disorders.

What Are the Symptoms of Autoimmune Hepatitis?

The most common symptoms of autoimmune hepatitis are

- fatigue

- joint pain

- nausea

- loss of appetite

- pain or discomfort over the liver

- skin rashes

- dark yellow urine

- light-colored stools

- jaundice, or yellowing of the skin and whites of the eyes

Symptoms of autoimmune hepatitis range from mild to severe. Some people may feel as if they have a mild case of the flu. Others may have no symptoms when a healthcare provider diagnoses the disease; however, they can develop symptoms later.

How Is Autoimmune Hepatitis Diagnosed?

A healthcare provider will make a diagnosis of autoimmune hepatitis based on symptoms, a physical exam, blood tests, and a liver biopsy.

A healthcare provider performs a physical exam and reviews the person's health history, including the use of alcohol and medications that can harm the liver. A person usually needs blood tests for an exact diagnosis because a person with autoimmune hepatitis can have the same symptoms as those of other liver diseases or metabolic disorders.

How Is Autoimmune Hepatitis Treated?

Treatment for autoimmune hepatitis includes medication to suppress, or slow down, an overactive immune system. Treatment may also include a liver transplant.

Treatment works best when autoimmune hepatitis is diagnosed early. People with autoimmune hepatitis generally respond to standard treatment and the disease can be controlled in most cases. Long-term response to treatment can stop the disease from getting worse and may even reverse some damage to the liver.

What Is a Possible Complication of Autoimmune Hepatitis and Cirrhosis?

People with autoimmune hepatitis and cirrhosis are at risk of developing liver cancer. A healthcare provider will monitor the person with a regular ultrasound examination of the liver. Ultrasound uses a device, called a transducer, that bounces safe, painless sound waves off organs to create an image of their structure. A specially trained technician performs the procedure in a healthcare provider's office, an outpatient center, or a hospital, and a radiologist—a doctor who specializes in medical imaging—interprets the images; anesthesia is not needed. The images can show the liver's size and the presence of cancerous tumors.

Eating, Diet, and Nutrition

Researchers have not found that eating, diet, and nutrition play a role in causing or preventing autoimmune hepatitis.

Chapter 44

Autoimmune Lymphoproliferative Syndrome (ALPS)

Autoimmune lymphoproliferative syndrome (ALPS) is a rare genetic disorder of the immune system that affects both children and adults. In ALPS, unusually high numbers of white blood cells called lymphocytes accumulate in the lymph nodes, liver, and spleen, which can lead to enlargement of these organs. ALPS can cause numerous autoimmune problems such as anemia (low count of red blood cells), thrombocytopenia (low count of platelets), and neutropenia (low count of neutrophils, the most common type of white blood cell in humans).

Causes

Genetics

Most cases of ALPS are caused by mutations in the *FAS* gene. The *FAS* gene produces a receptor that, when activated, leads to programmed cell death, or apoptosis. This is an important part of the

This chapter includes text excerpted from "Autoimmune Lymphoproliferative Syndrome (ALPS)," National Institute of Allergy and Infectious Diseases (NIAID), March 23, 2015.

normal cell lifecycle. When cells do not receive the message that it is time for them to die, an abnormal buildup of cells can result.

There are two types of *FAS* mutations:

1. Germline mutations, which are present in all the body's cells

2. Somatic, or acquired, mutations, which are present only in select groups of cells

Although germline mutations are more common than somatic mutations, people with germline and somatic *FAS* mutations generally have the same symptoms. Many different types of germline *FAS* mutations have been reported. These include missense, nonsense, insertion, deletion, and splice site mutations.

Less commonly, a person with ALPS may have a germline mutation in a gene other than *FAS*, such as *FASLG* or *CASP10*. Less information is available about ALPS due to *FASLG* or *CASP10* mutations because fewer families with these mutations have been identified. Approximately 25 percent of people with ALPS have no detectable mutation in any of these genes, suggesting that other undiscovered genes also are involved in ALPS.

Inheritance

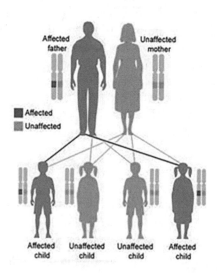

Figure 44.1. *Autosomal Dominant*

In this example, a man with an autosomal dominant disorder has two affected children and two unaffected children. Women also can pass on the mutation.

ALPS due to *FAS* mutations is inherited in an autosomal dominant manner, which means that a person only needs an abnormal gene from one parent to have ALPS. The abnormal *FAS* gene dominates the normal *FAS* gene from the other parent. This usually means that a parent or relative from the side of the family with the mutation also has ALPS. Importantly, however, not everyone with an abnormal *FAS* gene develops ALPS. In fact, up to 40 percent of people with a *FAS* mutation show no symptoms of ALPS. This is called incomplete penetrance. Among those with symptoms of ALPS, some are severely affected by the disorder, while others are not. These variations, called variable expressivity, can be striking, even within the same family.

In a family with a parent who has a *FAS* mutation, each child has a 50 percent chance of inheriting the mutated *FAS* gene. The chance of one child inheriting the mutation is independent of whether his or her siblings have the mutation. In other words, if the first three children in a family have the mutation, the fourth child still has a 50 percent chance of inheriting it. Children who do not inherit the abnormal gene will not develop ALPS or pass on the mutation.

Some germline mutations are not inherited but occur as a result of a mutation in the egg or sperm of one of the parents or in the fertilized egg itself. These are called *de novo* mutations. Approximately 10 percent of ALPS-FAS patients have *de novo* mutations. *De novo* mutations can be passed on to children.

Somatic *FAS* mutations are not inherited and cannot be passed on because the mutation is only present in the blood and not in a woman's ovaries or a man's testes.

Symptoms and Diagnosis

Symptoms

The major clinical symptoms of ALPS result from lymphoproliferation and autoimmune destruction of blood cells. Many, but not all, people with ALPS experience a lessening or complete resolution of their autoimmune and lymphoproliferative symptoms in adulthood.

Lymphoproliferation

The main lymphoproliferative symptoms are enlarged lymph nodes and spleen. While the spleen can be massive in some children, the National Institutes of Health (NIH) team is aware of only one case of splenic rupture. The swollen lymph nodes in the neck, armpit, and groin are usually most noticeable. Sometimes, these enlarged lymph nodes are confused with cancer of the lymph gland, or lymphoma. Large visible lymph nodes are normal for many people with ALPS. It also is normal for lymph nodes to change somewhat is size, shape, or feel over time. Such changes are usually not a lymphoma.

Autoimmunity

The main autoimmune issues are related to reactions against components of the blood:

- Anemia occurs when the body destroys its own red blood cells. This causes a feeling of weakness and fatigue.

- Thrombocytopenia occurs when the body attacks and destroys blood components called platelets. When platelet levels are low, the blood does not clot well, and bleeding cannot be stopped following minor injuries. Thrombocytopenia can lead to nosebleeds, gum bleeds, and bruises.

- Neutropenia occurs when the body destroys infection-fighting cells called neutrophils. A decrease in neutrophils increases the risk of infection, which can lead to symptoms such as mouth ulcers and slow wound healing.

ALPS-related autoimmunity sometimes targets other organs, leading to conditions such as

- hepatitis (inflammation of the liver)

- glomerulonephritis (inflammation of the kidneys)

- uveitis (inflammation of the iris in the eye)

Lymphoma

People with ALPS have an increased risk of developing lymphoma. Up to age 40, people with ALPS have an approximately 20 percent risk of developing lymphoma. In other words, about 1 in 5 patients will develop ALPS lymphoma by the time they are 40. The risk continues past age 40, although the data on older age groups are limited. Thus, doctors should monitor patients with ALPS for symptoms of lymphoma, such as night sweats, fever, fatigue, weight loss, loss of appetite, and sudden lymph node enlargement in one area. Although the lymphoma risk for people with ALPS is much higher than that of the general population, most people with ALPS never develop lymphoma.

Diagnosis

The diagnosis of ALPS is based on clinical findings, laboratory findings, and identification of mutations in genes, such as *FAS*, that affect the process of apoptosis, or the programmed destruction of cells. Clinical findings that suggest ALPS include

- Non-cancerous swelling of the lymph nodes (lymphadenopathy) that lasts for more than six months
- Autoimmune disease, especially against blood cells
- Cancer of the lymph nodes (lymphoma)
- Family history of ALPS or ALPS-like features

Laboratory Findings

One prominent finding is an elevated level of CD4- and CD8-negative T lymphocytes, called double-negative T cells. Lab tests can confirm defects in apoptosis of lymphocytes, which is highly suggestive of ALPS. Additionally, an increase in serum vitamin B12 can indicate lymphoproliferation in ALPS-FAS. People with ALPS-FAS tend to have B12 levels much higher than those of healthy people.

Doctors may perform additional blood tests to help diagnose ALPS. Other markers that may be elevated in ALPS include plasma interleukin-10; plasma interleukin-18; immunoglobulin subtypes IgG, IgA, and IgM; absolute monocyte count; absolute eosinophil count; anticardiolipin antibody; and antinuclear antibody. In contrast, people with ALPS often have abnormally low levels of HDL (high density lipoprotein) and total cholesterol.

Treatment

There currently is no standard cure for ALPS. The disorder can be managed by treating cytopenias and other autoimmune diseases that occur in people with ALPS, as well as monitoring for and treating lymphoproliferation, an enlarged spleen, and lymphoma.

Doctors closely observe lymphoproliferation in people with ALPS. They may conduct routine imaging tests to observe the lymph nodes. If lymphoma is suspected, the doctor may perform a biopsy—the removal of a small piece of tissue. Lymphomas in people with ALPS can be successfully treated with standard cancer-treatment protocols. The defective apoptosis underlying ALPS does not seem to hinder response to cancer treatment.

Doctors may prescribe corticosteroids and other immunosuppressive medications when lymphoproliferation causes complications such as airway obstruction. ALPS-related autoimmunity also can be treated by suppressing the immune system with medication. The corticosteroid prednisone is often given for this purpose. However, low blood counts frequently recur after a short course of treatment with prednisone, requiring repeated doses of corticosteroids or the use of different types of immune-suppressing medications. Chronic low blood counts often can be managed successfully with steroid-sparing approaches, including medications such as mycophenolate mofetil and sirolimus. In most cases, rare autoimmune complications of ALPS, such as hepatitis, glomerulonephritis, and uveitis, can be treated effectively with immune-suppressing medications.

Spleen removal, or splenectomy, may be necessary in rare cases of difficult-to-control cytopenias. Unfortunately, many patients still struggle with low blood counts after splenectomy. Additionally, lack of a spleen increases the risk of sepsis, a potentially fatal response to severe infection with common bacteria called pneumococcus.

Chapter 45

Autoimmune Polyglandular Syndrome Type 1 (APS-1)

Autoimmune polyglandular syndrome type 1 (APS-1) is a genetic immune disorder that causes a diverse range of symptoms, including autoimmunity against different types of organs and an increased susceptibility to candidiasis, a fungal infection caused by *Candida* yeast.

APS-1 has other names, including autoimmune polyendocrinopathy-candidiasis-ectodermal dystrophy (APECED); autoimmune polyendocrinopathy, type 1; and polyglandular autoimmune (PGA) syndrome, type 1.

Causes

APS-1 results from mutations in the *AIRE* gene, which trains the immune system to recognize the body's own cells and tissues as "self" and belonging to the body. When the immune system loses this state of tolerance and erroneously perceives the body as harmful, autoimmune attacks damage tissues and organs. In the case of APS-1, organs of the endocrine system, which regulate hormone production, and non-endocrine organs, including the liver, lungs, intestines, and kidneys, are disrupted.

This chapter includes text excerpted from "Autoimmune Polyglandular Syndrome Type 1 (APS-1)," National Institute of Allergy and Infectious Diseases (NIAID), June 21, 2016.

Mutations in *AIRE* also prevent immune cells from developing or functioning normally, and people become uniquely susceptible to fungal microbes that are typically harmless to those with healthy immune systems. People with APS-1 are especially vulnerable to *Candida*, a yeast fungus found on mucosal surfaces in approximately 50 percent of healthy individuals.

APS-1 is inherited in an autosomal recessive manner, meaning both parents must be carriers of the faulty gene in order to have an affected child.

Symptoms and Diagnosis

Signs and Symptoms

Most people with APS-1 develop symptoms during infancy, and the hallmark sign is chronic mucocutaneous candidiasis (CMC). CMC is caused by recurring *Candida* infections on mucosal surfaces like the mouth and genital areas.

Problems with the endocrine system caused by APS-1 may result in a number of conditions. Addison disease (also called adrenal insufficiency) is caused by deficient hormone production by the adrenal glands, and hypoparathyroidism is a failure of the parathyroid glands to produce hormones that regulate calcium and other minerals. These two endocrine deficiencies are the most common, affecting over 80 percent of people with APS-1.

Problems with non-endocrine organs are less common in APS-1. Autoimmune hepatitis and intestinal malabsorption are seen more often, while problems with autoimmunity in the lungs or the kidneys are seen in a minority of people.

Other symptoms include

- Alopecia

- Anemia

- Autoimmune thyroiditis

- Chronic gastritis

- Ectodermal dystrophy

- Hypogonadism

- Insulin-dependent diabetes

- Keratitis or keratoconjuctivitis

- Vitamin B12 deficiency
- Vitiligo
- Problems with dental enamel and nails

Diagnosis

APS-1 is diagnosed when a person exhibits at least two of the following symptoms: CMC, hypoparathyroidism, and adrenal insufficiency. Genetic testing can validate the presence of *AIRE* mutations.

Treatment

Treatment for APS-1 will depend on what symptoms a person exhibits. Endocrine problems may be treated with hormone replacement therapy, and CMC may be managed with anti-fungal medications. At present, there is no cure for APS-1 and no satisfactory treatment for the non-endocrine autoimmune symptoms of the syndrome. NIAID researchers are exploring how *AIRE* mutations impact the function of cells by studying people with APS-1, as well as using mouse models of *AIRE* deficiency.

Chapter 46

Behçet Disease

What Is Behçet Disease?

Behçet disease is now recognized as a chronic condition that causes canker sores or ulcers in the mouth and on the genitals, and inflammation in parts of the eye. In some people, the disease also results in arthritis (swollen, painful, stiff joints), skin problems, and inflammation of the digestive tract, brain, and spinal cord.

Who Gets Behçet Disease?

Behçet disease is common in the Middle East, Asia, and Japan; it is rare in the United States. In Middle Eastern and Asian countries, the disease affects more men than women. In the United States, the opposite is true. Behçet disease tends to develop in people in their twenties or thirties, but people of all ages can develop this disease.

What Causes Behçet Disease?

The exact cause of Behçet disease is unknown. Most symptoms of the disease are caused by inflammation of the blood vessels. Inflammation is a characteristic reaction of the body to injury or disease and is marked by four signs: swelling, redness, heat, and pain. Doctors

---

This chapter includes text excerpted from "Questions and Answers about Behçet Disease," National Institute of Arthritis and Musculoskeletal and Skin Diseases (NIAMS), August 2015.

think that an autoinflammatory reaction may cause the blood vessels to become inflamed, but they do not know what triggers this reaction. Under normal conditions, the immune system protects the body from diseases and infections by killing harmful "foreign" substances, such as germs, that enter the body. In an autoinflammatory reaction, the immune system mistakenly attacks and harms the body's own tissues.

Behçet disease is not contagious; it is not spread from one person to another. Researchers think that two factors are important for a person to get Behçet disease. First, it is believed that abnormalities of the immune system make some people susceptible to the disease. Scientists think that this susceptibility may be inherited; that is, it may be due to one or more specific genes. Second, something in the environment, possibly a bacterium or virus, might trigger or activate the disease in susceptible people.

What Are the Symptoms of Behçet Disease?

Behçet disease affects each person differently. Some people have only mild symptoms, such as canker sores or ulcers in the mouth or on the genitals. Others have more severe signs, such as meningitis, which is an inflammation of the membranes that cover the brain and spinal cord. Meningitis can cause fever, a stiff neck, and headaches. More severe symptoms usually appear months or years after a person notices the first signs of Behçet disease. Symptoms can last for a long time or may come and go in a few weeks. Typically, symptoms appear, disappear, and then reappear. The times when a person is having symptoms are called flares. Different symptoms may occur with each flare; the problems of the disease often do not occur together. To help the doctor diagnose Behçet disease and monitor its course, patients may want to keep a record of which symptoms occur and when. Because many conditions mimic Behçet disease, doctors must observe the lesions (injuries) caused by the disorder to make an accurate diagnosis.

Common symptoms of Behçet disease include:

- Mouth sores

- Genital sores

- Skin problems

- Uveitis (inflammation of parts of the eye)

- Arthritis

In addition, Behçet disease may also cause blood clots and inflammation in the central nervous system and digestive organs.

Vascular System

Some people with Behçet disease have blood clots resulting from inflammation in the veins (thrombophlebitis), usually in the legs. Symptoms include pain and tenderness in the affected area. The area may also be swollen and warm. Because thrombophlebitis can have severe complications, people should report symptoms to their doctor immediately. A few patients may experience artery problems such as aneurysms (balloon-like swelling of the artery wall).

Central Nervous System

In the United States, Behçet disease affects the central nervous system in an estimated one-fifth to one-quarter of people with the disease. The central nervous system includes the brain and spinal cord. Its function is to process information and coordinate thinking, behavior, sensation, and movement. Behçet disease can cause inflammation of the brain and the thin membrane that covers and protects the brain and spinal cord. This condition is called meningoencephalitis. People with meningoencephalitis may have fever, headache, stiff neck, and difficulty coordinating movement, and should report any of these symptoms to their doctor immediately. If this condition is left untreated, a stroke (blockage or rupture of blood vessels in the brain) can result.

Digestive Tract

Rarely, Behçet disease causes inflammation and ulceration (sores) throughout the digestive tract that are identical to the aphthous lesions in the mouth and genital area.

This leads to abdominal pain, diarrhea, and/or bleeding. Because these symptoms are very similar to symptoms of other diseases of the digestive tract, such as ulcerative colitis and Crohn's disease, careful evaluation is essential to rule out these other diseases.

How Is Behçet Disease Diagnosed?

Diagnosing Behçet disease is very difficult because no specific test confirms it. Less than half of people initially thought to have Behçet disease actually have it. When a patient reports symptoms, the doctor must conduct an examination and rule out other conditions with similar symptoms. Because it may take several months or even years for all the common symptoms to appear, the diagnosis may not be made for a long time. A patient may even visit several different kinds of doctors before the diagnosis is made.

These symptoms are key to a diagnosis of Behçet disease:

- mouth sores at least three times in 12 months

- any two of the following symptoms: recurring genital sores, eye inflammation with loss of vision, characteristic skin lesions, or positive pathergy (skin prick test)

Besides finding these signs, the doctor must rule out other conditions with similar symptoms, such as Crohn's disease and reactive arthritis. The doctor also may recommend that the patient see an eye specialist to identify possible complications related to eye inflammation. A dermatologist may perform a biopsy of mouth, genital, or skin lesions to help distinguish Behçet's from other disorders.

How Is Behçet Disease Treated?

Although there is no cure for Behçet disease, people usually can control symptoms with proper medication such as topical medicine and oral medicine that includes corticosteroids and immunosuppressive drugs, rest, exercise, and a healthy lifestyle. The goal of treatment is to reduce discomfort and prevent serious complications such as disability from arthritis or blindness. The type of medicine and the length of treatment depend on the person's symptoms and their severity. It is likely that a combination of treatments will be needed to relieve specific symptoms. Patients should tell each of their doctors about all of the medicines they are taking so that the doctors can coordinate treatment.

What Is the Prognosis for a Person with Behçet Disease?

Most people with Behçet disease can lead productive lives and control symptoms with proper medicine, rest, and exercise. Doctors can use many medicines to relieve pain, treat symptoms, and prevent complications. When treatment is effective, flares usually become less frequent. Many patients eventually enter a period of remission (a disappearance of symptoms). In some people, treatment does not relieve symptoms, and gradually more serious symptoms such as eye disease may occur. Serious symptoms may appear months or years after the first signs of Behçet disease.

Chapter 47

Celiac Disease

Definition and Facts for Celiac Disease

What is celiac disease?

Celiac disease is a digestive disorder that damages the small intestine. The disease is triggered by eating foods containing gluten. Gluten is a protein found naturally in wheat, barley, and rye, and is common in foods such as bread, pasta, cookies, and cakes. Many pre-packaged foods, lip balms and lipsticks, hair and skin products, toothpastes, vitamin and nutrient supplements, and, rarely, medicines, contain gluten.

Celiac disease can be very serious. The disease can cause long-lasting digestive problems and keep your body from getting all the nutrients it needs. Celiac disease can also affect the body outside the intestine.

Celiac disease is different from gluten sensitivity or wheat intolerance. If you have gluten sensitivity, you may have symptoms similar to those of celiac disease, such as abdominal pain and tiredness. Unlike celiac disease, gluten sensitivity does not damage the small intestine.

Celiac disease is also different from a wheat allergy. In both cases, your body's immune system reacts to wheat. However, some symptoms in wheat allergies, such as having itchy eyes or a hard time breathing, are different from celiac disease. Wheat allergies also do not cause long-term damage to the small intestine.

This chapter includes text excerpted from "Celiac Disease," National Institute of Diabetes and Digestive and Kidney Diseases (NIDDK), June 2016.

How Common Is Celiac Disease?

As many as one in 141 Americans has celiac disease, although most don't know it.

Who Is More Likely to Develop Celiac Disease?

Although celiac disease affects children and adults in all parts of the world, the disease is more common in Caucasians and more often diagnosed in females. You are more likely to develop celiac disease if someone in your family has the disease. Celiac disease also is more common among people with certain other diseases, such as Down syndrome, Turner syndrome, and type 1 diabetes.

What Other Health Problems Do People with Celiac Disease Have?

If you have celiac disease, you also may be at risk for

- Addison disease
- Hashimoto disease
- primary biliary cirrhosis
- type 1 diabetes

What Are the Complications of Celiac Disease?

Long-term complications of celiac disease include

- malnutrition, a condition in which you don't get enough vitamins, minerals, and other nutrients you need to be healthy
- accelerated osteoporosis or bone softening, known as osteomalacia
- nervous system problems
- problems related to reproduction

Rare complications can include

- intestinal cancer
- liver diseases
- lymphoma, a cancer of part of the immune system called the lymph system that includes the gut

In rare cases, you may continue to have trouble absorbing nutrients even though you have been following a strict gluten-free diet. If you have this condition, called refractory celiac disease, your intestines are severely damaged and can't heal. You may need to receive nutrients through an IV.

Symptoms and Causes of Celiac Disease

What Are the Symptoms of Celiac Disease?

Most people with celiac disease have one or more symptoms. However, some people with the disease may not have symptoms or feel sick. Sometimes health issues such as surgery, a pregnancy, childbirth, bacterial gastroenteritis, a viral infection, or severe mental stress can trigger celiac disease symptoms.

If you have celiac disease, you may have digestive problems or other symptoms. Digestive symptoms are more common in children and can include

- bloating, or a feeling of fullness or swelling in the abdomen
- chronic diarrhea
- constipation
- gas
- nausea
- pale, foul-smelling, or fatty stools that float
- stomach pain
- vomiting

For children with celiac disease, being unable to absorb nutrients when they are so important to normal growth and development can lead to

- damage to the permanent teeth's enamel
- delayed puberty
- failure to thrive in infants
- mood changes or feeling annoyed or impatient
- slowed growth and short height
- weight loss

Adults are less likely to have digestive symptoms and, instead, may have one or more of the following:

- anemia
- a red, smooth, shiny tongue
- bone or joint pain
- depression or anxiety
- dermatitis herpetiformis
- headaches
- infertility or repeated miscarriage
- missed menstrual periods
- mouth problems such a canker sores or dry mouth
- seizures
- tingling numbness in the hands and feet
- tiredness
- weak and brittle bones

Adults who have digestive symptoms with celiac disease may have

- abdominal pain and bloating
- intestinal blockages
- tiredness that lasts for long periods of time
- ulcers, or sores on the stomach or lining of the intestine

Celiac disease also can produce a reaction in which your immune system, or your body's natural defense system, attacks healthy cells in your body. This reaction can spread outside your digestive tract to other areas of your body, including your

- bones
- joints
- nervous system
- skin
- spleen

Diagnosis of Celiac Disease

How Do Doctors Diagnose Celiac Disease?

Celiac disease can be hard to diagnose because some of the symptoms are like symptoms of other diseases, such as irritable bowel syndrome (IBS) and lactose intolerance. Your doctor may diagnose celiac disease with a medical and family history, physical exam, and tests. Tests may include blood tests, genetic tests, and biopsy.

Medical and Famiy History

Your doctor will ask you for information about your family's health—specifically, if anyone in your family has a history of celiac disease.

Physical Exam

During a physical exam, a doctor most often

- checks your body for a rash or malnutrition, a condition that arises when you don't get enough vitamins, minerals, and other nutrients you need to be healthy

- listens to sounds in your abdomen using a stethoscope

- taps on your abdomen to check for pain and fullness or swelling

Dental Exam

For some people, a dental visit can be the first step toward discovering celiac disease. Dental enamel defects, such as white, yellow, or brown spots on the teeth, are a pretty common problem in people with celiac disease, especially children. These defects can help dentists and other healthcare professionals identify celiac disease.

Treatment for Celiac Disease

How Do Doctors Treat Celiac Disease?

A Gluten-Free Diet

Doctors treat celiac disease with a gluten-free diet. Gluten is a protein found naturally in wheat, barley, and rye that triggers a reaction if you have celiac disease. Symptoms greatly improve for most people with celiac disease who stick to a gluten-free diet. In recent years, grocery stores and restaurants have added many more gluten-free foods and products, making it easier to stay gluten free.

Your doctor may refer you to a dietitian who specializes in treating people with celiac disease. The dietitian will teach you how to avoid gluten while following a healthy diet. He or she will help you

- check food and product labels for gluten

- design everyday meal plans

- make healthy choices about the types of foods to eat

For most people, following a gluten-free diet will heal damage in the small intestine and prevent more damage. You may see symptoms improve within days to weeks of starting the diet. The small intestine usually heals in 3 to 6 months in children. Complete healing can take several years in adults. Once the intestine heals, the villi, which were damaged by the disease, regrow and will absorb nutrients from food into the bloodstream normally.

Gluten-Free Diet and Dermatitis Herpetiformis

If you have dermatitis herpetiformis—an itchy, blistering skin rash—skin symptoms generally respond to a gluten-free diet. However, skin symptoms may return if you add gluten back into your diet. Medicines such as dapsone, taken by mouth, can control the skin symptoms. People who take dapsone need to have regular blood tests to check for side effects from the medicine.

Dapsone does not treat intestinal symptoms or damage, which is why you should stay on a gluten-free diet if you have the rash. Even when you follow a gluten-free diet, the rash may take months or even years to fully heal—and often comes back over the years.

Avoiding Medicines and Nonfood Products That May Contain Gluten

In addition to prescribing a gluten-free diet, your doctor will want you to avoid all hidden sources of gluten. If you have celiac disease, ask a pharmacist about ingredients in

- herbal and nutritional supplements

- prescription and over-the-counter medicines

- vitamin and mineral supplements

You also could take in or transfer from your hands to your mouth other products that contain gluten without knowing it. Products that may contain gluten include

- children's modeling dough, such as Play-Doh

- cosmetics

- lipstick, lip gloss, and lip balm

- skin and hair products

- toothpaste and mouthwash

- communion wafers

Medications are rare sources of gluten. Even if gluten is present in a medicine, it is likely to be in such small quantities that it would not cause any symptoms.

Reading product labels can sometimes help you avoid gluten. Some product makers label their products as being gluten-free. If a product label doesn't list the product's ingredients, ask the maker of the product for an ingredients list.

Chapter 48

Type 1 Diabetes: Insulin Dependant

What Is Diabetes?

Diabetes is a complex group of diseases with a variety of causes. People with diabetes have high blood glucose, also called high blood sugar or hyperglycemia.

Diabetes is a disorder of metabolism—the way the body uses digested food for energy. The digestive tract breaks down carbohydrates—sugars and starches found in many foods—into glucose, a form of sugar that enters the bloodstream. With the help of the hormone insulin, cells throughout the body absorb glucose and use it for energy. Diabetes develops when the body doesn't make enough insulin or is not able to use insulin effectively, or both.

Insulin is made in the pancreas, an organ located behind the stomach. The pancreas contains clusters of cells called islets. Beta cells within the islets make insulin and release it into the blood.

If beta cells don't produce enough insulin, or the body doesn't respond to the insulin that is present, glucose builds up in the blood

This chapter contains text excerpted from the following sources: Text beginning with the heading "What is Diabetes?" is excerpted from "Causes of Diabetes," National Institute of Diabetes and Digestive and Kidney Diseases (NIDDK), August 2014; Text beginning with the heading "What Are the Signs and Symptoms of Diabetes?" is excerpted from "Types of Diabetes," National Institute of Diabetes and Digestive and Kidney Diseases (NIDDK), February 2014.

instead of being absorbed by cells in the body, leading to prediabetes or diabetes. Prediabetes is a condition in which blood glucose levels or A1C levels—which reflect average blood glucose levels—are higher than normal but not high enough to be diagnosed as diabetes. In diabetes, the body's cells are starved of energy despite high blood glucose levels.

Over time, high blood glucose damages nerves and blood vessels, leading to complications such as heart disease, stroke, kidney disease, blindness, dental disease, and amputations. Other complications of diabetes may include increased susceptibility to other diseases, loss of mobility with aging, depression, and pregnancy problems. No one is certain what starts the processes that cause diabetes, but scientists believe genes and environmental factors interact to cause diabetes in most cases.

The two main types of diabetes are type 1 diabetes and type 2 diabetes. A third type, gestational diabetes, develops only during pregnancy. Other types of diabetes are caused by defects in specific genes, diseases of the pancreas, certain drugs or chemicals, infections, and other conditions. Some people show signs of both type 1 and type 2 diabetes.

What Causes Type 1 Diabetes?

Type 1 diabetes is caused by a lack of insulin due to the destruction of insulin-producing beta cells in the pancreas. In type 1 diabetes—an autoimmune disease—the body's immune system attacks and destroys the beta cells. Normally, the immune system protects the body from infection by identifying and destroying bacteria, viruses, and other potentially harmful foreign substances. But in autoimmune diseases, the immune system attacks the body's own cells. In type 1 diabetes, beta cell destruction may take place over several years, but symptoms of the disease usually develop over a short period of time.

Type 1 diabetes typically occurs in children and young adults, though it can appear at any age. In the past, type 1 diabetes was called juvenile diabetes or insulin-dependent diabetes mellitus.

Latent autoimmune diabetes in adults (LADA) may be a slowly developing kind of type 1 diabetes. Diagnosis usually occurs after age 30. In LADA, as in type 1 diabetes, the body's immune system destroys the beta cells. At the time of diagnosis, people with LADA may still produce their own insulin, but eventually most will need insulin shots or an insulin pump to control blood glucose levels.

Genetic Susceptibility

Heredity plays an important part in determining who is likely to develop type 1 diabetes. Genes are passed down from biological parent to child. Genes carry instructions for making proteins that are needed for the body's cells to function. Many genes, as well as interactions among genes, are thought to influence susceptibility to and protection from type 1 diabetes. The key genes may vary in different population groups. Variations in genes that affect more than 1 percent of a population group are called gene variants.

Certain gene variants that carry instructions for making proteins called human leukocyte antigens (HLAs) on white blood cells are linked to the risk of developing type 1 diabetes. The proteins produced by HLA genes help determine whether the immune system recognizes a cell as part of the body or as foreign material. Some combinations of HLA gene variants predict that a person will be at higher risk for type 1 diabetes, while other combinations are protective or have no effect on risk.

While HLA genes are the major risk genes for type 1 diabetes, many additional risk genes or gene regions have been found. Not only can these genes help identify people at risk for type 1 diabetes, but they also provide important clues to help scientists better understand how the disease develops and identify potential targets for therapy and prevention.

Genetic testing can show what types of HLA genes a person carries and can reveal other genes linked to diabetes. However, most genetic testing is done in a research setting and is not yet available to individuals. Scientists are studying how the results of genetic testing can be used to improve type 1 diabetes prevention or treatment.

Autoimmune Destruction of Beta Cells

In type 1 diabetes, white blood cells called T cells attack and destroy beta cells. The process begins well before diabetes symptoms appear and continues after diagnosis. Often, type 1 diabetes is not diagnosed until most beta cells have already been destroyed. At this point, a person needs daily insulin treatment to survive. Finding ways to modify or stop this autoimmune process and preserve beta cell function is a major focus of current scientific research.

Recent research suggests insulin itself may be a key trigger of the immune attack on beta cells. The immune systems of people who are susceptible to developing type 1 diabetes respond to insulin as if it were a foreign substance, or antigen. To combat antigens, the body makes proteins called antibodies. Antibodies to insulin and other proteins produced by beta cells are found in people with type 1 diabetes. Researchers test for these antibodies to help identify people at increased risk of developing the disease. Testing the types and levels of antibodies in the blood can help determine whether a person has type 1 diabetes, LADA, or another type of diabetes.

Environmental Factors

Environmental factors, such as foods, viruses, and toxins, may play a role in the development of type 1 diabetes, but the exact nature of their role has not been determined. Some theories suggest that environmental factors trigger the autoimmune destruction of beta cells in people with a genetic susceptibility to diabetes. Other theories suggest that environmental factors play an ongoing role in diabetes, even after diagnosis.

Viruses and infections. A virus cannot cause diabetes on its own, but people are sometimes diagnosed with type 1 diabetes during or after a viral infection, suggesting a link between the two. Also, the onset of type 1 diabetes occurs more frequently during the winter when viral infections are more common. Viruses possibly associated with type 1 diabetes include coxsackievirus B, cytomegalovirus, adenovirus, rubella, and mumps. Scientists have described several ways these viruses may damage or destroy beta cells or possibly trigger an autoimmune response in susceptible people. For example, anti-islet antibodies have been found in patients with congenital rubella syndrome, and cytomegalovirus has been associated with significant beta cell damage and acute pancreatitis—inflammation of the pancreas. Scientists are trying to identify a virus that can cause type 1 diabetes so that a vaccine might be developed to prevent the disease.

Infant feeding practices. Some studies have suggested that dietary factors may raise or lower the risk of developing type 1 diabetes. For example, breastfed infants and infants receiving vitamin D supplements may have a reduced risk of developing type 1 diabetes, while early exposure to cow's milk and cereal proteins may increase risk. More research is needed to clarify how infant nutrition affects the risk for type 1 diabetes.

What Are the Signs and Symptoms of Diabetes?

The signs and symptoms of diabetes are

- being very thirsty

- urinating often
- feeling very hungry
- feeling very tired
- losing weight without trying
- sores that heal slowly
- dry, itchy skin
- feelings of pins and needles in your feet
- losing feeling in your feet
- blurry eyesight

Some people with diabetes don't have any of these signs or symptoms. The only way to know if you have diabetes is to have your doctor do a blood test.

Why Do You Need to Take Care of Your Diabetes?

Over time, diabetes can lead to serious problems with your blood vessels, heart, nerves, kidneys, mouth, eyes, and feet. These problems can lead to an amputation, which is surgery to remove a damaged toe, foot, or leg, for example.

The most serious problem caused by diabetes is heart disease. When you have diabetes, you are more than twice as likely as people without diabetes to have heart disease or a stroke. With diabetes, you may not have the usual signs or symptoms of a heart attack. The best way to take care of your health is to work with your healthcare team to keep your blood glucose, blood pressure, and cholesterol levels in your target range. Targets are numbers you aim for.

Chapter 49

Glomerular Diseases

Many diseases affect kidney function by attacking the glomeruli, the tiny units within the kidney where blood is cleaned. Glomerular diseases include many conditions with a variety of genetic and environmental causes, but they fall into two major categories:

- Glomerulonephritis describes the inflammation of the membrane tissue in the kidney that serves as a filter, separating wastes and extra fluid from the blood.

- Glomerulosclerosis describes the scarring or hardening of the tiny blood vessels within the kidney.

Although glomerulonephritis and glomerulosclerosis have different causes, they can both lead to kidney failure.

What Are the Kidneys and What Do They Do?

The two kidneys are bean-shaped organs located just below the rib cage, one on each side of the spine. Everyday, the two kidneys filter about 120 to 150 quarts of blood to produce about 1 to 2 quarts of urine, composed of wastes and extra fluid.

Blood enters the kidneys through arteries that branch inside the kidneys into tiny clusters of looping blood vessels. Each cluster is called a *glomerulus*, which comes from the Greek word meaning filter. The

This chapter includes text excerpted from "Glomerular Diseases," National Institute of Diabetes and Digestive and Kidney Diseases (NIDDK), April 2014.

plural form of the word is *glomeruli*. There are approximately 1 million glomeruli, or filters, in each kidney. The glomerulus is attached to the opening of a small fluid-collecting tube called a *tubule*. Blood is filtered in the glomerulus, and extra fluid and wastes pass into the tubule and become urine. Eventually, the urine drains from the kidneys into the bladder through larger tubes called *ureters*.

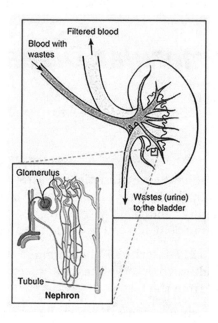

Figure 49.1. *Nephron*

In the nephron (left), tiny blood vessels intertwine with fluid-collecting tubes. Each kidney contains about 1 million nephrons.

Each glomerulus-and-tubule unit is called a *nephron*. Each kidney is composed of about 1 million nephrons. In healthy nephrons, the glomerular membrane that separates the blood vessel from the tubule allows waste products and extra water to pass into the tubule while keeping blood cells and protein in the bloodstream.

How Do Glomerular Diseases Interfere with Kidney Function?

Glomerular diseases damage the glomeruli, letting protein and sometimes red blood cells leak into the urine. Sometimes a glomerular disease also interferes with the clearance of waste products by the kidney, so they begin to build up in the blood. Furthermore, loss of blood proteins like albumin in the urine can result in a fall in their level in the bloodstream. In normal blood, albumin acts like a sponge, drawing extra fluid from the body into the bloodstream, where it remains until the kidneys remove it. But when albumin leaks into the urine, the blood loses its capacity to absorb extra fluid from the body. Fluid can accumulate outside the circulatory system in the face, hands, feet, or ankles and cause swelling.

What Are the Symptoms of Glomerular Disease?

The signs and symptoms of glomerular disease include

- **albuminuria:** large amounts of protein in the urine

- **hematuria:** blood in the urine

- **reduced glomerular filtration rate:** inefficient filtering of wastes from the blood

- **hypoproteinemia:** low blood protein

- **edema:** swelling in parts of the body

One or more of these symptoms can be the first sign of kidney disease. But how would you know, for example, whether you have proteinuria? Before seeing a doctor, you may not. But some of these symptoms have signs, or visible manifestations:

- Proteinuria may cause foamy urine.

- Blood may cause the urine to be pink or cola-colored.

- Edema may be obvious in hands and ankles, especially at the end of the day, or around the eyes when awakening in the morning, for example.

How Is Glomerular Disease Diagnosed?

Patients with glomerular disease have significant amounts of protein in the urine, which may be referred to as "nephrotic range" if levels are very high. Red blood cells in the urine are a frequent finding as well, particularly in some forms of glomerular disease. Urinalysis provides information about kidney damage by indicating levels of protein and red blood cells in the urine. Blood tests measure the levels of waste products such as creatinine and urea nitrogen to determine whether the filtering capacity of the kidneys is impaired. If these lab tests indicate kidney damage, the doctor may recommend ultrasound or an X-ray to see whether the shape or size of the kidneys is abnormal. These tests are called renal imaging. But since glomerular disease causes problems at the cellular level, the doctor will probably also recommend a kidney biopsy—a procedure in which a needle is used to extract small pieces of tissue for examination with different types of microscopes, each of which shows a different aspect of the tissue. A biopsy may be helpful in confirming glomerular disease and identifying the cause.

What Causes Glomerular Disease?

A number of different diseases can result in glomerular disease. It may be the direct result of an infection or a drug toxic to the kidneys, or it may result from a disease that affects the entire body, like diabetes or lupus. Many different kinds of diseases can cause swelling or scarring of the nephron or glomerulus. Sometimes glomerular disease is idiopathic, meaning that it occurs without an apparent associated disease.

Chapter 50

Goodpasture Syndrome

What Is Goodpasture Syndrome?

Goodpasture syndrome is a pulmonary-renal syndrome, which is a group of acute illnesses involving the kidneys and lungs. Goodpasture syndrome includes all of the following conditions:

- glomerulonephritis—inflammation of the glomeruli, which are tiny clusters of looping blood vessels in the kidneys that help filter wastes and extra water from the blood

- the presence of anti-glomerular basement membrane (GBM) antibodies; the GBM is part of the glomeruli and is composed of collagen and other proteins

- bleeding in the lungs

In Goodpasture syndrome, immune cells produce antibodies against a specific region of collagen. The antibodies attack the collagen in the lungs and kidneys.

Ernest Goodpasture first described the syndrome during the influenza pandemic of 1919 when he reported on a patient who died from bleeding in the lungs and kidney failure. Diagnostic tools to confirm Goodpasture syndrome were not available at that time, so it is not known whether the patient had true Goodpasture syndrome or vasculitis. Vasculitis is an autoimmune condition—a disorder in which the body's immune system

This chapter includes text excerpted from "Goodpasture Syndrome," National Institute of Diabetes and Digestive and Kidney Diseases (NIDDK), May 2012. Reviewed October 2016.

attacks the body's own cells and organs—that involves inflammation in the blood vessels and can cause similar lung and kidney problems.

Goodpasture syndrome is sometimes called anti-GBM disease. However, anti-GBM disease is only one cause of pulmonary-renal syndromes, including Goodpasture syndrome.

Goodpasture syndrome is fatal unless quickly diagnosed and treated.

What Causes Goodpasture Syndrome?

The causes of Goodpasture syndrome are not fully understood. People who smoke or use hair dyes appear to be at increased risk for this condition. Exposure to hydrocarbon fumes, metallic dust, and certain drugs, such as cocaine, may also raise a person's risk. Genetics may also play a part, as a small number of cases have been reported in more than one family member.

What Are the Symptoms of Goodpasture Syndrome?

The symptoms of Goodpasture syndrome may initially include fatigue, nausea, vomiting, and weakness. The lungs are usually affected before or at the same time as the kidneys, and symptoms can include shortness of breath and coughing, sometimes with blood. The progression from initial symptoms to the lungs being affected may be very rapid. Symptoms that occur when the kidneys are affected include blood in the urine or foamy urine, swelling in the legs, and high blood pressure.

How Is Goodpasture Syndrome Diagnosed?

A healthcare provider may order the following tests to diagnose Goodpasture syndrome:

- **Urinalysis.** Urinalysis is testing of a urine sample. The urine sample is collected in a special container in a healthcare provider's office or commercial facility and can be tested in the same location or sent to a lab for analysis. For the test, a nurse or technician places a strip of chemically treated paper, called a dipstick, into the urine. Patches on the dipstick change color when protein or blood are present in urine. A high number of red blood cells and high levels of protein in the urine indicate kidney damage.

- **Blood test.** A blood test involves drawing blood at a healthcare provider's office or commercial facility and sending the sample to a lab for analysis. The blood test can show the presence of anti-GBM antibodies.

- **Chest X-ray.** An X-ray of the chest is performed in a healthcare provider's office, outpatient center, or hospital by an X-ray technician, and the images are interpreted by a radiologist—a doctor who specializes in medical imaging. Abnormalities in the lungs, if present, can be seen on the X-ray.

- **Biopsy.** A biopsy is a procedure that involves taking a piece of kidney tissue for examination with a microscope. The biopsy is performed by a healthcare provider in a hospital with light sedation and local anesthetic. The healthcare provider uses imaging techniques such as ultrasound or a computerized tomography scan to guide the biopsy needle into the kidney. The tissue is examined in a lab by a pathologist—a doctor who specializes in diagnosing diseases. The test can show crescent-shaped changes in the glomeruli and lines of antibodies attached to the GBM.

How Is Goodpasture Syndrome Treated?

Goodpasture syndrome is usually treated with

- **immunosuppressive medications,** such as cyclophosphamide, to keep the immune system from making antibodies

- **corticosteroid medications** to suppress the body's autoimmune response

- **plasmapheresis**—a procedure that uses a machine to remove blood from the body, separate certain cells from the plasma, and return just the cells to the person's body; the anti-GBM antibodies remain in the plasma and are not returned to the person's body

Plasmapheresis is usually continued for several weeks, and immunosuppressive medications may be given for 6 to 12 months, depending on the response to therapy. In most cases, bleeding in the lungs stops and no permanent lung damage occurs. Damage to the kidneys, however, may be long lasting. If the kidneys fail, blood-filtering treatments called dialysis or kidney transplantation may become necessary.

Eating, Diet, and Nutrition

Eating, diet, and nutrition have not been shown to play a role in causing or preventing Goodpasture syndrome.

Chapter 51

Guillain-Barré Syndrome

What Is Guillain-Barré Syndrome?

Guillain-Barré syndrome (GBS) is a disorder in which the body's immune system attacks part of the peripheral nervous system. The first symptoms of this disorder include varying degrees of weakness or tingling sensations in the legs. In many instances the symmetrical weakness and abnormal sensations spread to the arms and upper body. These symptoms can increase in intensity until certain muscles cannot be used at all and, when severe, the person is almost totally paralyzed. In these cases the disorder is life threatening—potentially interfering with breathing and, at times, with blood pressure or heartrate—and is considered a medical emergency. Such an individual is often put on a ventilator to assist with breathing and is watched closely for problems such asanabnormalheart beat, infections, blood clots, and high or low blood pressure. Most individuals, however,have good recovery from even the most severe cases of Guillain-Barré syndrome, although some continue to have a certain degree of weakness.

Guillain-Barré syndrome can affect anybody. It can strike at any age and both sexes are equally prone to the disorder. The syndrome is rare, however, afflicting only about one person in 100,000. Usually Guillain-Barré occurs a few days or weeks after the patient has had symptoms of a respiratory or gastrointestinal viral infection.

This chapter includes text excerpted from "Guillain-Barré Syndrome Fact Sheet," National Institute of Neurological Disorders and Stroke (NINDS), June 1, 2016.

Occasionally surgery will trigger the syndrome. Recently, some countries worldwide have reported an increased incidence of GBS following infection with the Zika virus. In rare instances vaccinations may increase the risk of GBS.

After the first clinical manifestations of the disease, the symptoms can progress over the course of hours, days, or weeks. Most people reach the stage of greatest weakness within the first 2 weeks after symptoms appear, and by the third week of the illness 90 percent of all patients are at their weakest.

What Causes Guillain-Barré Syndrome?

No one yet knows why Guillain-Barré—which is not contagious—strikes some people and not others. Nor does anyone know exactly what sets the disease in motion.

What scientists do know is that the body's immune system begins to attack the body itself, causing what is known as an autoimmune disease. Usually the cells of the immune system attack only foreign material and invading organisms. In Guillain-Barré syndrome, however, the immune system starts to destroy the myelin sheath that surrounds the axons of many peripheral nerves, or even the axons themselves (axons are long, thin extensions of the nerve cells; they carry nerve signals). The myelin sheath surrounding the axon speeds up the transmission of nerve signals and allows the transmission of signals over long distances.

In diseases in which the peripheral nerves' myelin sheaths are injured or degraded, the nerves cannot transmit signals efficiently. That is why the muscles begin to lose their ability to respond to the brain's commands, commands that must be carried through the nerve network. The brain also receives fewer sensory signals from the rest of the body, resulting in an inability to feel textures, heat, pain, and other sensations. Alternately, the brain may receive inappropriate signals that result in tingling, "crawling-skin," or painful sensations. Because the signals to and from the arms and legs must travel the longest distances they are most vulnerable to interruption. Therefore, muscle weakness and tingling sensations usually first appear in the hands and feet and progress upwards.

When Guillain-Barré is preceded by a viral or bacterial infection, it is possible that the virus has changed the nature of cells in the nervous system so that the immune system treats them as foreign cells. It is also possible that the virus makes the immune system itself less discriminating about what cells it recognizes as its own, allowing some of the immune cells, such as certain kinds of lymphocytes and macrophages, to attack the myelin. Sensitized T lymphocytes cooperate with B lymphocytes to produce antibodies against components of the myelin sheath and may contribute to destruction of the myelin. In two forms of GBS, axons are attacked by antibodies against the bacteria Campylobacter jejuni, which react with proteins of the peripheral nerves. Acute motor axonal neuropathy is particularly common in Chinese children. Scientists are investigating these and other possibilities to find why the immune system goes awry in Guillain-Barré syndrome and other autoimmune diseases. The cause and course of Guillain-Barré syndrome is an active area of neurological investigation, incorporating the cooperative efforts of neurological scientists, immunologists, and virologists.

How Is Guillain-Barré Syndrome Diagnosed?

Guillain-Barré is called a syndrome rather than a disease because it is not clear that a specific disease-causing agent is involved. A syndrome is a medical condition characterized by a collection of symptoms (what the patient feels) and signs (what a doctor can observe or measure). The signs and symptoms of the syndrome can be quite varied, so doctors may, on rare occasions, find it difficult to diagnose Guillain-Barré in its earliest stages.

Several disorders have symptoms similar to those found in Guillain-Barré, so doctors examine and question patients carefully before making a diagnosis. Collectively, the signs and symptoms form a certain pattern that helps doctors differentiate Guillain-Barré from other disorders. For example, physicians will note whether the symptoms appear on both sides of the body (most common in Guillain-Barré) and the quickness with which the symptoms appear (in other disorders, muscle weakness may progress over months rather than days or weeks). In Guillain-Barré, reflexes such as knee jerks are usually lost. Because the signals traveling along the nerve are slower, a nerve conduction velocity (NCV) test can give a doctor clues to aid the diagnosis. In Guillain-Barré patients, the cerebrospinal fluid that bathes the spinal cord and brain contains more protein than usual. Therefore a physician may decide to perform a spinal tap, a procedure in which a needle is inserted into the patient's lower back and a small amount of cerebrospinal fluid from the spinal column is withdrawn for study.

How Is Guillain-Barré Treated?

There is no known cure for Guillain-Barré syndrome. However, there are therapies that lessen the severity of the illness and accelerate the recovery in most patients. There are also a number of ways to treat the complications of the disease.

What Is the Long-Term Outlook for Those with Guillain-Barré Syndrome?

Guillain-Barré syndrome can be a devastating disorder because of its sudden and unexpected onset. In addition, recovery is not necessarily quick. As noted above, patients usually reach the point of greatest weakness or paralysis days or weeks after the first symptoms occur. Symptoms then stabilize at this level for a period of days, weeks, or, sometimes, months. The recovery period may be as little as a few weeks or as long as a few years. About 30 percent of those with Guillain-Barré still have a residual weakness after 3 years. About 3 percent may suffer a relapse of muscle weakness and tingling sensations many years after the initial attack.

Guillain-Barré syndrome patients face not only physical difficulties, but emotionally painful periods as well. It is often extremely difficult for patients to adjust to sudden paralysis and dependence on others for help with routine daily activities. Patients sometimes need psychological counseling to help them adapt.

Chapter 52

Henoch-Schönlein Purpura

What Is Henoch-SchöNlein Purpura (HSP)?

Henoch-Schönlein purpura is a disease that causes small blood vessels in the body to become inflamed and leak. The primary symptom is a rash that looks like many small raised bruises. HSP can also affect the kidneys, digestive tract, and joints. HSP can occur any time in life, but it is most common in children between 2 and 6 years of age. Most people recover from HSP completely, though kidney damage is the most likely long-term complication. In adults, HSP can lead to chronic kidney disease (CKD) and kidney failure, described as end-stage renal disease when treated with blood-filtering treatments called dialysis or a kidney transplant.

What Are the Causes of HSP?

Henoch-Schönlein purpura is caused by an abnormal immune system response in which the body's immune system attacks the body's own cells and organs. Usually, the immune system makes antibodies, or proteins, to protect the body from foreign substances such as bacteria or viruses. In HSP, these antibodies attack the blood vessels. The factors that cause this immune system response are not known. However, in 30 to 50 percent of cases, people have an upper respiratory

This chapter includes text excerpted from "Henoch-Schönlein Purpura (HSP)," National Institute of Diabetes and Digestive and Kidney Diseases (NIDDK), September 2012. Reviewed October 2016.

tract infection, such as a cold, before getting HSP. HSP has also been associated with

- infectious agents such as chickenpox, measles, hepatitis, and HIV viruses

- medications

- foods

- insect bites

- exposure to cold weather

- trauma

Genetics may increase the risk of HSP, as it has occurred in different members of the same family, including in twins.

What Are the Symptoms of HSP?

The symptoms of HSP include the following:

- **Rash.** Leaking blood vessels in the skin cause a rash that looks like bruises or small red dots on the legs, arms, and buttocks. The rash may first look like hives and then change to look like bruises, and it may spread to the chest, back, and face. The rash does not disappear or turn pale when pressed.

- **Digestive tract problems.** HSP can cause vomiting and abdominal pain, which can range from mild to severe. Blood may also appear in the stool, though severe bleeding is rare.

- **Arthritis.** Pain and swelling can occur in the joints, usually in the knees and ankles and less frequently in the elbows and wrists.

- **Kidney involvement.** Hematuria—blood in the urine—is a common sign that HSP has affected the kidneys. Proteinuria—large amounts of protein in the urine—or development of high blood pressure suggests more severe kidney problems.

- **Other symptoms.** In some cases, boys with HSP develop swelling of the testicles. Symptoms affecting the central nervous system, such as seizures, and lungs, such as pneumonia, have been seen in rare cases.

Though the rash affects all people with HSP, pain in the joints or abdomen precedes the rash in about one-third of cases by as many as 14 days.

What Are the Complications of HSP?

In children, the risk of kidney damage leading to long-term problems may be as high as 15 percent, but kidney failure affects only about 1 percent of children with HSP. Up to 40 percent of adults with HSP will have CKD or kidney failure within 15 years after diagnosis.

A rare complication of HSP is intussusception of the bowel, which includes the small and large intestines. With this condition, a section of the bowel folds into itself like a telescope, causing the bowel to become blocked.

Women with a history of HSP who become pregnant are at higher risk for high blood pressure and proteinuria during pregnancy.

How Is HSP Diagnosed?

A diagnosis of HSP is suspected when a person has the characteristic rash and one of the following:

- abdominal pain

- joint pain

- antibody deposits on the skin

- hematuria or proteinuria

Antibody deposits on the skin can confirm the diagnosis of HSP. These deposits can be detected using a skin biopsy, a procedure that involves taking a piece of skin tissue for examination with a microscope. A skin biopsy is performed by a healthcare provider in a hospital with little or no sedation and local anesthetic. The skin tissue is examined in a lab by a pathologist—a doctor who specializes in diagnosing diseases.

A kidney biopsy may also be needed. A kidney biopsy is performed by a healthcare provider in a hospital with light sedation and local anesthetic. The healthcare provider uses imaging techniques such as ultrasound or a computerized tomography scan to guide the biopsy needle into the organ. The kidney tissue is examined in a lab by a pathologist. The test can confirm diagnosis and be used to determine the extent of kidney involvement, which will help guide treatment decisions.

Hematuria and proteinuria are detected using urinalysis, which is testing of a urine sample. The urine sample is collected in a special container in a healthcare provider's office or commercial facility and can be tested in the same location or sent to a lab for analysis. For the test, a nurse or technician places a strip of chemically treated paper, called a dipstick, into the urine sample. Patches on the dipstick change color when blood or protein are present in urine.

How Is HSP Treated?

No specific treatment for HSP exists. The main goal of treatment is to relieve symptoms such as joint pain, abdominal pain, and swelling. People with kidney involvement may receive treatment aimed at preventing long-term kidney disease.

Treatment is rarely required for the rash. Joint pain is often treated with nonsteroidal anti-inflammatory medications, such as aspirin or ibuprofen. Recent research has shown corticosteroids—medications that decrease swelling and reduce the activity of the immune system—to be even more effective in treating joint pain. Corticosteroids are also used to treat abdominal pain.

Though rare, surgery may be needed to treat intussusception or to determine the cause of swollen testicles.

HSP that affects the kidneys may be treated with corticosteroid and immunosuppressive medications. Immunosuppressive medications prevent the body from making antibodies. Adults with severe, acute kidney failure are treated with high-dose corticosteroids and the immunosuppressive cyclophosphamide (Cytoxan).

People with HSP that is causing high blood pressure may need to take medications that—when taken as prescribed by their healthcare provider—lower their blood pressure and can also significantly slow the progression of kidney disease. Two types of blood pressure lowering medications, angiotensin-converting enzyme (ACE) inhibitors and angiotensin receptor blockers (ARBs), have proven effective in slowing the progression of kidney disease. Many people require two or more medications to control their blood pressure. In addition to an ACE inhibitor or an ARB, a diuretic—a medication that helps the kidneys remove fluid from the blood—may be prescribed. Beta blockers, calcium channel blockers, and other blood pressure medications may also be needed.

Blood and urine tests are used to check the kidney function of people with HSP for at least 6 months after the main symptoms disappear.

Eating, Diet, and Nutrition

Eating, diet, and nutrition have not been shown to play a role in causing or preventing HSP.

Chapter 53

Immune Thrombocytopenia

What Is Immune Thrombocytopenia?

Immune thrombocytopenia, or ITP, is a bleeding disorder. In ITP, the blood doesn't clot as it should. This is due to a low number of blood cell fragments called platelets or thrombocytes.

Platelets are made in your bone marrow along with other kinds of blood cells. They stick together (clot) to seal small cuts or breaks on blood vessel walls and stop bleeding.

Types of Immune Thrombocytopenia

The two types of ITP are acute (temporary or short-term) and chronic (long-lasting).

Acute ITP generally lasts less than 6 months. It mainly occurs in children—both boys and girls—and is the most common type of ITP. Acute ITP often occurs after a viral infection.

Chronic ITP lasts 6 months or longer and mostly affects adults. However, some teenagers and children do get this type of ITP. Chronic ITP affects women two to three times more often than men.

Treatment depends on the severity of bleeding and the platelet count. In mild cases, treatment may not be needed.

This chapter includes text excerpted from "Immune Thrombocytopenia," National Heart, Lung, and Blood Institute (NHLBI), March 14, 2012. Reviewed October 2016.

Other Names for Immune Thrombocytopenia

- Idiopathic thrombocytopenic purpura

- Immune thrombocytopenic purpura

- Autoimmune thrombocytopenic purpura

What Causes Immune Thrombocytopenia?

In most cases, an autoimmune response is thought to cause immune thrombocytopenia (ITP).

Normally, your immune system helps your body fight off infections and diseases. In ITP, however, your immune system attacks and destroys your body's platelets by mistake. Why this happens isn't known.

In some people, ITP may be linked to viral or bacterial infections, such as HIV, hepatitis C, or *H. pylori*.

Children who have acute (short-term) ITP often have had recent viral infections. These infections may "trigger" or set off the immune reaction that leads to ITP.

Who Is at Risk for Immune Thrombocytopenia?

Immune thrombocytopenia (ITP) is a fairly common blood disorder. Both children and adults can develop ITP.

Children usually have the acute (short-term) type of ITP. Acute ITP often develops after a viral infection.

Adults tend to have the chronic (long-lasting) type of ITP. Women are two to three times more likely than men to develop chronic ITP.

The number of cases of ITP is rising because routine blood tests that can detect a low platelet count are being done more often.

ITP can't be passed from one person to another.

What Are the Signs and Symptoms of Immune Thrombocytopenia?

Immune thrombocytopenia (ITP) may not cause any signs or symptoms. However, ITP can cause bleeding inside the body (internal bleeding) or underneath or from the skin (external bleeding). Signs of bleeding may include:

- Bruising or purplish areas on the skin or mucous membranes (such as in the mouth). These bruises are called purpura.

They're caused by bleeding under the skin, and they may occur for no known reason.

- Pinpoint red spots on the skin called petechiae. These spots often are found in groups and may look like a rash. Bleeding under the skin causes petechiae.

- A collection of clotted or partially clotted blood under the skin that looks or feels like a lump. This is called a hematoma.

- Nosebleeds or bleeding from the gums (for example, during dental work).

- Blood in the urine or stool (bowel movement).

Any kind of bleeding that's hard to stop could be a sign of ITP. This includes menstrual bleeding that's heavier than normal. Bleeding in the brain is rare, and its symptoms may vary.

A low platelet count doesn't directly cause pain, problems concentrating, or other symptoms. However, a low platelet count might be associated with fatigue (tiredness).

How Is Immune Thrombocytopenia Diagnosed?

Your doctor will diagnose immune thrombocytopenia (ITP) based on your medical history, a physical exam, and test results.

Your doctor will want to make sure that your low platelet count isn't due to another condition (such as an infection) or medicines you're taking (such as chemotherapy medicines or aspirin).

Medical History

Your doctor may ask about:

- Your signs and symptoms of bleeding and any other signs or symptoms you're having

- Whether you have illnesses that could lower your platelet count or cause bleeding

- Medicines or any over-the-counter supplements or remedies you take that could cause bleeding or lower your platelet count

Physical Exam

During a physical exam, your doctor will look for signs of bleeding and infection. For example, your doctor may look for purplish areas on the skin or mucous membranes and pinpoint red spots on the skin. These are signs of bleeding under the skin.

Diagnostic Tests

You'll likely have blood tests to check your platelet count. These tests usually include:

- A complete blood count. This test checks the number of red blood cells, white blood cells, and platelets in your blood. In ITP, the red and white blood cell counts are normal, but the platelet count is low.

- A blood smear. For this test, some of your blood is put on a slide. A microscope is used to look at your platelets and other blood cells.

You also may have a blood test to check for the antibodies (proteins) that attack platelets.

If blood tests show that your platelet count is low, your doctor may recommend more tests to confirm a diagnosis of ITP. For example, bone marrow tests can show whether your bone marrow is making enough platelets.

If you're at risk for HIV, hepatitis C, or *H. pylori*, your doctor may screen you for these infections, which might be linked to ITP.

Some people who have mild ITP have few or no signs of bleeding. They may be diagnosed only if a blood test done for another reason shows that they have low platelet counts.

How Is Immune Thrombocytopenia Treated?

Treatment for immune thrombocytopenia (ITP) is based on how much and how often you're bleeding and your platelet count.

Adults who have mild ITP may not need any treatment, other than watching their symptoms and platelet counts. Adults who have ITP with very low platelet counts or bleeding problems often are treated.

The acute (short-term) type of ITP that occurs in children often goes away within a few weeks or months. Children who have bleeding symptoms, other than merely bruising (purpura), usually are treated.

Children who have mild ITP may not need treatment other than monitoring and follow up to make sure their platelet counts return to normal.

How Can Immune Thrombocytopenia Be Prevented?

You can't prevent immune thrombocytopenia (ITP), but you can prevent its complications.

- Talk with your doctor about which medicines are safe for you. Your doctor may advise you to avoid medicines that can affect your platelets and increase your risk of bleeding. Examples of such medicines include aspirin and ibuprofen.

- Protect yourself from injuries that can cause bruising or bleeding.

- Seek treatment right away if you develop any infections. Report any symptoms of infection, such as a fever, to your doctor. This is very important for people who have ITP and have had their spleens removed.

Chapter 54

Inflammatory Bowel Disease

Chapter Contents

Section 54.1

Crohn's Disease

This section includes text excerpted from "Crohn's Disease,"
National Institute of Diabetes and Digestive and Kidney
Diseases (NIDDK), July 2016.

Definition and Facts for Crohn's Disease

What Is Crohn's Disease?

Crohn's disease is a chronic disease that causes inflammation and irritation in your digestive tract. Most commonly, Crohn's affects your small intestine and the beginning of your large intestine. However, the disease can affect any part of your digestive tract, from your mouth to your anus.

Crohn's disease is an inflammatory bowel disease (IBD). Ulcerative colitis and microscopic colitis are other common types of IBD.

Crohn's disease most often begins gradually and can become worse over time. You may have periods of remission that can last for weeks or years.

How Common Is Crohn's Disease?

Researchers estimate that more than half a million people in the United States have Crohn's disease. Studies show that, over time, Crohn's disease has become more common in the United States and other parts of the world. Experts do not know the reason for this increase.

Who Is More Likely to Develop Crohn's Disease?

Crohn's disease can develop in people of any age and is more likely to develop in people

- between the ages of 20 and 29

- who have a family member, most often a sibling or parent, with IBD

- who smoke cigarettes

What Are the Complications of Crohn's Disease?

Complications of Crohn's disease can include the following:

- **Intestinal obstruction.** Crohn's disease can thicken the wall of your intestines. Over time, the thickened areas of your intestines can narrow, which can block your intestines. A partial or complete intestinal obstruction, also called a bowel blockage, can block the movement of food or stool through your intestines.

- **Fistulas.** In Crohn's disease, inflammation can go through the wall of your intestines and create tunnels, or fistulas. Fistulas are abnormal passages between two organs, or between an organ and the outside of your body. Fistulas may become infected.

- **Abscesses.** Inflammation that goes through the wall of your intestines can also lead to abscesses. Abscesses are painful, swollen, pus-filled pockets of infection.

- **Anal fissures.** Anal fissures are small tears in your anus that may cause itching, pain, or bleeding.

- **Ulcers.** Inflammation anywhere along your digestive tract can lead to ulcers or open sores in your mouth, intestines, anus, or perineum.

- **Malnutrition.** Malnutrition develops when your body does not get the right amount of vitamins, minerals, and nutrients it needs to maintain healthy tissues and organ function.

- **Inflammation in other areas of your body.** You may have inflammation in your joints, eyes, and skin.

Symptoms and Causes of Crohn's Disease

What Are the Symptoms of Crohn's Disease?

The most common symptoms of Crohn's disease are

- diarrhea
- cramping and pain in your abdomen
- weight loss

Other symptoms include

- anemia
- eye redness or pain

- feeling tired
- fever
- joint pain or soreness
- nausea or loss of appetite
- skin changes that involve red, tender bumps under the skin

Your symptoms may vary depending on the location and severity of your inflammation.

Some research suggests that stress, including the stress of living with Crohn's disease, can make symptoms worse. Also, some people may find that certain foods can trigger or worsen their symptoms.

Diagnosis of Crohn's Disease

Doctors typically use a combination of tests to diagnose Crohn's disease. Your doctor will also ask you about your medical history— including medicines you are taking—and your family history and will perform a physical exam.

Treatment for Crohn's Disease

Doctors treat Crohn's disease with medicines, bowel rest, and surgery.

No single treatment works for everyone with Crohn's disease. The goals of treatment are to decrease the inflammation in your intestines, to prevent flare-ups of your symptoms, and to keep you in remission.

Section 54.2

Ulcerative Colitis

This section includes text excerpted from "Ulcerative Colitis," National Institute of Diabetes and Digestive and Kidney Diseases (NIDDK), September 2014.

What Is Ulcerative Colitis?

Ulcerative colitis is a chronic, or long lasting, disease that causes inflammation—irritation or swelling—and sores called ulcers on the inner lining of the large intestine.

Ulcerative colitis is a chronic inflammatory disease of the gastrointestinal (GI) tract, called inflammatory bowel disease (IBD). Crohn's disease and microscopic colitis are the other common IBDs.

Ulcerative colitis most often begins gradually and can become worse over time. Symptoms can be mild to severe. Most people have periods of remission—times when symptoms disappear—that can last for weeks or years. The goal of care is to keep people in remission long term.

Most people with ulcerative colitis receive care from a gastroenterologist, a doctor who specializes in digestive diseases.

What Is the Large Intestine?

The large intestine is part of the GI tract, a series of hollow organs joined in a long, twisting tube from the mouth to the anus—an opening through which stool leaves the body. The last part of the GI tract, called the lower GI tract, consists of the large intestine—which includes the appendix, cecum, colon, and rectum—and anus. The intestines are sometimes called the bowel.

The large intestine is about 5 feet long in adults and absorbs water and any remaining nutrients from partially digested food passed from the small intestine. The large intestine changes waste from liquid to a solid matter called stool. Stool passes from the colon to the rectum. The rectum is located between the lower, or sigmoid, colon and the anus. The rectum stores stool prior to a bowel movement, when stool moves from the rectum to the anus and out of a person's body.

What Causes Ulcerative Colitis?

The exact cause of ulcerative colitis is unknown. Researchers believe the following factors may play a role in causing ulcerative colitis:

- overactive intestinal immune system
- genes
- environment

Overactive intestinal immune system. Scientists believe one cause of ulcerative colitis may be an abnormal immune reaction in the intestine. Normally, the immune system protects the body from infection by identifying and destroying bacteria, viruses, and other potentially harmful foreign substances. Researchers believe bacteria or viruses can mistakenly trigger the immune system to attack the inner lining of the large intestine. This immune system response causes the inflammation, leading to symptoms.

Genes. Ulcerative colitis sometimes runs in families. Research studies have shown that certain abnormal genes may appear in people with ulcerative colitis. However, researchers have not been able to show a clear link between the abnormal genes and ulcerative colitis.

Environment. Some studies suggest that certain things in the environment may increase the chance of a person getting ulcerative colitis, although the overall chance is low. Nonsteroidal anti-inflammatory drugs (NSAIDs), antibiotics, and oral contraceptives may slightly increase the chance of developing ulcerative colitis. A high-fat diet may also slightly increase the chance of getting ulcerative colitis.

Some people believe eating certain foods, stress, or emotional distress can cause ulcerative colitis. Emotional distress does not seem to cause ulcerative colitis. A few studies suggest that stress may increase a person's chance of having a flare-up of ulcerative colitis. Also, some people may find that certain foods can trigger or worsen symptoms.

Who Is More Likely to Develop Ulcerative Colitis?

Ulcerative colitis can occur in people of any age. However, it is more likely to develop in people

- between the ages of 15 and 30
- older than 60
- who have a family member with IBD
- of Jewish descent

What Are the Signs and Symptoms of Ulcerative Colitis?

The most common signs and symptoms of ulcerative colitis are diarrhea with blood or pus and abdominal discomfort. Other signs and symptoms include

- an urgent need to have a bowel movement

- feeling tired

- nausea or loss of appetite

- weight loss

- fever

- anemia—a condition in which the body has fewer red blood cells than normal

  Less common symptoms include

- joint pain or soreness

- eye irritation

- certain rashes

The symptoms a person experiences can vary depending on the severity of the inflammation and where it occurs in the intestine. When symptoms first appear,

- most people with ulcerative colitis have mild to moderate symptoms

- about 10 percent of people can have severe symptoms, such as frequent, bloody bowel movements; fevers; and severe abdominal cramping

How Is Ulcerative Colitis Diagnosed?

A healthcare provider diagnoses ulcerative colitis with the following:

- medical and family history

- physical exam

- lab tests

- endoscopies of the large intestine

The healthcare provider may perform a series of medical tests to rule out other bowel disorders, such as irritable bowel syndrome, Crohn's disease, or celiac disease, that may cause symptoms similar to those of ulcerative colitis.

Medical and Family History

Taking a medical and family history can help the healthcare provider diagnose ulcerative colitis and understand a patient's symptoms. The healthcare provider will also ask the patient about current and past medical conditions and medications.

Physical Exam

A physical exam may help diagnose ulcerative colitis. During a physical exam, the healthcare provider most often

- checks for abdominal distension, or swelling
- listens to sounds within the abdomen using a stethoscope
- taps on the abdomen to check for tenderness and pain

Lab Tests

A healthcare provider may order lab tests to help diagnose ulcerative colitis, including blood and stool tests.

Blood tests. A blood test involves drawing blood at a healthcare provider's office or a lab. A lab technologist will analyze the blood sample. A healthcare provider may use blood tests to look for

- anemia
- inflammation or infection somewhere in the body
- markers that show ongoing inflammation
- low albumin, or protein—common in patients with severe ulcerative colitis

Stool tests. A stool test is the analysis of a sample of stool. A healthcare provider will give the patient a container for catching and storing the stool at home. The patient returns the sample to the healthcare provider or to a lab. A lab technologist will analyze the stool sample. Healthcare providers commonly order stool tests to rule out other causes of GI diseases, such as infection.

Endoscopies of the Large Intestine

Endoscopies of the large intestine are the most accurate methods for diagnosing ulcerative colitis and ruling out other possible conditions, such as Crohn's disease, diverticular disease, or cancer. Endoscopies of the large intestine include

- colonoscopy
- flexible sigmoidoscopy

Colonoscopy. Colonoscopy is a test that uses a long, flexible, narrow tube with a light and tiny camera on one end, called a colonoscope or scope, to look inside the rectum and entire colon. In most cases, light anesthesia and pain medication help patients relax for the test. The medical staff will monitor a patient's vital signs and try to make him or her as comfortable as possible. A nurse or technician places an intravenous (IV) needle in a vein in the patient's arm or hand to give anesthesia.

For the test, the patient will lie on a table or stretcher while the gastroenterologist inserts a colonoscope into the patient's anus and slowly guides it through the rectum and into the colon. The scope inflates the large intestine with air to give the gastroenterologist a better view. The camera sends a video image of the intestinal lining to a monitor, allowing the gastroenterologist to carefully examine the tissues lining the colon and rectum. The gastroenterologist may move the patient several times and adjust the scope for better viewing. Once the scope has reached the opening to the small intestine, the gastroenterologist slowly withdraws it and examines the lining of the colon and rectum again.

A colonoscopy can show irritated and swollen tissue, ulcers, and abnormal growths such as polyps—extra pieces of tissue that grow on the inner lining of the intestine. If the gastroenterologist suspects ulcerative colitis, he or she will biopsy the patient's colon and rectum. A biopsy is a procedure that involves taking small pieces of tissue for examination with a microscope.

A healthcare provider will give patients written bowel prep instructions to follow at home before the test. The healthcare provider will also give patients information about how to care for themselves following the procedure.

Flexible sigmoidoscopy. Flexible sigmoidoscopy is a test that uses a flexible, narrow tube with a light and tiny camera on one end, called a sigmoidoscope or scope, to look inside the rectum, the sigmoid colon, and sometimes the descending colon. In most cases, a patient does not need anesthesia.

For the test, the patient will lie on a table or stretcher while the healthcare provider inserts the sigmoidoscope into the patient's anus and slowly guides it through the rectum, the sigmoid colon, and sometimes the descending colon. The scope inflates the large intestine with air to give the healthcare provider a better view. The camera sends a video image of the intestinal lining to a monitor, allowing the healthcare provider to examine the tissues lining the sigmoid colon and rectum. The healthcare provider may ask the patient to move several times and adjust the scope for better viewing. Once the scope reaches the end of the sigmoid colon, the healthcare provider slowly withdraws it while examining the lining of the colon and rectum again.

The healthcare provider will look for signs of bowel diseases and conditions such as irritated and swollen tissue, ulcers, and polyps.

If the healthcare provider suspects ulcerative colitis, he or she will biopsy the patient's colon and rectum.

A healthcare provider will give patients written bowel prep instructions to follow at home before the test. The healthcare provider will also give patients information about how to care for themselves following the procedure.

How Is Ulcerative Colitis Treated?

A healthcare provider treats ulcerative colitis with

- medications

- surgery

Which treatment a person needs depends on the severity of the disease and the symptoms. Each person experiences ulcerative colitis differently, so healthcare providers adjust treatments to improve the person's symptoms and induce, or bring about, remission.

What Are the Complications of Ulcerative Colitis?

Complications of ulcerative colitis can include

- **rectal bleeding**—when ulcers in the intestinal lining open and bleed. Rectal bleeding can cause anemia, which healthcare providers can treat with diet changes and iron supplements. People who have a large amount of bleeding in the intestine over a short period of time may require surgery to stop the bleeding. Severe bleeding is a rare complication of ulcerative colitis.

- **dehydration and malabsorbtion,** which occur when the large intestine is unable to absorb fluids and nutrients because of diarrhea and inflammation. Some people may need IV fluids to replace lost nutrients and fluids.

- **changes in bones.** Some corticosteroid medications taken to treat ulcerative colitis symptoms can cause

  - osteoporosis—the loss of bone

  - osteopenia—low bone density

Healthcare providers will monitor people for bone loss and can recommend calcium and vitamin D supplements and medications to help prevent or slow bone loss.

- **inflammation in other areas of the body.** The immune system can trigger inflammation in the

  - joints

  - eyes

  - skin

  - liver

Healthcare providers can treat inflammation by adjusting medications or prescribing new medications.

- **megacolon**—a serious complication that occurs when inflammation spreads to the deep tissue layers of the large intestine. The large intestine swells and stops working. Megacolon can be a life-threatening complication and most often requires surgery. Megacolon is a rare complication of ulcerative colitis.

Points to Remember

- Ulcerative colitis is a chronic, or long lasting, disease that causes inflammation—irritation or swelling—and sores called ulcers on the inner lining of the large intestine.

- The exact cause of ulcerative colitis is unknown. Researchers believe that factors such as an overactive intestinal immune system, genes, and environment may play a role in causing ulcerative colitis.

315

- Ulcerative colitis can occur in people of any age. However, it is more likely to develop in people

  - between the ages of 15 and 30

  - older than 60

  - who have a family member with inflammatory bowel disease (IBD)

  - of Jewish descent

- The most common signs and symptoms of ulcerative colitis are diarrhea with blood or pus and abdominal discomfort.

- A health care provider diagnoses ulcerative colitis with the following:

  - medical and family history

  - physical exam

  - lab tests

  - endoscopies of the large intestine

- Which treatment a person needs depends on the severity of the disease and symptoms.

- Good nutrition is important in the management of ulcerative colitis. A health care provider may recommend that a person make dietary changes.

- People with ulcerative colitis should talk with their health care provider about how often they should get screened for colon cancer.

Chapter 55

Inflammatory Myopathies

Chapter Contents

Section 55.1

Inflammatory Myopathies Explained

This section includes text excerpted from "Inflammatory
Myopathies Fact Sheet," National Institute of Neurological
Disorders and Stroke (NINDS), July 27, 2015.

What Are the Inflammatory Myopathies?

Myopathy is a term used to describe muscle disease. The *inflammatory myopathies* are a group of diseases that involve chronic muscle inflammation, accompanied by muscle weakness. Another word for chronic inflammation of muscle tissue is *myositis*.

The three main types of chronic, or persistent, inflammatory myopathy are polymyositis, dermatomyositis, and inclusion body myositis (IBM).

What Causes These Disorders?

Muscle inflammation may be caused by an allergic reaction, exposure to a toxic substance or medicine, another disease such as cancer or rheumatic conditions, or a virus or other infectious agent. The chronic inflammatory myopathies are idiopathic, meaning they have no known cause. They are thought to be autoimmune disorders, in which the body's white blood cells (that normally fight disease) attack blood vessels, normal muscle fibers, and connective tissue in organs, bones, and joints.

Who Is at Risk?

These rare disorders may affect both adults and children, although dermatomyositis is the most common chronic form in children. Polymyositis and dermatomyositis are more common in women than in men. A rare childhood onset form of polymyositis and dermatomyositis can occur in children between the ages of 2 and 15 years. Inclusion body myositis usually affects individuals over age 50.

What Are the Signs and Symptoms?

General symptoms of chronic inflammatory myopathy include slow but progressive muscle weakness that starts in the proximal muscles—those muscles closest to the trunk of the body. Inflammation damages the muscle fibers, causing weakness, and may affect the arteries and blood vessels that run through the muscle. Other symptoms include fatigue after walking or standing, tripping or falling, and difficulty swallowing or breathing. Some individuals may have slight muscle pain or muscles that are tender to touch.

How Are the Inflammatory Myopathies Diagnosed?

Diagnosis is based on the individual's medical history, results of a physical exam and tests of muscle strength, and blood samples that show elevated levels of various muscle enzymes and autoantibodies. Diagnostic tools include electromyography to record the electrical activity that controls muscles during contraction and at rest, ultrasound to look for muscle inflammation, and magnetic resonance imaging to reveal abnormal muscle and evaluate muscle disease. A muscle biopsy can be examined by microscopy for signs of chronic inflammation, muscle fiber death, vascular deformities, or the changes specific to the diagnosis of IBM. A skin biopsy can show changes in the skin layer in patients with dermatomyositis.

How Are the Inflammatory Myopathies Treated?

The chronic inflammatory myopathies cannot be cured in most adults but many of the symptoms can be treated. Options include medication, physical therapy, exercise, heat therapy (including microwave and ultrasound), orthotics and assistive devices, and rest. Inflammatory myopathies that are caused by medicines, a virus or other infectious agents, or exposure to a toxic substance usually abate when the harmful substance is removed or the infection is treated. If left untreated, inflammatory myopathy can cause permanent disability.

Polymyositis and dermatomyositis are first treated with high doses of corticosteroid drug. This is most often given as an oral medication but can be delivered intravenously. Immunosuppressant drugs, such as azathioprine and methotrexate, may reduce inflammation in individuals who do not respond well to prednisone. Periodic treatment using intravenous immunoglobulin can increase the chance for recovery in individuals with dermatomyositis or polymyositis. Other immuno-suppressive agents that may treat the inflammation associated with dermatomyositis and polymyositis include cyclosporine A, cyclophosphamide, and tacrolimus. Physical therapy is usually recommended to prevent muscle atrophy and to regain muscle strength and range of motion. Bed rest for an extended period of time should be avoided, as people may develop muscle atrophy, decreased muscle function, and joint contractures. A low-sodium diet may help to counter edema and cardiovascular complications.

Many individuals with dermatomyositis may need a topical ointment (such as topical corticosteroids or tacrolimus or pimecrolimus) or additional treatment for their skin disorder. A high-protection sunscreen and protective clothing should be worn by all affected individuals, particularly those who are sensitive to light. Surgery may be required to remove calcium deposits that cause nerve pain and recurrent infections.

There is no standard course of treatment for IBM. The disease is generally unresponsive to corticosteroids and immunosuppressive drugs. Some evidence suggests that immunosuppressive medications or intravenous immunoglobulin may have a slight, but short-lasting, beneficial effect in a small number of cases. Physical therapy may be helpful in maintaining mobility. Other therapy is symptomatic and supportive.

What Is the Prognosis for the Inflammatory Myopathies?

Most cases of dermatomyositis respond to therapy. The disease is usually more severe and resistant to therapy in individuals with cardiac or pulmonary problems.

The prognosis for polymyositis varies. Most individuals respond fairly well to therapy, but some patients have a more severe disease that does not respond adequately to therapies and are left with significant disability. In rare cases people with severe and progressive muscle weakness can have respiratory failure or pneumonia. Difficulty swallowing can lead to becoming malnourished. Falls leading to fractures (particularly of the hip) should be guarded against because of the high rate of disability or death that can result.

IBM is generally resistant to all therapies and its rate of progression appears to be unaffected by currently available treatments.

Approximately one-third of individuals with juvenile-onset dermatomyositis recover from their illness, one-third have a relapsing-remitting course of disease, and the other third have a more chronic course of illness.

Section 55.2

Dermatomyositis

This section includes text excerpted from "Dermatomyositis," Genetic and Rare Diseases Information Center (GARD), National Center for Advancing Translational Sciences (NCATS) August 26, 2013.

What Is Dermatomyositis?

Dermatomyositis is one of a group of acquired muscle diseases called inflammatory myopathies (disorder of muscle tissue or muscles), which are characterized by chronic muscle inflammation accompanied by muscle weakness. The cardinal symptom is a skin rash that precedes or accompanies progressive muscle weakness. Dermatomyositis may occur at any age, but is most common in adults in their late 40s to early 60s, or children between 5 and 15 years of age. There is no cure for dermatomyositis, but the symptoms can be treated. Options include medication, physical therapy, exercise, heat therapy (including microwave and ultrasound), orthotics and assistive devices, and rest. The cause of dermatomyositis is unknown.

Symptoms

The signs and symptoms of dermatomyositis may appear suddenly or develop gradually, over weeks or months. The cardinal symptom of dermatomyositis is a skin rash that precedes or accompanies progressive muscle weakness. The rash looks patchy, with bluish-purple or red discolorations, and characteristically develops on the eyelids and on muscles used to extend or straighten joints, including knuckles, elbows, heels, and toes. Red rashes may also occur on the face, neck, shoulders, upper chest, back, and other locations, and there may be swelling in the affected areas. The rash sometimes occurs without obvious muscle involvement.

Adults with dermatomyositis may experience weight loss or a low-grade fever, have inflamed lungs, and be sensitive to light. Children and adults with dermatomyositis may develop calcium deposits, which appear as hard bumps under the skin or in the muscle (called calcinosis). Calcinosis most often occurs 1–3 years after the disease begins.

These deposits are seen more often in children with dermatomyositis than in adults. In some cases of dermatomyositis, distal muscles (muscles located away from the trunk of the body, such as those in the forearms and around the ankles and wrists) may be affected as the disease progresses. Dermatomyositis may be associated with collagen-vascular or autoimmune diseases, such as lupus.

Signs and Symptoms

- Abnormality of the eye
- Autoimmunity
- EMG abnormality
- Muscle weakness
- Myalgia
- Periorbital edema
- Abnormal hair quantity
- Abnormality of the nail
- Acrocyanosis
- Arthralgia
- Arthritis
- Chondrocalcinosis
- Dry skin
- Muscular hypotonia
- Poikiloderma
- Pruritus
- Pulmonary fibrosis
- Recurrent respiratory infections
- Respiratory insufficiency
- Restrictive ventilatory defect
- Skin ulcer
- Weight loss

- Abnormality of eosinophils
- Abnormality of temperature regulation
- Abnormality of the myocardium
- Abnormality of the pericardium
- Abnormality of the voice
- Aplasia/Hypoplasia of the skin
- Arrhythmia
- Cellulitis
- Coronary artery disease
- Cutaneous photosensitivity
- Feeding difficulties in infancy
- Gangrene
- Gastrointestinal stroma tumor
- Lymphoma
- Neoplasm of the breast
- Neoplasm of the lung
- Neurological speech impairment
- Ovarian neoplasm

- Pulmonary hypertension
- Telangiectasia of the skin
- Vasculitis

Cause

The cause of this disorder is unknown. It is theorized that an auto-immune reaction (reactions caused by an immune response against the body's own tissues) or a viral infection of the skeletal muscle may cause the disease. In addition, some doctors think certain people may have a genetic susceptibility to the disease.

Treatment

While there is no cure for dermatomyositis, the symptoms can be treated. Options include medication, physical therapy, exercise, heat therapy (including microwave and ultrasound), orthotics and assistive devices, and rest. The standard treatment for dermatomyositis is a corticosteroid drug, given either in pill form or intravenously. Immunosuppressant drugs, such as azathioprine and methotrexate, may reduce inflammation in people who do not respond well to predni-sone. Periodic treatment using intravenous immunoglobulin can also improve recovery. Other immunosuppressive agents used to treat the inflammation associated with dermatomyositis include cyclosporine A, cyclophosphamide, and tacrolimus. Physical therapy is usually recom-mended to prevent muscle atrophy and to regain muscle strength and range of motion. Many individuals with dermatomyositis may need a topical ointment, such as topical corticosteroids, for their skin disorder. They should wear a high-protection sunscreen and protective clothing. Surgery may be required to remove calcium deposits that cause nerve pain and recurrent infections.

Prognosis

Most cases of dermatomyositis respond to therapy. Some people may recover and have symptoms completely disappear. This is more common in children. In adults, death may result from severe and pro-longed muscle weakness, malnutrition, pneumonia, or lung failure. The outcome is usually worse if the heart or lungs are involved.

Section 55.3

Inclusion-Body Myositis

This section includes text excerpted from "Inclusion Body Myositis," National Institute of Neurological Disorders and Stroke (NINDS), July 27, 2015.

What Is Inclusion Body Myositis?

Inclusion body myositis (IBM) is one of a group of muscle diseases known as the inflammatory myopathies, which are characterized by chronic, progressive muscle inflammation accompanied by muscle weakness. The onset of muscle weakness in IBM is generally gradual (over months or years) and affects both proximal (close to the trunk of the body) and distal (further away from the trunk) muscles. Muscle weakness may affect only one side of the body. Falling and tripping are usually the first noticeable symptoms of IBM. For some individuals, the disorder begins with weakness in the wrists and fingers that causes difficulty with pinching, buttoning, and gripping objects. There may be weakness of the wrist and finger muscles and atrophy (thinning or loss of muscle bulk) of the forearm muscles and quadricep muscles in the legs. Difficulty swallowing occurs in approximately half of IBM cases. Symptoms of the disease usually begin after the age of 50, although the disease can occur earlier. IBM occurs more frequently in men than in women.

Is There Any Treatment?

There is no cure for IBM, nor is there a standard course of treatment. The disease is generally unresponsive to corticosteroids and immunosuppressive drugs. Some evidence suggests that intravenous immunoglobulin may have a slight, but short-lasting, beneficial effect in a small number of cases. Physical therapy may be helpful in maintaining mobility. Other therapy is symptomatic and supportive.

What Is the Prognosis?

IBM is generally resistant to all therapies and its rate of progression appears to be unaffected by currently available treatments.

Section 55.4

Polymyositis

This section includes text excerpted from "Polymyositis," Genetic and Rare Diseases Information Center (GARD), National Center for Advancing Translational Sciences (NCATS), September 9, 2015.

What Is Polymyositis?

Polymyositis is a type of inflammatory myopathy, which refers to a group of muscle diseases characterized by chronic muscle inflammation and weakness. It involves skeletal muscles (those involved with making movement) on both sides of the body. Although it can affect people of all ages, most cases are seen in adults between the ages of 31 and 60. The exact cause of polymyositis is unknown; however, the disease shares many characteristics with autoimmune disorders which occur when the immune system mistakenly attacks healthy body tissues. It some cases, the condition may be associated with viral infections, malignancies, or connective tissue disorders. Although there is no cure for polymyositis, treatment can improve muscle strength and function.

Symptoms

Polymyositis is characterized by chronic muscle inflammation and weakness involving the skeletal muscles (those involved with making movement) on both sides of the body. Weakness generally starts in the proximal muscles which can eventually cause difficulties climbing stairs, rising from a sitting position, lifting objects, or reaching overhead. In some cases, distal muscles may also be affected as the disease progresses.

Other symptoms may include arthritis; shortness of breath; difficulty swallowing and speaking; mild joint or muscle tenderness; fatigue, and heart arrhythmias.

Diagnosis

A diagnosis of polymyositis is often suspected in people with proximal muscle weakness and other associated signs and symptoms.

Additional testing can then be ordered to confirm the diagnosis and rule out other conditions that may cause similar features. This testing may include:

- Blood tests to measure the levels of certain muscle enzymes (i.e., creatine kinase and aldolase) and detect specific autoantibodies associated with different symptoms of polymyositis

- Electromyography to check the health of the muscles and the nerves that control them

- Imaging studies such as an MRI scan to detect muscle inflammation

- A muscle biopsy to diagnose muscle abnormalities such as inflammation, damage and/or infection

Treatment

The treatment of polymyositis is based on the signs and symptoms present in each person. Although there is currently no cure, symptoms of the condition may be managed with the following:

- Medications such as corticosteroids, corticosteroid-sparing agents, immunosuppressive drugs

- Physical therapy to improve muscle strength and flexibility

- Speech therapy to address difficulties with swallowing and speech

- Intravenous immunoglobulin (healthy antibodies are given to block damaging autoantibodies that attack muscle)

Prognosis

The long-term outlook (prognosis) for people with polymyositis varies. Most affected people respond well to treatment and regain muscle strength, although a certain degree of muscle weakness may persist in some cases. If the treatment is not effective, people may develop significant disability.

In rare cases, people with severe and progressive muscle weakness will develop respiratory failure or pneumonia. Difficulty swallowing may cause weight loss and malnutrition.

Chapter 56

Lambert-Eaton Myasthenic Syndrome (LEMS)

What Is Lambert Eaton Myasthenic Syndrome (LEMS)?

Lambert Eaton myasthenic syndrome (LEMS) is a disorder of the neuromuscular junction. The neuromuscular junction is the site where nerve cells meet muscle cells and help activate the muscles. This syndrome occurs when antibodies interfere with electrical impulses between the nerve and muscle cells. It may be associated with other autoimmune diseases, or more commonly coincide with or precede a diagnosis of cancer such as small cell lung cancer. Symptoms may include muscle weakness, a tingling sensation in the affected areas, fatigue, and dry mouth. Treatment of a underlying disorder or cancer is the first priority of treatment.

Symptoms

Signs and symptoms of Lambert-Eaton myasthenic syndrome may include:
Weakness or loss of movement that varies in severity:

- difficulty climbing stairs

This chapter includes text excerpted from "Lambert Eaton Myasthenic Syndrome," Genetic and Rare Diseases Information Center (GARD), National Center for Advancing Translational Sciences (NCATS), April 22, 2011. Reviewed October 2016.

- difficulty lifting objects
- need to use hands to arise from sitting or lying positions
- difficulty talking
- difficulty chewing
- drooping head
- swallowing difficulty, gagging, or choking

Vision changes:

- blurry vision
- double vision
- difficulty maintaining a steady gaze

Other symptoms may include blood pressure changes, dizziness upon rising, and dry mouth.

Cause

Lambert Eaton myasthenic syndrome is the result of an autoimmune process which causes a disruption of electrical impulses between nerve cells and muscle fibers. In cases where Lambert Eaton myasthenic syndrome appears in association with cancer, the cause may be that the body's attempt to fight the cancer inadvertently causes it to attack nerve fiber endings, especially the voltage-gated calcium channels found there. The trigger for the cases not associated with cancer is unknown.

Treatment

Medications and therapies used to treat Lambert-Eaton myasthenic syndrome may include anticholinesterase agents (e.g., Pyridostigmine), guanidine hydrochloride, plasmapheresis (where blood plasma is removed and replaced with fluid, protein, or donated plasma) or IV immunoglobulins, steroids (e.g., prednisone), azathioprine or cyclosporine, and/or 3,4-diaminopyridine.

3,4-diaminopyridine is available in Europe and may be available in the United States on a compassionate use basis. While there has been some evidence that either 3,4-diaminopyridine or IV immunoglobulin can improve muscle strength and nerve to muscle cell communication, the degree of benefit (i.e., how much symptoms are improved) still needs to be determined.

Prognosis

The prognosis for individuals with LEMS varies. The symptoms of Lambert-Eaton syndrome may improve with treatment of an underlying tumor and/or with suppressing the immune system. However, not all people respond well to treatment.

Chapter 57

Lupus

What Is Lupus?

Lupus is one of many disorders of the immune system known as autoimmune diseases. In autoimmune diseases, the immune system turns against parts of the body it is designed to protect. This leads to inflammation and damage to various body tissues. Lupus can affect many parts of the body, including the joints, skin, kidneys, heart, lungs, blood vessels, and brain.

Typically, lupus is characterized by periods of illness, called flares, and periods of wellness, or remission. Understanding how to prevent flares and how to treat them when they do occur helps people with lupus maintain better health.

Who Gets Lupus?

We know that many more women than men have lupus. Lupus is more common in African American women than in Caucasian women and is also more common in women of Hispanic, Asian, and Native American descent. African American and Hispanic women are also more likely to have active disease and serious organ system involvement. In addition, lupus can run in families, but the risk that a child or a brother or sister of a patient will also have lupus is still quite low.

This chapter includes text excerpted from "Lupus," National Institute of Arthritis and Musculoskeletal and Skin Diseases (NIAMS), June 2016.

It is difficult to estimate how many people in the United States have the disease, because its symptoms vary widely and its onset is often hard to pinpoint. Although Systemic Lupus Erythematosus (SLE) usually first affects people between the ages of 15 and 45 years, it can occur in childhood or later in life as well.

Understanding What Causes Lupus

Lupus is a complex disease, and its cause is not fully understood. Research suggests that genetics plays an important role, but it also shows that genes alone do not determine who gets lupus, and that other factors play a role. Some of the factors scientists are studying include sunlight, stress, hormones, cigarette smoke, certain drugs, and infectious agents such as viruses. Studies have confirmed that one virus, Epstein-Barr virus (EBV), which causes mononucleosis, is a cause of lupus in genetically susceptible people.

Scientists believe there is no single gene that predisposes people to lupus. Rather, studies suggest that a number of different genes may be involved in determining a person's likelihood of developing the disease, which tissues and organs are affected, and the severity of disease.

In lupus, the body's immune system does not work as it should. A healthy immune system produces proteins called antibodies and specific cells called lymphocytes that help fight and destroy viruses, bacteria, and other foreign substances that invade the body. In lupus, the immune system produces antibodies against the body's healthy cells and tissues. These antibodies, called autoantibodies, contribute to the inflammation of various parts of the body and can cause damage to organs and tissues. The most common type of autoantibody that develops in people with lupus is called an antinuclear antibody (ANA) because it reacts with parts of the cell's nucleus (command center). Doctors and scientists do not yet understand all of the factors that cause inflammation and tissue damage in lupus, and researchers are actively exploring them.

Common Symptoms of Lupus

- Painful or swollen joints and muscle pain
- Unexplained fever
- Red rashes, most commonly on the face
- Chest pain upon deep breathing
- Unusual loss of hair

- Pale or purple fingers or toes from cold or stress (Raynaud phenomenon)

- Sensitivity to the sun

- Swelling (edema) in legs or around eyes

- Mouth ulcers

- Swollen glands

- Extreme fatigue

Symptoms of Lupus

Each person with lupus has slightly different symptoms that can range from mild to severe and may come and go over time. However, some of the most common symptoms of lupus include painful or swollen joints (arthritis), unexplained fever, and extreme fatigue. A characteristic red skin rash—the so-called butterfly or malar rash—may appear across the nose and cheeks. Rashes may also occur on the face and ears, upper arms, shoulders, chest, and hands and other areas exposed to the sun. Because many people with lupus are sensitive to sunlight (called photosensitivity), skin rashes often first develop or worsen after sun exposure.

Other symptoms of lupus include chest pain, hair loss, anemia (a decrease in red blood cells), mouth ulcers, and pale or purple fingers and toes from cold and stress. Some people also experience headaches, dizziness, depression, confusion, or seizures. New symptoms may continue to appear years after the initial diagnosis, and different symptoms can occur at different times. In some people with lupus, only one system of the body, such as the skin or joints, is affected. Other people experience symptoms in many parts of their body. Just how seriously a body system is affected varies from person to person. The following systems in the body also can be affected by lupus.

- **Kidneys:** Inflammation of the kidneys (nephritis) can impair their ability to get rid of waste products and other toxins from the body effectively. There is usually no pain associated with kidney involvement. Most often, the only indication of kidney disease is an abnormal urine or blood test; however, some patients may notice dark urine and swelling around their eyes, legs, ankles, or fingers. Because the kidneys are so important to overall health, lupus affecting the kidneys generally requires intensive drug treatment to prevent permanent damage.

- **Lungs:** Some people with lupus develop pleuritis, an inflammation of the lining of the chest cavity that causes chest pain, particularly with breathing. Patients with lupus also may get pneumonia.

- **Central nervous system:** In some patients, lupus affects the brain or central nervous system. This can cause headaches, dizziness, depression, memory disturbances, vision problems, seizures, stroke, or changes in behavior.

- **Blood vessels:** Blood vessels may become inflamed (vasculitis), affecting the way blood circulates through the body. The inflammation may be mild and may not require treatment or may be severe and require immediate attention. People with lupus are also at increased risk for atherosclerosis (hardening of the arteries).

- **Blood:** People with lupus may develop anemia, leukopenia (a decreased number of white blood cells), or thrombocytopenia (a decrease in the number of platelets in the blood, which assist in clotting). People with lupus who have a type of autoantibody called antiphospholipid antibodies have an increased risk of blood clots.

- **Heart:** In some people with lupus, inflammation can occur in the heart itself (myocarditis and endocarditis) or the membrane that surrounds it (pericarditis), causing chest pain or other symptoms. Endocarditis can damage the heart valves, causing the valve surface to thicken and develop growths, which can cause heart murmurs. However, this usually doesn't affect the valves' function.

Diagnosing Lupus

Diagnosing lupus can be difficult. It may take months or even years for doctors to piece together the symptoms to diagnose this complex disease accurately. Making a correct diagnosis of lupus requires knowledge and awareness on the part of the doctor and good communication on the part of the patient. Giving the doctor a complete, accurate medical history (for example, what health problems you have had and for how long) is critical to the process of diagnosis. This information, along with a physical examination and the results of laboratory tests, helps the doctor consider other diseases that may mimic lupus, or determine if you truly have the disease. Reaching a diagnosis may take time as new symptoms appear.

No single test can determine whether a person has lupus, but several laboratory tests may help the doctor to confirm a diagnosis of lupus or rule out other causes for a person's symptoms. The most useful tests identify certain autoantibodies often present in the blood of people with lupus. For example, the antinuclear antibody (ANA) test is commonly used to look for autoantibodies that react against components of the nucleus, or "command center," of the body's cells. Most people with lupus test positive for ANA; however, there are a number of other causes of a positive ANA besides lupus, including infections and other autoimmune diseases. Occasionally, it is also found in healthy people. The ANA test simply provides another clue for the doctor to consider in making a diagnosis. In addition, there are blood tests for individual types of autoantibodies that are more specific to people with lupus, although not all people with lupus test positive for these and not all people with these antibodies have lupus. These antibodies include anti-DNA, anti-Sm, anti-RNP, anti-Ro (SSA), and anti-La (SSB). The doctor may use these antibody tests to help make a diagnosis of lupus.

Some tests are used less frequently but may be helpful if the cause of a person's symptoms remains unclear. The doctor may order a biopsy of the skin or kidneys if those body systems are affected. Some doctors may order a test for anticardiolipin (or antiphospholipid) antibody. The presence of this antibody may indicate increased risk for blood clotting and increased risk for miscarriage in pregnant women with lupus. Again, all these tests merely serve as tools to give the doctor clues and information in making a diagnosis. The doctor will look at the entire picture—medical history, symptoms, and test results—to determine if a person has lupus.

Diagnostic Tools for Lupus

- Medical history
- Complete physical examination
- Laboratory tests:
    - Complete blood count (CBC)
    - Erythrocyte sedimentation rate (ESR)
    - Urinalysis
    - Blood chemistries
    - Complement levels
    - Antinuclear antibody test (ANA)

- Other autoantibody tests (anti-DNA, anti-Sm, anti-RNP, anti-Ro [SSA], antiLa [SSB])
- Anticardiolipin antibody test
- Skin biopsy
- Kidney biopsy

Other laboratory tests are used to monitor the progress of the disease once it has been diagnosed. A complete blood count, urinalysis, blood chemistries, and the erythrocyte sedimentation rate test (a test to measure inflammation) can provide valuable information. Another common test measures the blood level of a group of substances called complement, which help antibodies fight invaders. A low level of complement could mean the substance is being used up because of an immune response in the body, such as that which occurs during a flare of lupus.

Treating Lupus

Diagnosing and treating lupus often require a team effort between the patient and several types of healthcare professionals. Most people will see a rheumatologist for their lupus treatment. A rheumatologist is a doctor who specializes in rheumatic diseases (arthritis and and other inflammatory disorders, often involving the immune system). Clinical immunologists (doctors specializing in immune system disorders) may also treat people with lupus. As treatment progresses, other professionals often help. These may include nurses, psychologists, social workers, nephrologists (doctors who treat kidney disease), cardiologists (doctors specializing in the heart and blood vessels), hematologists (doctors specializing in blood disorders), endocrinologists (doctors specializing in problems related to the glands and hormones), dermatologists (doctors who treat skin disease), and neurologists (doctors specializing in disorders of the nervous system). It is also important for people with lupus to have a primary care doctor—usually a family physician or internist (internal medicine specialist)—who can coordinate care between their different health providers and treat other problems as they arise.

The range and effectiveness of treatments for lupus have increased dramatically in recent decades, giving doctors more choices in how to manage the disease.

What You Can Do: The Importance of Self-Care

Despite the symptoms of lupus and the potential side effects of treatment, people with lupus can maintain a high quality of life overall. One key to managing lupus is to understand the disease and its impact. Learning to recognize the warning signs of a flare can help the patient take steps to ward it off or reduce its intensity. Many people with lupus experience increased fatigue, pain, a rash, fever, abdominal discomfort, headache, or dizziness just before a flare. Developing strategies to prevent flares can also be helpful, such as learning to recognize your warning signals and maintaining good communication with your doctor.

It is also important for people with lupus to receive regular healthcare, instead of seeking help only when symptoms worsen. Results from a medical exam and laboratory work on a regular basis allow the doctor to note any changes and to identify and treat flares early. The treatment plan, which is tailored to the individual's specific needs and circumstances, can be adjusted accordingly. If new symptoms are identified early, treatments may be more effective. Other concerns also can be addressed at regular checkups.

People with lupus should also be aware of their increased risk of premature cardiovascular disease. This makes healthy lifestyle choices such as eating well, exercising regularly, and not smoking particularly important for people with lupus.

Warning Signs of a Flare

- Increased fatigue
- Pain
- Rash
- Fever
- Abdominal discomfort
- Headache
- Dizziness

Preventing a Flare

- Learn to recognize your warning signals.
- Maintain good communication with your doctor.

Staying healthy requires extra effort and care for people with lupus, so it becomes especially important to develop strategies for maintaining wellness. One of the primary goals of wellness for people with lupus is coping with the stress of having a chronic disorder. Some approaches that may help include exercise, relaxation techniques such as meditation, and setting priorities for spending time and energy.

Developing and maintaining a good support system is also important. A support system may include family, friends, medical professionals, community organizations, and support groups.

Learning more about lupus may also help. Studies have shown that patients who are well-informed and participate actively in their own care experience less pain, make fewer visits to the doctor, build self-confidence, and remain more active.

Pregnancy and Contraception for Women with Lupus

Although pregnancy in women with lupus is considered high risk, NIAMS-supported research suggests that most women with mild to moderate lupus can expect to have healthy pregnancies. Pregnancy counseling and planning before pregnancy are important. Ideally, a woman should have no signs or symptoms of lupus and be taking no medications for several months before she becomes pregnant.

Some women may experience a mild to moderate flare during or after their pregnancy; others do not. Pregnant women with lupus, especially those taking corticosteroids, also are more likely to develop high blood pressure, diabetes, hyperglycemia (high blood sugar), and kidney complications, so regular care and good nutrition during pregnancy are essential.

For women with lupus who do not wish to become pregnant or who are taking drugs that could be harmful to an unborn baby, reliable birth control is important. Oral contraceptives (birth control pills) were once not an option for women with lupus because doctors feared the hormones in the pill would cause a flare of the disease. However, a large National Institutes of Health (NIH)-supported study called Safety of Estrogens in Lupus Erythematosus National Assessment (SELENA) found that severe flares were no more common among women with lupus taking oral contraceptives than those taking a placebo (inactive pill). As a result of this study, doctors are increasingly prescribing oral contraceptives to women with inactive or stable disease.

Chapter 58

Multiple Sclerosis

Multiple sclerosis (MS) is the most common disabling neurological disease of young adults. It most often appears when people are between 20 to 40 years old. However, it can also affect children and older people.

The course of MS is unpredictable. A small number of those with MS will have a mild course with little to no disability, while another smaller group will have a steadily worsening disease that leads to increased disability over time. Most people with MS, however, will have short periods of symptoms followed by long stretches of relative relief, with partial or full recovery. There is no way to predict, at the beginning, how an individual person's disease will progress.

Researchers have spent decades trying to understand why some people get MS and others don't, and why some individuals with MS have symptoms that progress rapidly while others do not. How does the disease begin? Why is the course of MS so different from person to person? Is there anything we can do to prevent it? Can it be cured?

This brochure includes information about why MS develops, how it progresses, and what new therapies are being used to treat its symptoms and slow its progression. New treatments can reduce long-term disability for many people with MS. However, there are still no cures and no clear ways to prevent MS from developing.

This chapter includes text excerpted from "Multiple Sclerosis," National Institute of Neurological Disorders and Stroke (NINDS), November 19, 2015.

What Is Multiple Sclerosis?

Multiple sclerosis (MS) is a neuroinflammatory disease that affects myelin, a substance that makes up the membrane (called the myelin sheath) that wraps around nerve fibers (axons). Myelinated axons are commonly called *white matter*. Researchers have learned that MS also damages the nerve cell bodies, which are found in the brain's *gray matter*, as well as the axons themselves in the brain, spinal cord, and optic nerve (the nerve that transmits visual information from the eye to the brain). As the disease progresses, the brain's cortex shrinks (cortical atrophy).

The term multiple sclerosis refers to the distinctive areas of scar tissue (sclerosis or *plaques*) that are visible in the white matter of people who have MS. Plaques can be as small as a pinhead or as large as the size of a golf ball. Doctors can see these areas by examining the brain and spinal cord using a type of brain scan called *magnetic resonance imaging* (MRI).

While MS sometimes causes severe disability, it is only rarely fatal and most people with MS have a normal life expectancy.

What Are Plaques Made of and Why Do They Develop?

Plaques, or *lesions*, are the result of an inflammatory process in the brain that causes immune system cells to attack myelin. The myelin sheath helps to speed nerve impulses traveling within the nervous system. Axons are also damaged in MS, although not as extensively, or as early in the disease, as myelin.

Under normal circumstances, cells of the immune system travel in and out of the brain patrolling for infectious agents (viruses, for example) or unhealthy cells. This is called the "surveillance" function of the immune system.

Surveillance cells usually won't spring into action unless they recognize an infectious agent or unhealthy cells. When they do, they produce substances to stop the infectious agent. If they encounter unhealthy cells, they either kill them directly or clean out the dying area and produce substances that promote healing and repair among the cells that are left.

Researchers have observed that immune cells behave differently in the brains of people with MS. They become active and attack what appears to be healthy myelin. It is unclear what triggers this attack. MS is one of many *autoimmune* disorders, such as rheumatoid arthritis and lupus, in which the immune system mistakenly attacks a person's healthy tissue as opposed to performing its normal role of attacking foreign invaders like viruses and bacteria. Whatever the reason, during these periods of immune system activity, most of the myelin within the affected area is damaged or destroyed. The axons also may be damaged. The symptoms of MS depend on the severity of the immune reaction as well as the location and extent of the plaques, which primarily appear in the brain stem, cerebellum, spinal cord, optic nerves, and the white matter of the brain around the brain ventricles (fluid-filled spaces inside of the brain).

What Are the Signs and Symptoms of MS?

The symptoms of MS usually begin over one to several days, but in some forms, they may develop more slowly. They may be mild or severe and may go away quickly or last for months. Sometimes the initial symptoms of MS are overlooked because they disappear in a day or so and normal function returns. Because symptoms come and go in the majority of people with MS, the presence of symptoms is called an attack, or in medical terms, an *exacerbation*. Recovery from symptoms is referred to as remission, while a return of symptoms is called a relapse. This form of MS is therefore called *relapsing-remitting* MS, in contrast to a more slowly developing form called primary progressive MS. Progressive MS can also be a second stage of the illness that follows years of relapsing-remitting symptoms.

A diagnosis of MS is often delayed because MS shares symptoms with other neurological conditions and diseases.

The first symptoms of MS often include:

- vision problems such as blurred or double vision or *optic neuritis*, which causes pain in the eye and a rapid loss of vision.

- weak, stiff muscles, often with painful muscle spasms

- tingling or numbness in the arms, legs, trunk of the body, or face

- clumsiness, particularly difficulty staying balanced when walking

- bladder control problems, either inability to control the bladder or urgency

- dizziness that doesn't go away

MS may also cause later symptoms such as:

- mental or physical *fatigue* which accompanies the above symptoms during an attack

341

- mood changes such as depression or euphoria

- changes in the ability to concentrate or to multitask effectively

- difficulty making decisions, planning, or prioritizing at work or in private life.

Some people with MS develop transverse *myelitis*, a condition caused by inflammation in the spinal cord. Transverse myelitis causes loss of spinal cord function over a period of time lasting from several hours to several weeks. It usually begins as a sudden onset of lower back pain, muscle weakness, or abnormal sensations in the toes and feet, and can rapidly progress to more severe symptoms, including paralysis. In most cases of transverse myelitis, people recover at least some function within the first 12 weeks after an attack begins. Transverse myelitis can also result from viral infections, arteriovenous malformations, or neuroinflammatory problems unrelated to MS. In such instances, there are no plaques in the brain that suggest previous MS attacks.

Neuro-myelitis optica is a disorder associated with transverse myelitis as well as optic nerve inflammation. Patients with this disorder usually have *antibodies* against a particular protein in their spinal cord, called the aquaporin channel. These patients respond differently to treatment than most people with MS.

How Many People Have MS?

No one knows exactly how many people have MS. Experts think there are currently 250,000 to 350,000 people in the United States diagnosed with MS. This estimate suggests that approximately 200 new cases are diagnosed every week. Studies of the prevalence (the proportion of individuals in a population having a particular disease) of MS indicate that the rate of the disease has increased steadily during the twentieth century.

As with most autoimmune disorders, twice as many women are affected by MS as men. MS is more common in colder climates. People of Northern European descent appear to be at the highest risk for the disease, regardless of where they live. Native Americans of North and South America, as well as Asian American populations, have relatively low rates of MS.

What Causes MS?

The ultimate cause of MS is damage to myelin, nerve fibers, and neurons in the brain and spinal cord, which together make up the central nervous system (CNS). But how that happens, and why, are questions that challenge researchers. Evidence appears to show that MS is a disease caused by genetic vulnerabilities combined with environmental factors.

Although there is little doubt that the immune system contributes to the brain and spinal cord tissue destruction of MS, the exact target of the immune system attacks and which immune system cells cause the destruction isn't fully understood.

Researchers have several possible explanations for what might be going on. The immune system could be:

- fighting some kind of infectious agent (for example, a virus) that has components which mimic components of the brain (molecular mimickry)

- destroying brain cells because they are unhealthy

- mistakenly identifying normal brain cells as foreign.

The last possibility has been the favored explanation for many years. Research now suggests that the first two activities might also play a role in the development of MS. There is a special barrier, called the *blood-brain barrier*, which separates the brain and spinal cord from the immune system. If there is a break in the barrier, it exposes the brain to the immune system for the first time. When this happens, the immune system may misinterpret the brain as "foreign."

How Is MS Diagnosed?

There is no single test used to diagnose MS. Doctors use a number of tests to rule out or confirm the diagnosis. There are many other disorders that can mimic MS. Some of these other disorders can be cured, while others require different treatments than those used for MS. Therefore it is very important to perform a thorough investigation before making a diagnosis.

In addition to a complete medical history, physical examination, and a detailed neurological examination, a doctor will order an MRI scan of the head and spine to look for the characteristic lesions of MS. MRI is used to generate images of the brain and/or spinal cord. Then a special dye or contrast agent is injected into a vein and the MRI is repeated. In regions with active inflammation in MS, there is disruption of the blood-brain barrier and the dye will leak into the active MS lesion.

Doctors may also order evoked potential tests, which use electrodes on the skin and painless electric signals to measure how quickly and accurately the nervous system responds to stimulation. In addition, they may request a lumbar puncture (sometimes called a "spinal tap") to obtain a sample of *cerebrospinal fluid*. This allows them to look for proteins and inflammatory cells associated with the disease and to rule out other diseases that may look similar to MS, including some infections and other illnesses. MS is confirmed when positive signs of the disease are found in different parts of the nervous system at more than one time interval and there is no alternative diagnosis.

What Is the Course of MS?

The course of MS is different for each individual, which makes it difficult to predict. For most people, it starts with a first attack, usually (but not always) followed by a full to almost-full recovery. Weeks, months, or even years may pass before another attack occurs, followed again by a period of relief from symptoms. This characteristic pattern is called relapsing-remitting MS.

Primary-progressive MS is characterized by a gradual physical decline with no noticeable remissions, although there may be temporary or minor relief from symptoms. This type of MS has a later onset, usually after age 40, and is just as common in men as in women.

Secondary-progressive MS begins with a relapsing-remitting course, followed by a later primary-progressive course. The majority of individuals with severe relapsing-remitting MS will develop secondary progressive MS if they are untreated.

Finally, there are some rare and unusual variants of MS. One of these is Marburg variant MS (also called malignant MS), which causes a swift and relentless decline resulting in significant disability or even death shortly after disease onset. Balo's concentric sclerosis, which causes concentric rings of demyelination that can be seen on an MRI, is another variant type of MS that can progress rapidly.

Determining the particular type of MS is important because the current disease modifying drugs have been proven beneficial only for the relapsing-remitting types of MS.

What Is an Exacerbation or Attack of MS?

An exacerbation—which is also called a relapse, flare-up, or attack—is a sudden worsening of MS symptoms, or the appearance of new symptoms that lasts for at least 24 hours. MS relapses are thought to be associated with the development of new areas of damage in the brain. Exacerbations are characteristic of relapsing-remitting MS, in which attacks are followed by periods of complete or partial recovery with no apparent worsening of symptoms.

An attack may be mild or its symptoms may be severe enough to significantly interfere with life's daily activities. Most exacerbations last from several days to several weeks, although some have been known to last for months.

When the symptoms of the attack subside, an individual with MS is said to be in remission. However, MRI data have shown that this is somewhat misleading because MS lesions continue to appear during these remission periods. Patients do not experience symptoms during remission because the inflammation may not be severe or it may occur in areas of the brain that do not produce obvious symptoms. Research suggests that only about 1 out of every 10 MS lesions is perceived by a person with MS. Therefore, MRI examination plays a very important role in establishing an MS diagnosis, deciding when the disease should be treated, and determining whether treatments work effectively or not. It also has been a valuable tool to test whether an experimental new therapy is effective at reducing exacerbations.

Are There Treatments Available for MS?

There is still no cure for MS, but there are treatments for initial attacks, medications and therapies to improve symptoms, and recently developed drugs to slow the worsening of the disease. These new drugs have been shown to reduce the number and severity of relapses and to delay the long term progression of MS.

How Do Doctors Treat the Symptoms of MS?

MS causes a variety of symptoms that can interfere with daily activities but which can usually be treated or managed to reduce their impact. Many of these issues are best treated by neurologists who have advanced training in the treatment of MS and who can prescribe specific medications to treat the problems.

Complementary and Alternative Therapies

Many people with MS use some form of complementary or alternative medicine. These therapies come from many disciplines, cultures, and traditions and encompass techniques as different as acupuncture, aromatherapy, ayurvedic medicine, touch and energy therapies, physical movement disciplines such as yoga and tai chi, herbal supplements, and biofeedback.

Because of the risk of interactions between alternative and more conventional therapies, people with MS should discuss all the therapies they are using with their doctor, especially herbal supplements. Although herbal supplements are considered "natural," they have biologically-active ingredients that could have harmful effects on their own or interact harmfully with other medications.

Chapter 59

Myasthenia Gravis

What Is Myasthenia Gravis?

Myasthenia gravis is a chronic autoimmune neuromuscular disease characterized by varying degrees of weakness of the skeletal (voluntary) muscles of the body. The name myasthenia gravis, which is Latin and Greek in origin, literally means "grave muscle weakness." With current therapies, however, most cases of myasthenia gravis are not as "grave" as the name implies. In fact, most individuals with myasthenia gravis have a normal life expectancy.

The hallmark of myasthenia gravis is muscle weakness that increases during periods of activity and improves after periods of rest. Certain muscles such as those that control eye and eyelid movement, facial expression, chewing, talking, and swallowing are often, but not always, involved in the disorder. The muscles that control breathing and neck and limb movements may also be affected.

What Causes Myasthenia Gravis?

Myasthenia gravis is caused by a defect in the transmission of nerve impulses to muscles. It occurs when normal communication between the nerve and muscle is interrupted at the neuromuscular junction—the place where nerve cells connect with the muscles they control. Normally when impulses travel down the nerve, the nerve

This chapter includes text excerpted from "Myasthenia Gravis Fact Sheet," National Institute of Neurological Disorders and Stroke (NINDS), May 10, 2016.

endings release a neurotransmitter substance called acetylcholine. Acetylcholine travels from the neuromuscular junction and binds to acetylcholine receptors which are activated and generate a muscle contraction.

In myasthenia gravis, antibodies block, alter, or destroy the receptors for acetylcholine at the neuromuscular junction, which prevents the muscle contraction from occurring. These antibodies are produced by the body's own immune system. Myasthenia gravis is an autoimmune disease because the immune system—which normally protects the body from foreign organisms—mistakenly attacks itself.

What Is the Role of the Thymus Gland in Myasthenia Gravis?

The thymus gland, which lies in the chest area beneath the breastbone, plays an important role in the development of the immune system in early life. Its cells form a part of the body's normal immune system. The gland is somewhat large in infants, grows gradually until puberty, and then gets smaller and is replaced by fat with age. In adults with myasthenia gravis, the thymus gland remains large and is abnormal. It contains certain clusters of immune cells indicative of lymphoid hyperplasia—a condition usually found only in the spleen and lymph nodes during an active immune response. Some individuals with myasthenia gravis develop thymomas (tumors of the thymus gland). Thymomas are generally benign, but they can become malignant.

The relationship between the thymus gland and myasthenia gravis is not yet fully understood. Scientists believe the thymus gland may give incorrect instructions to developing immune cells, ultimately resulting in autoimmunity and the production of the acetylcholine receptor antibodies, thereby setting the stage for the attack on neuromuscular transmission.

What Are the Symptoms of Myasthenia Gravis?

Although myasthenia gravis may affect any voluntary muscle, muscles that control eye and eyelid movement, facial expression, and swallowing are most frequently affected. The onset of the disorder may be sudden and symptoms often are not immediately recognized as myasthenia gravis.

In most cases, the first noticeable symptom is weakness of the eye muscles. In others, difficulty in swallowing and slurred speech may be the first signs. The degree of muscle weakness involved in myasthenia gravis varies greatly among individuals, ranging from a localized form limited to eye muscles (ocular myasthenia), to a severe or generalized form in which many muscles—sometimes including those that control breathing—are affected. Symptoms, which vary in type and severity, may include a drooping of one or both eyelids (ptosis), blurred or double vision (diplopia) due to weakness of the muscles that control eye movements, unstable or waddling gait, a change in facial expression, difficulty in swallowing, shortness of breath, impaired speech (dysarthria), and weakness in the arms, hands, fingers, legs, and neck.

Who Gets Myasthenia Gravis?

Myasthenia gravis occurs in all ethnic groups and both genders. It most commonly affects young adult women (under 40) and older men (over 60), but it can occur at any age.

In neonatal myasthenia, the fetus may acquire immune proteins (antibodies) from a mother affected with myasthenia gravis. Generally, cases of neonatal myasthenia gravis are temporary and the child's symptoms usually disappear within 2-3 months after birth. Other children develop myasthenia gravis indistinguishable from adults. Myasthenia gravis in juveniles is uncommon.

Myasthenia gravis is not directly inherited nor is it contagious. Occasionally, the disease may occur in more than one member of the same family.

Rarely, children may show signs of congenital myasthenia or congenital myasthenic syndrome. These are not autoimmune disorders, but are caused by defective genes that produce abnormal proteins instead of those which normally would produce acetylcholine, acetylcholinesterase (the enzyme that breaks down acetylcholine), or the acetylcholine receptor and other proteins present along the muscle membrane.

How Is Myasthenia Gravis Diagnosed?

Because weakness is a common symptom of many other disorders, the diagnosis of myasthenia gravis is often missed or delayed (sometimes up to two years) in people who experience mild weakness or in those individuals whose weakness is restricted to only a few muscles.

The first steps of diagnosing myasthenia gravis include a review of the individual's medical history, and physical and neurological examinations. The physician looks for impairment of eye movements or muscle weakness without any changes in the individual's ability to feel things. If the doctor suspects myasthenia gravis, several tests are available to confirm the diagnosis.

How Is Myasthenia Gravis Treated?

Today, myasthenia gravis can generally be controlled. There are several therapies available to help reduce and improve muscle weakness. Medications used to treat the disorder include anticholinesterase agents such as neostigmine and pyridostigmine, which help improve neuromuscular transmission and increase muscle strength. Immunosuppressive drugs such as prednisone, azathioprine, cyclosporin, mycophenolate mofetil, and tacrolimus may also be used. These medications improve muscle strength by suppressing the production of abnormal antibodies. Their use must be carefully monitored by a physician because they may cause major side effects.

Thymectomy, the surgical removal of the thymus gland (which often is abnormal in individuals with myasthenia gravis), reduces symptoms in some individuals without thymoma and may cure some people, possibly by re-balancing the immune system. Thymectomy is recommended for individuals with thymoma. Other therapies used to treat myasthenia gravis include plasmapheresis, a procedure in which serum containing the abnormal antibodies is removed from the blood while cells are replaced, and high-dose intravenous immune globulin, which temporarily modifies the immune system by infusing antibodies from donated blood. These therapies may be used to help individuals during especially difficult periods of weakness. A neurologist will determine which treatment option is best for each individual depending on the severity of the weakness, which muscles are affected, and the individual's age and other associated medical problems.

What Are Myasthenic Crises?

A myasthenic crisis occurs when the muscles that control breathing weaken to the point that ventilation is inadequate, creating a medical emergency and requiring a respirator for assisted ventilation. In individuals whose respiratory muscles are weak, crises—which generally call for immediate medical attention—may be triggered by infection, fever, or an adverse reaction to medication.

What Is the Prognosis?

With treatment, most individuals with myasthenia can significantly improve their muscle weakness and lead normal or nearly normal lives. Some cases of myasthenia gravis may go into remission—either temporarily or permanently—and muscle weakness may disappear completely so that medications can be discontinued. Stable, long-lasting complete remissions are the goal of thymectomy and may occur in about 50 percent of individuals who undergo this procedure. In a few cases, the severe weakness of myasthenia gravis may cause respiratory failure, which requires immediate emergency medical care.

Chapter 60

Myocarditis

Myocarditis is a disease characterized by inflammation of the heart muscle, called the myocardium. It is estimated to affect thousands of Americans each year and is caused by a wide variety of factors, including viral and bacterial infections, environmental toxins, autoimmune diseases, and allergic reactions to certain toxins and medications. Myocarditis often produces no symptoms, and because it is relatively uncommon, the best ways to diagnose and treat the condition are still being studied. It usually affects people who are otherwise healthy, including a significant number of young adults. The best way to prevent myocarditis is by seeking immediate medical attention for infections.

What Are the Causes?

Myocarditis is primarily caused by viral infections, the most common among them being those that affect the upper respiratory tract. Other less common causes include contagious infections, such as Lyme disease.

Some of the viral infections that can cause myocarditis include hepatitis C, herpes, HIV, and parvovirus. Bacterial infections that can lead to myocarditis include chlamydia (a common sexually transmitted disease), streptococcus (strep), staphylococcus (staph), mycoplasma (bacteria that cause a lung infection), and treponema

"Myocarditis," © 2016 Omnigraphics. Reviewed June 2016.

(the cause of syphilis). The condition can also be brought on by such factors as allergic reactions to certain medicines and toxins like drugs, alcohol, spider or snake bites, wasp stings, lead, radiation, and chemotherapy.

Myocarditis can also be caused by autoimmune diseases (in which the immune system attacks the body), such as lupus or rheumatoid arthritis.

What Are the Signs and Symptoms?

Some of the symptoms of myocarditis include:

- Shortness of breath during exercise, which may lead to breathing troubles at night, as well

- Irregular heartbeat and, in some cases, fainting

- Heart palpitations

- Light-headedness

- Sharp or stabbing chest pain or pressure

- Fatigue

- Swelling in joints, legs, or neck veins

- Indications of infection, such as fever, sore throat, muscle aches, headache, or diarrhea

These symptoms often follow a respiratory infection, and if they occur it is important to seek medical attention promptly.

What Are the Complications?

Not treating myocarditis can cause the heart to work harder to pump blood. This can lead to symptoms of heart failure and in serious cases may be fatal. Cardiomyopathy and pericarditis are other possible complications of this infection, both of which are leading causes of heart transplants in the United States. Cardiomyopathy is an increase in size, thickness, or rigidity of the heart muscle. Pericarditis is the inflammation of pericardium, or the sac covering the heart.

How Is It Diagnosed?

In many cases, myocarditis has no symptoms and is not diagnosed. However, when there are symptoms, the doctor will conduct a physical exam to check for abnormal heartbeat, fluid in lungs, or swelling in legs. Some of the following tests may also be conducted:

- **Blood test** to analyze blood cell count and check for infection or antibodies

- An **electrocardiogram** to evaluate the electrical activity of the heart

- A **chest X-ray** to study the shape and size of the heart

- An **echocardiogram** to inspect the structure of the heart and measure blood flow

- Occasionally, a **cardiac magnetic resonance imaging (MRI)** scan or a **heart biopsy** may be performed to confirm the diagnosis

How Is It Treated?

When a person has myocarditis, treatment will be provided for its underlying cause. This will typically include medication to take the load off the heart, improve heart function, and prevent or control further complications.

In the presence of an abnormal heart rhythm, additional treatment such as a pacemaker or defibrillator could be required. Hospitalization may be necessary in case of serious complications, such as a blood clots or a weakened heart. ACE (Angiotensin Converting Enzyme) inhibitors, calcium channel blockers, and diuretics are some medicines that may be prescribed to help the heart function better. Steroids and other medications may also be used to treat heart inflammation. Often, reduced physical activity for at least six months, rest, and a low-salt diet are recommended.

The cause of myocarditis, overall health of the person, and complications, if any, determine the outlook. The infected person could either recover completely or develop a chronic condition. There is a small possibility that myocarditis may recur and could, in rare cases, lead to dilated cardiomyopathy, an enlargement and weakening of the ventricles, the heart's pumping chambers.

References

1. "Discover Myocarditis Causes, Symptoms, Diagnosis and Treatment," Myocarditis Foundation, n.d.

2. Beckerman, James. "Myocarditis," WebMD, July 14, 2014.

Chapter 61

Neuromyelitis Optica

What Is Neuromyelitis Optica?

Neuromyelitis optica, is an autoimmune condition that affects the spinal cord and optic nerves (the nerves that carry information regarding sight from the eye). In Devic disease, the body's immune system attacks and destroys myelin, a fatty substance that surrounds nerves and helps nerve signals move from cell to cell. Signs and symptoms worsen with time and include optic neuritis; transverse myelitis; pain in spine and limbs; and bladder and bowel dysfunction. The exact cause of Devic disease is unknown. Most affected people do not have other family members with the condition. Currently there is no cure for Devic disease, but there are therapies to treat an attack while it is happening, to reduce symptoms, and to prevent relapses.

Symptoms

The most common signs and symptoms of neuromyelitis optica are optic neuritis and/or transverse myelitis. Optic neuritis (inflammation of the optic nerve) can cause pain and sudden, reduced vision in the affected eye. In most cases, only one eye is affected; however, some people may develop optic neuritis in both eyes at the same time.

This chapter includes text excerpted from "Neuromyelitis Optica," Genetic and Rare Diseases Information Center (GARD), National Center for Advancing Translational Sciences (NCATS), December 5, 2014.

357

Signs and symptoms of transverse myelitis (inflammation of the spinal cord) include pain in the spine or limbs (arms and legs); mild to severe paralysis of the legs; paresthesias (abnormal sensations such as burning, tickling, pricking, or tingling) in the legs; and loss of bowel or bladder control. Depending on which section of the spinal cord is affected, breathing problems may be present, as well. Some affected people may also experience muscle spasms, a stiff neck, a general feeling of discomfort, headache, fever, and loss of appetite. Progression of transverse myelitis leads to full paralysis of the legs, requiring the patient to use a wheelchair.

In rare cases, neuromyelitis optica can also affect the brainstem (the part of the brain connected to the spinal cord). This can lead to symptoms such as uncontrollable vomiting and hiccups.

Cause

In most cases, the exact cause of neuromyelitis optica is unknown. However, studies of affected nerves have improved our understanding of the disease process. In neuromyelitis optica, certain immune proteins (autoantibodies) attach themselves to specialized proteins in the spinal cord and optical nerve called "water channel proteins." The autoantibodies signal immune cells to attack, resulting in damage to myelin and the breakdown of healthy nerves and tissues.

There is a strong link between neuromyelitis optica and a personal or family history of other autoimmune conditions. In fact, 50 percent of people with neuromyelitis optica are also affected by other autoimmune conditions and/or have family members with an autoimmune condition.

There have been a few cases of neuromyelitis optica occurring in association with certain infectious conditions (e.g., syphilis, HIV, chlamydia, varicella, cytomegalovirus, and Epstein Barr virus). The nature of this link isn't clear. It is possible that certain infections may trigger neuromyelitis optica in people who are predisposed to the condition.

Inheritance

Neuromyelitis optica is not thought to be inherited in most cases, and only 3 percent of affected people have a family member with the condition.

Diagnosis

A diagnosis of neuromyelitis optica is based on a physical examination; identification of characteristic signs and symptoms; and a variety of specialized imaging and laboratory tests. For example, magnetic resonance imaging (MRI scan) or computed tomography (CT scan) of the brain and spinal cord and optical coherence tomography (specialized pictures of the retina) can be used to locate areas of nerve damage. Special blood tests that are used to detect autoimmune conditions and/or examination of the cerebrospinal fluid may also be necessary to confirm a diagnosis.

Treatment

There is no cure for neuromyelitis optica, but there are therapies to treat an attack while it is happening, to reduce symptoms, and to prevent relapses. Doctors usually treat an initial attack of neuromyelitis optica with a combination of corticosteroid drugs to stop the attack and immunosuppressive drugs to prevent additional attacks. If frequent relapses occur, some people may need to continue a low dose of steroids for longer periods. Plasma exchange (plasmapheresis) is a technique that separates antibodies out of the blood stream and is used with people who do not respond to corticosteroid therapy. Pain, stiffness, muscle spasms, and bladder and bowel control problems can be managed with the appropriate medications and therapies. People with neuromyelitis optica may require the combined efforts of occupational therapists, physical therapists, and social services professionals to address their complex rehabilitation needs.

Prognosis

The onset of neuromyelitis optica varies from childhood to adulthood, with two peaks: one in childhood and the other in adults in their 40s. Most people with neuromyelitis optica have a relapsing form of the disease and experience clusters of attacks months or years apart, followed by partial recovery during periods of remission (a decrease or disappearance of symptoms). Disability is cumulative, the result of each attack damaging new areas of myelin. In rare cases, neuromyelitis optica is characterized by a single, severe attack extending over a month or two, with little recurrence after the initial onset of symptoms. Some people are severely affected by neuromyelitis optica and can lose vision in both eyes and the use of their arms and legs. Most people experience a moderate degree of permanent limb weakness from myelitis. Muscle weakness can cause breathing difficulties and may require the use of artificial ventilation. The death of an individual with neuromyelitis optica is most often caused by respiratory (breathing) complications from myelitis attacks.

Chapter 62

Pediatric Autoimmune Neuropsychiatric Disorders (PANDAS)

What Is PANDAS?

PANDAS is short for Pediatric Autoimmune Neuropsychiatric Disorders Associated with Streptococcal Infections. A child may be diagnosed with PANDAS when:

- Obsessive compulsive disorder (OCD) and/or tic disorders suddenly appear following a strep infection (such as strep throat or scarlet fever); or

- The symptoms of OCD or tic symptoms suddenly become worse following a strep infection.

The symptoms are usually dramatic, happen "overnight and out of the blue," and can include motor and/or vocal tics, obsessions, and/or compulsions. In addition to these symptoms, children may also become moody, irritable, experience anxiety attacks, or show concerns about separating from parents or loved ones.

This chapter includes text excerpted from "PANDAS Frequently Asked Questions," National Institute of Mental Health (NIMH), April 2016.

What Causes PANDAS?

The strep bacteria is a very ancient organism which survives in its human host by hiding from the immune system as long as possible. It does this by putting molecules on its cell wall that look nearly identical to molecules found on the child's heart, joints, skin, and brain tissues. This is called "molecular mimicry" and allows the strep bacteria to evade detection for a time.

However, the molecules on the strep bacteria are eventually recognized as foreign to the body and the child's immune system reacts to them by producing antibodies. Because of the molecular mimicry, the antibodies react not only with the strep molecules, but also with the human host molecules that were mimicked.

The cross-reactive antibodies then trigger an immune reaction that "attacks" the mimicked molecules in the child's own tissues. Studies at the National Institute of Mental Health (NIMH) and elsewhere showed that some cross-reactive "anti-brain" antibodies target the brain, causing OCD, tics, and the other neuropsychiatric symptoms of PANDAS.

Could an Adult Develop PANDAS?

PANDAS is considered a pediatric disorder and typically first appears in childhood from age 3 to puberty. Reactions to strep infections are rare after age 12, but the investigators recognize that PANDAS could occur (rarely) among adolescents. It is unlikely that someone would experience these poststrep neuropsychiatric symptoms for the first time as an adult, but it has not been fully studied.

It is possible that adolescents and adults may have immune-mediated OCD, but this is not known. The research studies at the NIMH are restricted to children.

Symptoms

How is PANDAS diagnosed?

The diagnosis of PANDAS is a clinical diagnosis, which means that there are no lab tests that can diagnose PANDAS. Instead, clinicians use 6 diagnostic criteria for the diagnosis of PANDAS (see below). At the present time the clinical features of the illness are the only means of determining whether or not a child might have PANDAS.

The diagnostic criteria are:

- Presence of OCD and/or a tic disorder

- Pediatric onset of symptoms (age 3 years to puberty)

- Episodic course of symptom severity
- Association with group A beta-hemolytic streptococcal infection (a positive throat culture for strep or history of scarlet fever)
- Association with neurological abnormalities (for example, physical hyperactivity, or unusual, jerky movements that are not in the child's control)
- Very abrupt onset or worsening of symptoms

If the symptoms have been present for more than a week, blood tests (antistreptococcal titers) may be done to document a preceding streptococcal infection.

Are There Any Other Symptoms Associated with PANDAS Episodes?

Yes. Children with PANDAS often experience one or more of the following symptoms in conjunction with their OCD and/or tics:

- Attention deficit hyperactivity disorder (ADHD) symptoms (hyperactivity, inattention, fidgety)
- Separation anxiety (child is "clingy" and has difficulty separating from his/her caregivers; for example, the child may not want to be in a different room in the house from his/her parents)
- Mood changes (irritability, sadness, emotional lability)
- Sleep disturbance
- Night-time bed wetting and/or day-time urinary frequency
- Fine/gross motor changes (e.g., changes in handwriting)
- Joint pains

What Is an Episodic Course of Symptoms?

Children with PANDAS seem to have dramatic ups and downs in their OCD and/or tic severity. Tics or OCD which are almost always present at a relatively consistent level do not represent an episodic course. Many kids with OCD or tics have good days and bad days, or even good weeks and bad weeks. However, patients with PANDAS have a very sudden onset or worsening of their symptoms, followed by a slow, gradual improvement. If they get another strep infection, their symptoms suddenly worsen again. The increased symptom severity usually persists for at least several weeks, but may last for several months or longer. The tics or OCD then seem to gradually fade away, and the children often enjoy a few weeks or several months without problems. When they have another strep throat infection, the tics or OCD may return just as suddenly and dramatically as they did previously.

My Child Has Had Strep Throat before, and He Has Tics and / or OCD. Does That Mean He Has PANDAS?

No. Many children have OCD and/or tics, and almost all school aged children get strep throat at some point. In fact, the average grade-school student will have 2–3 strep throat infections each year.

PANDAS is considered as a diagnosis when there is a very close relationship between the abrupt onset or worsening or OCD and/or tics, and a preceding strep infection. If strep is found in conjunction with two or three episodes of OCD/tics, then it may be that the child has PANDAS.

What Is an Anti-Streptococcal Antibody Titer?

The anti-streptococcal antibody titer determines whether the child has had a previous strep infection. Two different strep tests are commercially available:

1. Antistrepolysin O (ASO) titer*, which rises 3–6 weeks after a strep infection, and

2. Antistreptococcal DNAse B (AntiDNAse-B) titer, which rises 6–8 weeks after a strep infection.

Titer refers to the amount of something, in this case biological molecules in blood that indicate a previous infection.

What Does an Elevated Anti-Streptococcal Antibody Titer Mean? Is This Bad for My Child?

An elevated anti-strep titer (such as ASO or AntiDNAse-B) means the child has had a strep infection sometime within the past few months, and his body created antibodies to fight the strep bacteria. Some grade-school aged children have chronically "elevated" titers. These may actually be in the normal range for that child, as there is a lot of individual variability in titer values.

Some children create lots of antibodies and have very high titers (up to 2,000), while others have more modest elevations. The height of the titer elevation doesn't matter. Further, elevated titers are not a bad thing. They are measuring a normal, healthy response—the production of antibodies to fight off an infection. The antibodies stay in the body for some time after the infection is gone, but the amount of time that the antibodies persist varies greatly between different individuals. Some children have "positive" antibody titers for many months after a single infection.

When Is a Strep Titer Considered to Be Abnormal, Or "Elevated"?

The lab at National Institutes of Health (NIH) considers strep titers between 0–400 to be normal. Other labs set the upper limit at 150 or 200. Since each lab measures titers in different ways, it is important to know the range used by the laboratory where the test was done—just ask where they draw the line between negative or positive titers.

It is important to note that some grade-school aged children have chronically "elevated" titers. These may actually be in the normal range for that child, as there is a lot of individual variability in titer values. Because of this variability, doctors will often draw a titer when the child is sick, or shortly thereafter, and then draw another titer several weeks later to see if the titer is "rising"—if so, this is strong evidence that the illness was due to strep. (Of course, a less expensive and more reliable way to make this determination is to take a throat culture at the time that the child is ill.)

Treatment

What Are the Treatment Options for Children with PANDAS?

Treatment with Antibiotics

The best treatment for acute episodes of PANDAS is to treat the strep infection causing the symptoms (if it is still present) with antibiotics.

- A throat culture should be done to document the presence of strep bacteria in the throat (oropharynx).

- If the throat culture is positive, a single course of antibiotics will usually get rid of the strep infection and allow the PANDAS symptoms to subside.

If a properly obtained throat culture is negative, the clinician should make sure that the child doesn't have an occult strep infection, such as a sinus infection (often caused by strep bacteria) or strep bacteria infecting the anus, vagina, or urethral opening of the penis. Although the latter infections are rare, they have been reported to trigger PANDAS symptoms in some patients and can be particularly problematic because they will linger for longer periods of time and continue to provoke the production of cross-reactive antibodies.

The strep bacteria can be harder to eradicate in the sinuses and other sites, so the course of antibiotic treatment may need to be longer than that used for strep throat.

Tips for Parents or Caregivers

- Sterilize or replace toothbrushes during/following the antibiotics treatment, to make sure that the child isn't re-infected with strep.

- It might also be helpful to check throat cultures on child's family members to make sure that none are "strep carriers" who could serve as a source of strep bacteria.

Management of Neuropsychiatric Symptoms

Children with PANDAS-related obsessive-compulsive symptoms will benefit from standard medications and/or behavioral therapies, such as cognitive behavioral therapy (CBT). OCD symptoms are treated best with a combination of CBT and an selective serotonin reuptake inhibitor (SSRI) medication, and tics respond to a variety of medications.

Children with PANDAS appear to be unusually sensitive to the side-effects of SSRIs and other medications, so it is important to "START LOW AND GO SLOW!" when using these medications. In other words, clinicians should prescribe a very small starting dose of the medication and increase it slowly enough that the child experiences as few side-effects as possible. If symptoms worsen, the dosage should be decreased promptly. However, SSRIs and other medications should not be stopped abruptly, as that could also cause difficulties.

What about Treating PANDAS with Plasma Exchange or Immunoglobulin (IVIG)?

Plasma exchange or immunoglobulin (IVIG) may be a consideration for acutely and severely affected children with PANDAS. Research suggests that both active treatments can improve global functioning, depression, emotional ups and downs, and obsessive-compulsive symptoms. However, there were a number of side-effects associated with the research treatments, including nausea, vomiting, headaches, and dizziness.

In addition, there is a risk of infection with any invasive procedure, such as these. Thus, the treatments should be reserved for severely ill patients, and administered by a qualified team of healthcare professionals.

Should an Elevated Strep Titer Be Treated with Antibiotics?

No. Elevated titers indicate that a patient has had a past strep exposure but the titers can't tell you precisely when the strep infection occurred. Children may have "positive" titers for many months after one infection. Since these elevated titers are merely a marker of a prior infection and not proof of an ongoing infection it is not appropriate to give antibiotics for elevated titers. Antibiotics are recommended only when a child has a positive rapid strep test or positive strep throat culture.

Can Penicillin Be Used to Treat PANDAS or Prevent Future PANDAS Symptom Exacerbations?

Penicillin and other antibiotics kill streptococcus and other types of bacteria. The antibiotics treat the sore throat or pharyngitis caused by the strep by getting rid of the bacteria. However, in PANDAS, it appears that antibodies produced by the body in response to the strep infection are the cause of the problem, not the bacteria themselves. Therefore one could not expect penicillin to treat the symptoms of PANDAS.

Researchers at the NIMH have been investigating the use of antibiotics as a form of prophylaxis or prevention of future problems. At this time, however, there isn't enough evidence to recommend the long-term use of antibiotics.

My Child Has PANDAS. Should He Have His Tonsils Removed?

The NIH does not recommend tonsillectomies for children with PANDAS, as there is no evidence that they are helpful. If a tonsillectomy is recommended because of frequent episodes of tonsillitis, it would be useful to discuss the pros and cons of the procedure with your child's doctor because of the role that the tonsils play in fighting strep infections.

Chapter 63

Pemphigus Diseases

What Is Pemphigus?

Pemphigus is a group of rare autoimmune diseases that cause blistering of the skin and mucous membranes (mouth, nose, throat, eyes, and genitals). Some forms of the disease, including the most common form, may be fatal if left untreated.

What Causes Pemphigus?

Normally, our immune system produces antibodies that attack viruses and harmful bacteria to keep us healthy. In people with pemphigus, however, the immune system mistakenly attacks the cells in the epidermis, or top layer of the skin, and the mucous membranes. The immune system produces antibodies against proteins in the skin known as desmogleins. These proteins form the glue that keeps skin cells attached and the skin intact. When desmogleins are attacked, skin cells separate from each other and fluid can collect between the layers of skin, forming blisters that do not heal. In some cases, these blisters can cover a large area of skin.

It is unclear what triggers the disease, although it appears that some people have a genetic susceptibility. Environmental agents may trigger the development of pemphigus in people who are likely to be affected by the disease because of their genes. In rare cases, it may be

This chapter includes text excerpted from "Pemphigus," National Institute of Arthritis and Musculoskeletal and Skin Diseases (NIAMS), June 2015.

triggered by certain medications. In those cases, the disease usually goes away when the medication is stopped.

Is Pemphigus Contagious?

Pemphigus is not contagious. It does not spread from person to person.

Who Gets Pemphigus?

Pemphigus affects people across racial and ethnic lines. Research has shown that certain ethnic groups (such as the eastern European Jewish community and people of Mediterranean descent) are more susceptible to pemphigus. A particular type of pemphigus occurs more frequently in people who live in the rain forests of Brazil.

Men and women are equally affected. Research studies suggest a genetic predisposition to the disease. Although the onset usually occurs in middle-aged and older adults, all forms of the disease may occur in young adults and children.

What Are the Different Types of Pemphigus?

There are several types of pemphigus and other similar blistering disorders. The type of disease depends on where (what layer) in the skin the blisters form and where they are located on the body. Blisters always occur on or near the surface of the skin, which is called the epidermis. People with pemphigus vulgaris, for example, have blisters that occur within the lower layer of the epidermis, while people with pemphigus foliaceus have blisters that form in the topmost layer. The type of antibody that is attacking the skin cells may also define the type of disease present.

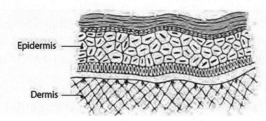

Figure 63.1. *Skin Structure*

- *Pemphigus vulgaris* is the most common type of pemphigus in the United States. Soft and limp blisters appear on healthy-looking skin and mucous membranes. The sores almost always start in the mouth. The blisters of pemphigus vulgaris form within the deep layer of the epidermis and are often painful. Blistered skin becomes so fragile that it may peel off by rubbing a finger on it. The blisters normally heal without scarring, but pigmented spots (spots where skin appears darker than the surrounding skin) may remain for a number of months.

- *Pemphigus vegetans* is a form of pemphigus with thick sores in the groin and under the arms.

- *Pemphigus foliaceus* involves crusted sores or fragile blisters that often appear first on the face and scalp and later on the chest and other parts of the body. Unlike pemphigus vulgaris, blisters do not form in the mouth. The sores are superficial and often itchy, and are rarely as painful as pemphigus vulgaris blisters. There may also be loose, moist scales on the skin.

- *IgA pemphigus* is a blistering disorder in which a different type of antibody binds to the cell surface of epidermal cells. This disease is different from other forms of pemphigus because it involves a different type of antibody (called immunoglobulin A or IgA) than other types. The disease may result in blisters similar to those seen in pemphigus foliaceus, or it may involve many small bumps containing pus. This is the most benign, or least harmful, form of pemphigus.

- *Paraneoplastic pemphigus* is a rare disease that is distinct from pemphigus, but shares some features of it. It occurs in people with certain types of cancer, including some lymphomas and leukemias. It often involves severe ulcers of the mouth and lips, cuts and scarring of the lining of the eye and eyelids, and skin blisters. Because the antibodies also target the membranes lining the airways, patients may develop life-threatening problems in the lungs. This disease is different from pemphigus, and the antibodies in the blood are different. Special tests may be needed to identify paraneoplastic pemphigus.

What Is Pemphigoid, and How Is It Different from Pemphigus?

Pemphigoid is also a blistering disorder caused by autoimmune problems that result in an attack on the skin cells by a person's own antibodies. Pemphigoid produces a split in the cells where the epidermis and the dermis (the layer below the epidermis) meet, causing deep, tense (taut or rigid) blisters that do not break easily. Pemphigus, on the other hand, causes a separation within the epidermis, and the blisters are soft, limp, and easily broken. Pemphigoid is seen most often in the elderly and may be fatal. Usually, both pemphigus and pemphigoid are treated with similar medications. Severe cases may require different treatment.

How Is Pemphigus Diagnosed?

A diagnosis of pemphigus has several parts:

- **A visual examination by a dermatologist.** The doctor will take a complete history and physical exam, noting the appearance and location of the blisters.

- **A blister biopsy.** A sample of a blister is removed and examined under the microscope. The doctor will look for cell separation that is characteristic of pemphigus, and will also determine the layer of skin in which the cells are separated.

- **Direct immunofluorescence.** A biopsy of a skin sample is treated in the laboratory with a chemical compound to find the abnormal desmoglein antibodies that attack the skin. The specific type of antibodies that form may indicate what type of pemphigus exists.

- **Indirect immunofluorescence.** Sometimes called an antibody titre test, a sample of blood is tested to measure pemphigus antibody levels in the blood and to help determine the severity of the disease. Once treatment begins, this blood test may also be used to find out if treatment is working.

Pemphigus is a serious disease, and it is important to do all of these tests to confirm a diagnosis. No single test is right all of the time.

Because it is rare, pemphigus is often the last disease considered during diagnosis. Early diagnosis may permit successful treatment with only low levels of medication, so consult a doctor if you have persistent blisters on the skin or in the mouth. In the most common form of pemphigus (pemphigus vulgaris), the mouth is often the first place that blisters or sores appear.

What Type of Doctor Treats Pemphigus?

Pemphigus is a rare disease of the skin; therefore, dermatologists are the doctors best equipped to diagnose and treat people with pemphigus. If you have blisters in the mouth, a dentist can provide guidance for maintaining good oral health. This is important for preventing gum disease and tooth loss.

How Is Pemphigus Treated?

Treatment for pemphigus vulgaris may involve using one or more drugs. The main goal is to suppress the immune system so that it will stop attacking the tissues. Commonly prescribed drugs include corticosteroids, immunosuppressive drugs, and biologics.

Antibiotics, antivirals, and antifungal medications may be prescribed to control or prevent infections. Many patients will go into complete remission with treatment, although this may take a number of years. Other patients will need to continue to take small doses of medication to keep the disease under control. Be sure to report any problems or side effects you experience to the doctor.

People with severe pemphigus that cannot be controlled with medicine may undergo plasmapheresis, a treatment in which the blood containing the damaging antibodies is removed and replaced with blood that is free of antibodies. Such patients are sometimes treated with intravenous (IV) immunoglobulin (Ig). Plasmapheresis and IV Ig are both very expensive treatments, since they require large amounts of donated and specially processed blood. The treatment prescribed will depend on the type of pemphigus and the severity of the disease.

A dentist can offer approaches that help you to maintain healthy teeth and gums, because blisters in the mouth may make brushing and flossing your teeth painful. Avoiding certain foods may help minimize irritation of the blisters in the mouth.

What Is the Prognosis for People Who Have Pemphigus?

The outlook for people with pemphigus has changed dramatically in the past decades. A person diagnosed with pemphigus vulgaris in the 1960s faced the reality that they had a disease that was rare, usually fatal, poorly understood, and with no good treatment options. Today, through medical research supported by the National Institutes of Health (NIH), the picture is dramatically better. The disease is now rarely fatal, and the majority of deaths occur from infections. For most people with pemphigus, the disease can be controlled with corticosteroids and other medications, and these medications can eventually be completely discontinued. However, these medications can cause side effects that may sometimes be serious. Pemphigus and its treatments can be debilitating and cause lost time at work, weight loss, loss of sleep, and emotional distress. Support groups may help patients cope with the disease.

Chapter 64

Polyarteritis Nodosa

What Is Polyarteritis Nodosa?

Polyarteritis nodosa is a serious blood vessel disease in which medium-sized arteries become swollen and damaged. It occurs when certain immune cells attack the affected arteries preventing vital oxygen and nourishment. Signs and symptoms may include fever, fatigue, weakness, loss of appetite, weight loss, muscle and joint aches, and abdominal pain. The skin may show rashes, swelling, ulcers, and lumps. When nerve cells are involved numbness, pain, burning, and weakness may be present. Polyarteritis nodosa can cause serious health complications including strokes, seizures, and kidney failure. Treatment often includes steroids and other drugs to suppress the immune system.

Symptoms

The signs and symptoms are mentioned below:

- abdominal pain
- abnormal pyramidal signs
- abnormality of extrapyramidal motor function
- abnormality of temperature regulation
- abnormality of the pericardium

This chapter includes text excerpted from "Polyarteritis Nodosa," Genetic and Rare Diseases Information Center (GARD), National Center for Advancing Translational Sciences (NCATS), January 10, 2016.

- abnormality of the retinal vasculature
- acrocyanosis
- aneurysm
- arrhythmia
- arterial thrombosis
- arthralgia
- arthritis
- ascites
- asthma
- autoimmunity
- behavioral abnormality
- congestive heart failure
- coronary artery disease
- cutis marmorata
- edema of the lower limbs
- encephalitis
- gangrene
- gastrointestinal hemorrhage
- gastrointestinal infarctions
- hemiplegia/hemiparesis
- hemobilia
- hypertensive crisis
- hypertrophic cardiomyopathy

- inflammatory abnormality of the eye
- leukocytosis
- malabsorption
- migraine
- myalgia
- myositis
- nephropathy
- orchitis
- osteolysis
- osteomyelitis
- pancreatitis
- paresthesia
- polyneuropathy
- renal insufficiency
- retinal detachment
- seizures
- skin rash
- skin ulcer
- subcutaneous hemorrhage
- ureteral stenosis
- urticaria
- vasculitis
- weight loss

Treatment

Few people with polyarteritis nodosa have mild disease that remains stable with nonaggressive therapy; because of the risk for serious health complications, aggressive therapy is often recommended. Treatment may include prednisone in divided doses. Additional therapy, such as cyclophosphamide, chlorambucil, azathioprine, methotrexate, dapsone, cyclosporine, or plasma exchange, may also be recommended. The goal of therapy is remission (to have no active disease) within 6 months or so. At this point the person may be maintained on cyclophosphamide (or other therapy) for a year, before it is tapered and withdrawn over the course of 3 to 6 months.

It is very important that people undergoing treatment for polyarteritis nodosa be monitored closely for toxic effects of the drugs or for signs of worsening disease. This monitoring may involve blood counts, urinalyses, serum chemistries, and the erythrocyte sedimentation rate (ESR) on at least monthly intervals.

Prognosis

A description of the average life expectancy for individuals with polyarteritis nodosa is not available. However, one study examined the overall mortality of a group of individuals with this condition. Mortality is a measure of the proportion of individuals in a group who die in a given time period. Of 348 individual with polyarteritis nodosa, approximately 20 percent had died within 5 years of initial diagnosis and treatment; approximately 32 percent had died within 10 years. Only a third of these deaths was directly caused by severe symptoms of polyarteritis nodosa. Factors which increased the risk of death included being older than 65 years, being recently diagnosed with high blood pressure (hypertension), or having gastrointestinal symptoms that required surgery at the time of diagnosis (for example, abdominal pain, internal bleeding, pancreatitis, cholecystitis, appendicitis).

Chapter 65

Polymyalgia Rheumatica and Giant Cell Arteritis

What Is Polymyalgia Rheumatica?

Polymyalgia rheumatica is a rheumatic disorder associated with moderate-to-severe musculoskeletal pain and stiffness in the neck, shoulder, and hip area. Stiffness is most noticeable in the morning or after a period of inactivity. This disorder may develop rapidly; in some people it comes on literally overnight. But for most people, polymyalgia rheumatica develops more gradually.

The cause of polymyalgia rheumatica is not known. But it is associated with immune system problems, genetic factors, and an event, such as an infection, that triggers symptoms. The fact that polymyalgia rheumatica is rare in people under the age of 50 and becomes more common as age increases, suggests that it may be linked to the aging process.

Polymyalgia rheumatica usually resolves within 1 to several years. The symptoms of polymyalgia rheumatica are quickly controlled by treatment with corticosteroids, but symptoms return if treatment is stopped too early. Corticosteroid treatment does not appear to influence the length of the disease.

This chapter includes text excerpted from "Polymyalgia Rheumatica and Giant Cell Arteritis," National Institute of Arthritis and Musculoskeletal and Skin Diseases (NIAMS), May 2016.

What Is Giant Cell Arteritis?

Giant cell arteritis is a form of vasculitis, a group of disorders that results in inflammation of blood vessels. This inflammation causes the arteries to narrow, impeding adequate blood flow. In giant cell arteritis, the vessels most involved are those of the head, especially the temporal arteries (located on each side of the head). For this reason, the disorder is sometimes called temporal arteritis. However, other blood vessels can also become inflamed in giant cell arteritis. For a good prognosis, it is critical to receive early treatment, before irreversible tissue damage occurs.

How Are Polymyalgia Rheumatica and Giant Cell Arteritis Related?

It is unclear how or why polymyalgia rheumatica and giant cell arteritis frequently occur together. But some people with polymyalgia rheumatica also develop giant cell arteritis either simultaneously, or after the musculoskeletal symptoms have disappeared. Other people with giant cell arteritis also have polymyalgia rheumatica at some time while the arteries are inflamed.

When undiagnosed or untreated, giant cell arteritis can cause potentially serious problems, including permanent vision loss and stroke. So regardless of why giant cell arteritis might occur along with polymyalgia rheumatica, it is important that doctors look for symptoms of the arteritis in anyone diagnosed with polymyalgia rheumatica.

Patients, too, must learn and watch for symptoms of giant cell arteritis, because early detection and proper treatment are key to preventing complications. Any symptoms should be reported to your doctor immediately.

What Are the Symptoms of Polymyalgia Rheumatica?

In addition to the musculoskeletal stiffness mentioned earlier, people with polymyalgia rheumatica also may have flu-like symptoms, including fever, weakness, and weight loss.

What Are the Symptoms of Giant Cell Arteritis?

Early symptoms of giant cell arteritis may resemble flu symptoms such as fatigue, loss of appetite, and fever. Symptoms specifically related to the inflamed arteries of the head include headaches, pain and tenderness over the temples, double vision or visual loss, dizziness or problems with coordination, and balance. Pain may also affect the jaw and tongue, especially when eating, and opening the mouth wide may become difficult. In rare cases, giant cell arteritis causes ulceration of the scalp.

Who Is at Risk for These Conditions?

Caucasian women over the age of 50 have the highest risk of developing polymyalgia rheumatica and giant cell arteritis. Although women are more likely than men to develop the conditions, research suggests that men with giant cell arteritis are more likely to suffer potentially blinding eye involvement. Both conditions almost exclusively affect people over the age of 50. The incidence of both peaks between 70 and 80 years of age.

Polymyalgia rheumatica and giant cell arteritis are both quite common. It is estimated that 711,000 Americans have polymyalgia rheumatica and 228,000 have giant cell arteritis.

How Are Polymyalgia Rheumatica and Giant Cell Arteritis Diagnosed?

A diagnosis of polymyalgia rheumatica is based primarily on the patient's medical history and symptoms, and on a physical examination. No single test is available to definitively diagnose polymyalgia rheumatica. However, doctors often use lab tests to confirm a diagnosis or rule out other diagnoses or possible reasons for the patient's symptoms.

The most typical laboratory finding in people with polymyalgia rheumatica is an elevated erythrocyte sedimentation rate, commonly referred to as the sed rate. This test measures inflammation by determining how quickly red blood cells fall to the bottom of a test tube of unclotted blood. Rapidly descending cells (an elevated sed rate) indicate inflammation in the body. Although the sed rate measurement is a helpful diagnostic tool, it alone does not confirm polymyalgia rheumatica. An abnormal result indicates only that tissue is inflamed, but this is also a symptom of many forms of arthritis and other rheumatic diseases.

Before making a diagnosis of polymyalgia rheumatica, the doctor may order additional tests. For example, the C-reactive protein test is another common means of measuring inflammation. There is also a common test for rheumatoid factor, an antibody (a protein made by the immune system) that is sometimes found in the blood of people with rheumatoid arthritis. Although polymyalgia rheumatica and rheumatoid arthritis share many symptoms, those with polymyalgia rheumatica rarely test positive for rheumatoid factor. Therefore, a positive rheumatoid factor might suggest a diagnosis of rheumatoid arthritis instead of polymyalgia rheumatica.

As with polymyalgia rheumatica, a diagnosis of giant cell arteritis is based largely on symptoms and a physical examination. The exam may reveal that the temporal artery is inflamed and tender to the touch, and that it has a reduced pulse.

When a doctor suspects giant cell arteritis a temporal artery biopsy is typically ordered. In this procedure, a small section of the artery is removed through an incision in the skin over the temple area and examined under a microscope. A biopsy that is positive for giant cell arteritis will show abnormal cells in the artery walls. Some patients showing symptoms of giant cell arteritis will have negative biopsy results. In such cases, the doctor may suggest a second biopsy.

How Are They Treated?

The treatment of choice for both polymyalgia rheumatica and giant cell arteritis is corticosteroid medication, such as prednisone.

Polymyalgia rheumatica responds to a low daily dose of corticosteroids that is increased as needed until symptoms disappear. At this point, the doctor may gradually reduce the dosage to determine the lowest amount needed to alleviate symptoms. Most patients can discontinue medication after 6 months to 2 years. If symptoms recur, corticosteroid treatment is required again.

Nonsteroidal anti-inflammatory drugs (NSAIDs), such as aspirin and ibuprofen, also may be used to treat polymyalgia rheumatica. The medication must be taken daily, and long-term use may cause stomach irritation. For most patients, NSAIDs alone are not enough to relieve symptoms.

Even without treatment, polymyalgia rheumatica usually disappears in 1 to several years. With treatment, however, symptoms disappear quickly, usually in 24 to 48 hours. If corticosteroids don't bring improvement, the doctor is likely to consider other possible diagnoses.

Giant cell arteritis is treated with high doses of corticosteroids. If not treated promptly, the condition carries a small but definite risk of blindness, so corticosteroids should be started as soon as possible, perhaps even before confirming the diagnosis with a temporal artery biopsy.

As with polymyalgia rheumatica, the symptoms of giant cell arteritis quickly disappear with treatment; however, high doses of corticosteroids are typically maintained for 1 month.

Once symptoms disappear and the sed rate is normal, there is much less risk of blindness. At that point, the doctor can begin to gradually reduce the corticosteroid dose.

In both polymyalgia rheumatica and giant cell arteritis, an increase in symptoms may develop when the corticosteroid dose is reduced to lower levels. The doctor may need to hold the lower dose for a longer period of time or even modestly increase it again, temporarily, to control the symptoms. Once the symptoms are in remission and the corticosteroid has been discontinued for several months, recurrence is less common.

Whether taken on a long-term basis for polymyalgia rheumatica or for a shorter period for giant cell arteritis, corticosteroids carry a risk of side effects. Although long-term use and/or higher doses carry the greatest risk, people taking the drug at any dose or for any length of time should be aware of the potential side effects, which include:

- fluid retention and weight gain

- rounding of the face

- delayed wound healing

- bruising easily

- diabetes

- myopathy (muscle wasting)

- glaucoma

- increased blood pressure

- decreased calcium absorption in the bones, which can lead to osteoporosis

- irritation of the stomach

- increase in infections.

People taking corticosteroids may have some side effects or none at all. Anyone who experiences side effects should report them to his or her doctor. When the medication is stopped, the side effects disappear. Because corticosteroid drugs reduce the body's natural production of corticosteroid hormones, which are necessary for the body to function properly, it is important not to stop taking the medication unless instructed by a doctor to do so. The patient and doctor must work together to gradually reduce the medication.

What Is the Outlook?

Most people with polymyalgia rheumatica and giant cell arteritis lead productive, active lives. The duration of drug treatment differs by patient. Once treatment is discontinued, polymyalgia may recur; but once again, symptoms respond rapidly to prednisone. When properly treated, giant cell arteritis rarely recurs.

Chapter 66

Primary Biliary Cirrhosis

What Is Primary Biliary Cirrhosis?

Primary biliary cirrhosis is a chronic, or long lasting, disease that causes the small bile ducts in the liver to become inflamed and damaged and ultimately disappear.

The bile ducts carry a fluid called bile from the liver to the gallbladder, where it is stored. When food enters the stomach after a meal, the gallbladder contracts, and the bile ducts carry bile to the duodenum, the first part of the small intestine, for use in digestion. The liver makes bile, which is made up of bile acids, cholesterol, fats, and fluids. Bile helps the body absorb fats, cholesterol, and fat-soluble vitamins. Bile also carries cholesterol, toxins, and waste products to the intestines, where the body removes them. When chronic inflammation, or swelling, damages the bile ducts, bile and toxic wastes build up in the liver, damaging liver tissue.

This damage to the liver tissue can lead to cirrhosis, a condition in which the liver slowly deteriorates and is unable to function normally. In cirrhosis, scar tissue replaces healthy liver tissue, partially blocking the flow of blood through the liver.

The liver is the body's largest internal organ. The liver is called the body's metabolic factory because of the important role it plays in metabolism—the way cells change food into energy after food is

This chapter includes text excerpted from "Primary Biliary Cirrhosis," National Institute of Diabetes and Digestive and Kidney Diseases (NIDDK), April 2014.

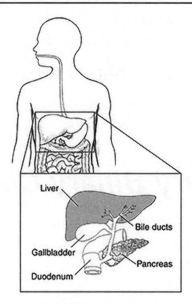

Figure 66.1. *Primary Biliary Cirrhosis*

Primary biliary cirrhosis causes the small bile ducts in the liver to become inflamed and damaged and ultimately disappear.

digested and absorbed into the blood. The liver has many functions, including

- taking up, storing, and processing nutrients from food—including fat, sugar, and protein—and delivering them to the rest of the body when needed

- making new proteins, such as clotting factors and immune factors

- producing bile

- removing waste products the kidneys cannot remove, such as fats, cholesterol, toxins, and medications

A healthy liver is necessary for survival. The liver can regenerate most of its own cells when they become damaged. However, if injury to the liver is too severe or long lasting, regeneration is incomplete, and the liver creates scar tissue. Scarring of the liver may lead to cirrhosis.

The buildup of scar tissue that causes cirrhosis is usually a slow and gradual process. In the early stages of cirrhosis, the liver continues to function. However, as cirrhosis gets worse and scar tissue replaces more healthy tissue, the liver will begin to fail. Chronic liver failure, which is also called end-stage liver disease, progresses over months, years, or even decades. With end-stage liver disease, the liver can no longer perform important functions or effectively replace damaged cells.

Primary biliary cirrhosis usually occurs between the ages of 30 and 65 and affects women more often than men.

What Causes Primary Biliary Cirrhosis?

The causes of primary biliary cirrhosis are unknown. Most research suggests it is an autoimmune disease. The immune system protects people from infection by identifying and destroying bacteria, viruses, and other potentially harmful foreign substances. An autoimmune disease is a disorder in which the body's immune system attacks the body's own cells and organs. In primary biliary cirrhosis, the immune system attacks the small bile ducts in the liver.

Genetics, or inherited genes, can make a person more likely to develop primary biliary cirrhosis. Primary biliary cirrhosis is more common in people who have a parent or sibling—particularly an identical twin—with the disease. In people who are genetically more likely to develop primary biliary cirrhosis, environmental factors may trigger or worsen the disease, including

- exposure to toxic chemicals
- smoking
- infections

Genetics can also make some people more likely to develop other autoimmune diseases, such as

- autoimmune hepatitis, a disease in which the body's immune system attacks liver cells
- Sjögren syndrome, a condition in which the immune system attacks the glands that produce tears and saliva
- autoimmune thyroid dysfunctions, conditions in which the immune system attacks the thyroid gland

What Are the Symptoms of Primary Biliary Cirrhosis?

The first and most common symptoms of primary biliary cirrhosis are

- fatigue, or feeling tired

- itching skin, and darkened skin in itching areas due to scratching

- dry eyes and mouth

Some people may have jaundice, a condition that causes the skin and whites of the eyes to turn yellow. Healthcare providers diagnose up to 60 percent of people with primary biliary cirrhosis before symptoms begin. Routine blood tests showing abnormal liver enzyme levels may lead a healthcare provider to suspect that a person without symptoms has primary biliary cirrhosis.

What Are the Complications of Primary Biliary Cirrhosis?

Most complications of primary biliary cirrhosis are related to cirrhosis and start after primary biliary cirrhosis progresses to cirrhosis. In some cases, portal hypertension and esophageal varices may develop before cirrhosis.

Portal hypertension. The portal vein carries blood from the stomach, intestines, spleen, gallbladder, and pancreas to the liver. In cirrhosis, scar tissue partially blocks the normal flow of blood, which increases the pressure in the portal vein. This condition is called portal hypertension. Portal hypertension is a common complication of cirrhosis. This condition may lead to other complications, such as

- edema—swelling due to a buildup of fluid—in the feet, ankles, or legs, and ascites—a buildup of fluid in the abdomen

- enlarged blood vessels, called varices, in the esophagus, stomach, or both

- an enlarged spleen, called splenomegaly

- mental confusion due to a buildup of toxins that are ordinarily removed by the liver, a condition called hepatic encephalopathy

Edema and ascites. Liver failure causes fluid buildup that results in edema and ascites. Ascites can lead to spontaneous bacterial peritonitis, a serious infection that requires immediate medical attention.

Varices. Portal hypertension may cause enlarged blood vessels in the esophagus, stomach, or both. These enlarged blood vessels, called esophageal or gastric varices, cause the vessel walls to become thin and blood pressure to increase, making the blood vessels more likely to burst. If they burst, serious bleeding can occur in the esophagus or upper stomach, requiring immediate medical attention.

Splenomegaly. Portal hypertension may cause the spleen to enlarge and retain white blood cells and platelets, reducing the numbers of these cells and platelets in the blood. A low platelet count may be the first evidence that a person has developed cirrhosis.

Hepatic encephalopathy. A failing liver cannot remove toxins from the blood, so they eventually accumulate in the brain. The buildup of toxins in the brain is called hepatic encephalopathy. This condition can decrease mental function and cause stupor and even coma. Stupor is an unconscious, sleeplike state from which a person can only be aroused briefly by a strong stimulus, such as a sharp pain. Coma is an unconscious, sleeplike state from which a person cannot be aroused. Signs of decreased mental function include

- confusion
- personality changes
- memory loss
- trouble concentrating
- a change in sleep habits

Metabolic bone diseases. Some people with cirrhosis develop a metabolic bone disease, which is a disorder of bone strength usually caused by abnormalities of vitamin D, bone mass, bone structure, or minerals, such as calcium and phosphorous. Osteopenia is a condition in which the bones become less dense, making them weaker. When bone loss becomes more severe, the condition is referred to as osteoporosis. People with these conditions are more likely to develop bone fractures.

Gallstones and bile duct stones. If cirrhosis prevents bile from flowing freely to and from the gallbladder, the bile hardens into gallstones. Symptoms of gallstones include abdominal pain and recurrent bacterial cholangitis—irritated or infected bile ducts. Stones may also form in and block the bile ducts, causing pain, jaundice, and bacterial cholangitis.

Steatorrhea. Steatorrhea is a condition in which the body cannot absorb fat, causing a buildup of fat in the stool and loose, greasy, and foul-smelling bowel movements. Steatorrhea may be caused by impairment of bile delivery to the small intestine or by the pancreas not producing enough digestive enzymes.

Liver cancer. Liver cancer is common in people with cirrhosis. Liver cancer has a high mortality rate. Current treatments are limited and only fully successful if a healthcare provider detects the cancer early, before the tumor is too large. For this reason, healthcare providers should check people with cirrhosis for signs of liver cancer every 6 to 12 months. Healthcare providers use blood tests, ultrasound, or both to check for signs of liver cancer.

How Is Primary Biliary Cirrhosis Diagnosed?

A healthcare provider may use the following tests to diagnose primary biliary cirrhosis:

- a medical and family history
- a physical exam
- blood tests
- imaging tests
- a liver biopsy

A healthcare provider usually bases a diagnosis of primary biliary cirrhosis on two out of three of the following criteria:

- a blood test showing elevated liver enzymes
- a blood test showing the presence of anti-mitochondrial antibodies (AMA)
- a liver biopsy showing signs of the disease

How Is Primary Biliary Cirrhosis Treated?

Treatment for primary biliary cirrhosis depends on how early a healthcare provider diagnoses the disease and whether complications are present. In the early stages of primary biliary cirrhosis, treatment can slow the progression of liver damage to cirrhosis. In the early stages of cirrhosis, the goals of treatment are to slow the progression of tissue scarring in the liver and prevent complications. As cirrhosis progresses, a person may need additional treatments and hospitalization to manage complications.

When Is a Liver Transplant Considered for Primary Biliary Cirrhosis?

A healthcare provider may consider a liver transplant when cirrhosis leads to liver failure or treatment for complications is ineffective. Liver transplantation is surgery to remove a diseased or an injured liver and replace it with a healthy liver or part of a liver from another person, called a donor.

Chapter 67

Psoriasis

What Is Psoriasis?

Psoriasis is a chronic (long-lasting) skin disease of scaling and inflammation that affects greater than 3.1 percent of the U.S. population, or more than 6.7 million adults. Although the disease occurs in all age groups, it primarily affects adults. It appears about equally in males and females.

Psoriasis occurs when skin cells quickly rise from their origin below the surface of the skin and pile up on the surface before they have a chance to mature. Usually this movement (also called turnover) takes about a month, but in psoriasis it may occur in only a few days.

In its typical form, psoriasis results in patches of thick, red (inflamed) skin covered with silvery scales. These patches, which are sometimes referred to as plaques, usually itch or feel sore. They most often occur on the elbows, knees, other parts of the legs, scalp, lower back, face, palms, and soles of the feet, but they can occur on skin anywhere on the body. The disease may also affect the fingernails, the toenails, and the soft tissues of the genitals, and inside the mouth.

How Does Psoriasis Affect Quality of Life?

Individuals with psoriasis may experience significant physical discomfort and some disability. Itching and pain can interfere with basic

This chapter includes text excerpted from "Psoriasis," National Institute of Arthritis and Musculoskeletal and Skin Diseases (NIAMS), July 2016.

functions, such as self-care, walking, and sleep. Plaques on hands and feet can prevent individuals from working at certain occupations, playing some sports, and caring for family members or a home. The frequency of medical care is costly and can interfere with an employment or school schedule. People with moderate to severe psoriasis may feel self-conscious about their appearance. Psychological distress can lead to depression and social isolation.

What Causes Psoriasis?

Psoriasis is a skin disorder driven by the immune system, especially involving a type of white blood cell called a T cell. Normally, T cells help protect the body against infection and disease. In the case of psoriasis, T cells are put into action by mistake and become so active that they trigger other immune responses, which lead to inflammation and to rapid turnover of skin cells.

In many cases, there is a family history of psoriasis. Researchers have studied a large number of families affected by psoriasis and identified genes linked to the disease.

People with psoriasis may notice that there are times when their skin worsens, called flares, then improves. Conditions that may cause flares include infections, stress, and changes in climate that dry the skin. Also, certain medicines may trigger an outbreak or worsen the disease. Sometimes people who have psoriasis notice that lesions will appear where the skin has experienced trauma. The trauma could be from a cut, scratch, sunburn, or infection.

How Is Psoriasis Diagnosed?

Occasionally, doctors may find it difficult to diagnose psoriasis, because it often looks like other skin diseases. It may be necessary to confirm a diagnosis by examining a small skin sample under a microscope.

There are several forms of psoriasis. Some of these include:

- **Plaque psoriasis.** Skin lesions are red at the base and covered by silvery scales.

- **Guttate psoriasis.** Small, drop-shaped lesions appear on the trunk, limbs, and scalp. Guttate psoriasis is most often triggered by upper respiratory infections (for example, a sore throat caused by streptococcal bacteria).

- **Pustular psoriasis.** Blisters of noninfectious pus appear on the skin. Attacks of pustular psoriasis may be triggered by medications, infections, stress, or exposure to certain chemicals.

- **Inverse psoriasis.** Smooth, red patches occur in the folds of the skin near the genitals, under the breasts, or in the armpits. The symptoms may be worsened by friction and sweating.

- **Erythrodermic psoriasis.** Widespread reddening and scaling of the skin may be a reaction to severe sunburn or to taking corticosteroids (cortisone) or other medications. It can also be caused by a prolonged period of increased activity of psoriasis that is poorly controlled. Erythrodermic psoriasis can be very serious and requires immediate medical attention.

Another condition in which people may experience psoriasis is **psoriatic arthritis.** This is a form of arthritis that produces the joint inflammation common in arthritis and the lesions common in psoriasis. The joint inflammation and the skin lesions don't necessarily have to occur at the same time.

How Is Psoriasis Treated?

Doctors generally treat psoriasis in steps based on the severity of the disease, size of the areas involved, type of psoriasis, where the psoriasis is located, and the patient's response to initial treatments. Treatment can include:

- medicines applied to the skin (topical treatment)
- light treatment (phototherapy)
- medicines by mouth or injection (systemic therapy)

Chapter 68

Sarcoidosis

What Is Sarcoidosis?

Sarcoidosis is a disease of unknown cause that leads to inflammation. This disease affects your body's organs.

Normally, your immune system defends your body against foreign or harmful substances. For example, it sends special cells to protect organs that are in danger.

These cells release chemicals that recruit other cells to isolate and destroy the harmful substance. Inflammation occurs during this process. Once the harmful substance is gone, the cells and the inflammation go away.

In people who have sarcoidosis, the inflammation doesn't go away. Instead, some of the immune system cells cluster to form lumps called granulomas in various organs in your body.

What Causes Sarcoidosis?

The cause of sarcoidosis isn't known. More than one factor may play a role in causing the disease.

Some researchers think that sarcoidosis develops if your immune system responds to a trigger, such as bacteria, viruses, dust, or chemicals.

This chapter includes text excerpted from "Sarcoidosis," National Heart, Lung, and Blood Institute (NHLBI), June 14, 2013.

Normally, your immune system defends your body against foreign or harmful substances. For example, it sends special cells to protect organs that are in danger.

These cells release chemicals that recruit other cells to isolate and destroy the harmful substance. Inflammation occurs during this process. Once the harmful substance is gone, the cells and the inflammation go away.

In people who have sarcoidosis, the inflammation doesn't go away. Instead, some of the immune system cells cluster to form lumps called granulomas in various organs in your body.

Genetics also may play a role in sarcoidosis. Researchers believe that sarcoidosis occurs if:

- you have a certain gene or genes that raise your risk for the disease, and

- you're exposed to something that triggers your immune system

Triggers may vary depending on your genetic makeup. Certain genes may influence which organs are affected and the severity of your symptoms.

Who Is at Risk for Sarcoidosis?

Sarcoidosis affects people of all ages and races. However, it's more common among African Americans and Northern Europeans. In the United States, the disease affects African Americans somewhat more often and more severely than Whites.

Studies have shown that sarcoidosis tends to vary amongst ethnic groups. For example, eye problems related to the disease are more common in Japanese people.

Lofgren syndrome, a type of sarcoidosis, is more common in people of European descent. Lofgren syndrome may involve fever, enlarged lymph nodes, arthritis (usually in the ankles), and/or erythema nodosum. Erythema nodosum is a rash of red or reddish-purple bumps on your ankles and shins. The rash may be warm and tender to the touch.

Sarcoidosis is somewhat more common in women than in men. The disease usually develops between the ages of 20 and 50. People who have a family history of sarcoidosis also are at higher risk for the disease.

What Are the Signs and Symptoms of Sarcoidosis?

Many people who have sarcoidosis have no signs or symptoms or mild ones. Often, the disease is found when a chest X-ray is done for another reason (for example, to diagnose pneumonia).

The signs and symptoms of sarcoidosis vary depending on which organs are affected. Signs and symptoms also may vary depending on your gender, age, and ethnic background.

In both adults and children, sarcoidosis most often affects the lungs. If granulomas (inflamed lumps) form in your lungs, you may wheeze, cough, feel short of breath, or have chest pain. Or, you may have no symptoms at all.

Some people who have sarcoidosis feel very tired, uneasy, or depressed. Night sweats and weight loss are common symptoms of the disease.

Common signs and symptoms in children are fatigue (tiredness), loss of appetite, weight loss, bone and joint pain, and anemia.

Children who are younger than 4 years old may have a distinct form of sarcoidosis. It may cause enlarged lymph nodes in the chest (which can be seen on chest X-ray pictures), skin lesions, and eye swelling or redness.

How Is Sarcoidosis Diagnosed?

Your doctor will diagnose sarcoidosis based on your medical history, a physical exam, and test results. He or she will look for granulomas (inflamed lumps) in your organs. Your doctor also will try to rule out other possible causes of your symptoms.

How Is Sarcoidosis Treated?

Not everyone who has sarcoidosis needs treatment. Sometimes the disease goes away on its own. Whether you need treatment and what type of treatment you need depend on your signs and symptoms, which organs are affected, and whether those organs are working well.

If the disease affects certain organs—such as your eyes, heart, or brain—you'll need treatment even if you don't have any symptoms.

In either case, whether you have symptoms or not, you should see your doctor for ongoing care. He or she will want to check to make sure that the disease isn't damaging your organs. For example, you may need routine lung function tests to make sure that your lungs are working well.

If the disease isn't worsening, your doctor may watch you closely to see whether the disease goes away on its own. If the disease does start to get worse, your doctor can prescribe treatment.

The goals of treatment include:

• relieving symptoms

- improving organ function
- controlling inflammation and reducing the size of granulomas (inflamed lumps)
- preventing pulmonary fibrosis (lung scarring) if your lungs are affected

Your doctor may prescribe topical treatments and/or medicines to treat the disease.

Chapter 69

Scleroderma

What Is Scleroderma?

Derived from the Greek words *"sklerosis,"* meaning hardness, and *"derma,"* meaning skin, scleroderma literally means "hard skin." Although it is often referred to as if it were a single disease, scleroderma is really a symptom of a group of diseases that involve the abnormal growth of connective tissue, which supports the skin and internal organs. It is sometimes used, therefore, as an umbrella term for these disorders. In some forms of scleroderma, hard, tight skin is the extent of this abnormal process. In other forms, however, the problem goes much deeper, affecting blood vessels and internal organs, such as the heart, lungs, and kidneys.

Scleroderma is called both a rheumatic disease and a connective tissue disease. The term rheumatic disease refers to a group of conditions characterized by inflammation or pain in the muscles, joints, or fibrous tissue. A connective tissue disease is one that affects tissues such as skin, tendons, and cartilage.

What Are the Different Types of Scleroderma?

The group of diseases we call scleroderma falls into two main classes: localized scleroderma and systemic sclerosis. (Localized

This chapter includes text excerpted from "Scleroderma," National Institute of Arthritis and Musculoskeletal and Skin Diseases (NIAMS), February 2015.

diseases affect only certain parts of the body; systemic diseases can affect the whole body.)

What Causes Scleroderma?

Although scientists don't know exactly what causes scleroderma, they are certain that people cannot catch it from or transmit it to others. Studies of twins suggest it is also not inherited. Scientists suspect that scleroderma comes from several factors that may include:

Abnormal immune or inflammatory activity: Like many other rheumatic disorders, scleroderma is believed to be an autoimmune disease. An autoimmune disease is one in which the immune system, for unknown reasons, turns against one's own body.

In scleroderma, the immune system is thought to stimulate cells called fibroblasts so they produce too much collagen. The collagen forms thick connective tissue that builds up within the skin and internal organs and can interfere with their functioning. Blood vessels and joints can also be affected.

Genetic makeup: Although genes seem to put certain people at risk for scleroderma and play a role in its course, the disease is not passed from parent to child like some genetic diseases.

Environmental triggers: Research suggests that exposure to some environmental factors may trigger scleroderma-like disease (which is not actually scleroderma) in people who are genetically predisposed to it. Suspected triggers include viral infections, certain adhesive and coating materials, and organic solvents such as vinyl chloride or trichloroethylene. But no environmental agent has been shown to cause scleroderma. In the past, some people believed that silicone breast implants might have been a factor in developing connective tissue diseases such as scleroderma. But several studies have not shown evidence of a connection.

Hormones: Women develop scleroderma more often than men. Scientists suspect that hormonal differences between women and men play a part in the disease. However, the role of estrogen or other female hormones has not been proven.

Who Gets Scleroderma?

Although scleroderma is more common in women, the disease also occurs in men and children. It affects people of all races and ethnic groups. However, there are some patterns by disease type. For example:

- **Localized forms** of scleroderma are more common in people of European descent than in African Americans. Morphea usually appears between the ages of 20 and 40, and linear scleroderma usually occurs in children or teenagers.

- **Systemic scleroderma,** whether limited or diffuse, typically occurs in people from 30 to 50 years old. It affects more women of African American than European descent.

Because scleroderma can be hard to diagnose and it overlaps with or resembles other diseases, scientists can only estimate how many cases there actually are. It is estimated that 49,000 adults in the United States have systemic sclerosis.

For some people, scleroderma (particularly the localized forms) is fairly mild and resolves with time. But for others, living with the disease and its effects day to day has a significant impact on their quality of life.

How Is Scleroderma Diagnosed?

Depending on your particular symptoms, a diagnosis of scleroderma may be made by:

- A **general internist.**

- A **dermatologist,** who specializes in treating diseases of the skin, hair, and nails.

- An **orthopaedist,** who treats bone and joint disorders.

- A **pulmonologist,** who is trained to treat lung problems.

- A **rheumatologist,** who specializes in treating musculoskeletal disorders and rheumatic diseases.

A diagnosis of scleroderma is based largely on the medical history and findings from the physical exam. To make a diagnosis, your doctor will ask you a lot of questions about what has happened to you over time and about any symptoms you may be experiencing. Are you having a problem with heartburn or swallowing? Are you often tired or achy? Do your hands turn white in response to anxiety or cold temperatures?

Once your doctor has taken a thorough medical history, he or she will perform a physical exam.

How Is Scleroderma Treated?

Because scleroderma can affect many different organs and organ systems, you may have several different doctors involved in your care. Typically, care will be managed by a rheumatologist (a doctor specializing in treatment of musculoskeletal disorders and rheumatic diseases). Your rheumatologist may refer you to other specialists, depending on the specific problems you are having. For example, you may see a dermatologist for the treatment of skin symptoms, a nephrologist for kidney complications, a cardiologist for heart complications, a gastroenterologist for problems of the digestive tract, and a pulmonary specialist for lung involvement.

In addition to doctors, professionals such as nurse practitioners, physician assistants, physical or occupational therapists, psychologists, and social workers may play a role in your care. Dentists, orthodontists, and even speech therapists can treat oral complications that arise from thickening of tissues in and around the mouth and on the face.

How Can Scleroderma Affect My Life?

Having a chronic disease can affect almost every aspect of your life, from family relationships to holding a job. For people with scleroderma, there may be other concerns about appearance or even the ability to dress, bathe, or handle the most basic daily tasks. Here are some areas in which scleroderma could intrude.

Appearance and self-esteem: Aside from the initial concerns about health and longevity, people with scleroderma quickly become concerned with how the disease will affect their appearance. Thick, hardened skin can be difficult to accept, particularly on the face. Systemic scleroderma may result in facial changes that eventually cause the opening to the mouth to become smaller and the upper lip to virtually disappear. Linear scleroderma may leave its mark on the forehead. Although these problems can't always be prevented, their effects may be minimized with proper treatment. Also, special cosmetics—and in some cases plastic surgery—can help conceal scleroderma's damage.

Caring for yourself: Tight, hard connective tissue in the hands can make it difficult to do what were once simple tasks, such as brushing your teeth and hair, pouring a cup of coffee, using a knife and fork, unlocking a door, or buttoning a jacket. If you have trouble using your hands, consult an occupational therapist, who can recommend new ways of doing things or devices to make tasks easier. Devices as simple as Velcro fasteners and built-up brush handles can help you be more independent.

Family relationships: Spouses, children, parents, and siblings may have trouble understanding why you don't have the energy to keep house, drive to soccer practice, prepare meals, or hold a job the way you used to. If your condition isn't that visible, they may even suggest you are just being lazy. On the other hand, they may be overly concerned and eager to help you, not allowing you to do the things you are able to do or giving up their own interests and activities to be with you. It's important to learn as much about your form of the disease as you can and to share any information you have with your family. Involving them in counseling or a support group may also help them better understand the disease and how they can help you.

Sexual relations: Sexual relationships can be affected when systemic scleroderma enters the picture. For men, the disease's effects on the blood vessels can lead to problems achieving an erection. For women, damage to the moisture-producing glands can cause vaginal dryness that makes intercourse painful. People of either sex may find they have difficulty moving the way they once did. They may be self-conscious about their appearance or afraid that their sexual partner will no longer find them attractive. With communication between partners, good medical care, and perhaps counseling, many of these changes can be overcome or at least worked around.

How Can I Play a Role in My Healthcare?

Although your doctors direct your treatment, you are the one who must take your medicine regularly, follow your doctor's advice, and report any problems promptly. In other words, the relationship between you and your doctors is a partnership, and you are the most important partner. Here's what you can do to make the most of this important role.

- Get educated.
- Seek support.
- Assemble a healthcare team.
- Be patient.

- Speak up.
- Don't accept depression.
- Learn coping skills.
- Ask the experts.

Chapter 70

Sjögren Syndrome

What Is Sjögren Syndrome?

Sjögren syndrome is an autoimmune disease; that is, a disease in which the immune system turns against the body's own cells. Normally, the immune system works to protect us from disease by destroying harmful invading organisms like viruses and bacteria. In the case of Sjögren syndrome, disease-fighting cells attack various organs, most notably the glands that produce tears and saliva. Damage to these glands causes a reduction in both the quantity and quality of their secretions. This results in symptoms that include dry eyes and dry mouth.

Sjögren syndrome is also a rheumatic disease. These are diseases characterized by inflammation (signs include redness or heat, swelling, and symptoms such as pain) and loss of function of one or more connecting or supporting structures of the body. They especially affect joints, tendons, ligaments, bones, and muscles.

Classifications of Sjögren Syndrome

Sjögren syndrome is classified as either primary or secondary. The primary form occurs in people who do not have other rheumatic disesaes. The secondary form occurs in people who already have another rheumatic disease, most commonly rheumatoid arthritis (RA) or

This chapter includes text excerpted from "Sjögren's Syndrome," National Institute of Arthritis and Musculoskeletal and Skin Diseases (NIAMS), April 2016.

systemic lupus erythematosus (SLE). These people then develop dry eyes or dry mouth.

What Are the Symptoms of Sjögren Syndrome?

Sjögren syndrome can cause many symptoms. The main ones are:

- **Dry eyes.** Eyes affected by Sjögren syndrome may burn or itch. Some people say it feels like they have sand in their eyes. Others have trouble with blurry vision, or are bothered by bright light, especially fluorescent lighting.

- **Dry mouth.** Dry mouth may feel chalky or like your mouth is full of cotton. It may be difficult to swallow, speak, or taste. Because you lack the protective effects of saliva, you may develop more dental decay (cavities) and mouth infections.

Sjögren syndrome can also affect other parts of the body, causing symptoms such as:

- multiple sites of joint and muscle pain
- prolonged dry skin
- skin rashes on the extremities
- chronic dry cough
- vaginal dryness
- numbness or tingling in the extremities
- prolonged fatigue that interferes with daily life

Who Gets Sjögren Syndrome?

Sjögren syndrome can affect people of either sex and of any age, but most cases occur in women. The average age for onset is late forties, but in rare cases, Sjögren syndrome is diagnosed in children.

What Causes Sjögren Syndrome?

Researchers think Sjögren syndrome is caused by a combination of genetic and environmental factors. Several different genes appear to be involved, but scientists are not certain exactly which ones are linked to the disease, because different genes seem to play a role in different people.

Scientists think that the trigger may be a viral or bacterial infection. The possibility that the endocrine and nervous systems play a role in the disease is also under investigation.

How Is Sjögren Syndrome Diagnosed?

Your doctor will diagnose Sjögren syndrome based on your medical history, a physical exam, and results from clinical or laboratory tests. During the exam, your doctor will check for clinical signs of Sjögren syndrome, such as indications of mouth dryness or signs of other connective tissue diseases.

Depending on what your doctor finds during the history and exam, he or she may want to perform some tests or refer you to a specialist to establish the diagnosis of Sjögren syndrome and/or to see how severe the problem is and whether the disease is affecting other parts of the body as well.

Because there are many causes of dry eyes and dry mouth (including many common medications, other diseases, or previous treatment such as radiation of the head or neck), the doctor needs a thorough history from the patient, and additional tests to see whether other parts of the body are affected.

Blood tests can determine the presence of antibodies common in Sjogren syndrome, including anti-SSA and anti-SSB antibodies or rheumatoid factor. Other tests can identify decreases in tear and saliva production. Biopsy of the saliva glands and other specialized tests can also help to confirm the diagnosis.

What Type of Doctor Diagnoses and Treats Sjögren Syndrome?

Because the symptoms of Sjögren syndrome develop gradually and are similar to those of many other diseases, getting a diagnosis can take time. A person could see a number of doctors, any of whom could diagnose the disease and be involved in its treatment. These might include a rheumatologist (a doctor who specializes in diseases of the joints, muscles, and bones), a primary care physician, internist, ophthalmologist (eye specialist), otolaryngologist (ear, nose, and throat specialist), or another specialist. Usually a rheumatologist will coordinate treatment among a number of specialists.

How Is Sjögren Syndrome Treated?

Treatment can vary from person to person, depending on what parts of the body are affected.

Treatments for Dry Eyes

There are many treatments you can try or your doctor can prescribe for dry eyes. Here are some that might help:

- **Artificial tears.** Available by prescription or over the counter under many brand names, these products keep eyes moist by replacing natural tears. Artificial tears come in different thicknesses, so you may have to experiment to find the right one. Some drops contain preservatives that might irritate your eyes. Drops without preservatives usually don't bother the eyes.

- **Ointments.** Ointments are thicker than artificial tears. Because they moisturize and protect the eye for several hours, and may blur your vision, they are most effective during sleep.

- **Other therapies.** Other therapies such as plugging or blocking the tear ducts, anti-inflammatory medication, or surgery may be needed in more severe cases.

Treatments for Dry Mouth

There are many remedies for dry mouth. You can try some of them on your own. Your doctor may prescribe others. Here are some many people find useful:

- **Chewing gum and hard candy.** If your salivary glands still produce some saliva, you can stimulate them to make more by chewing gum or sucking on hard candy. However, gum and candy **must** be sugar-free, because dry mouth makes you extremely prone to progressive dental decay (cavities).

- **Water.** Take sips of water or another sugar-free, noncarbonated drink throughout the day to wet your mouth, especially when you are eating or talking. Note that drinking large amounts of liquid throughout the day will not make your mouth any less dry and will make you urinate more often. You should only take small sips of liquid, but not too often. If you sip liquids every few minutes, it may reduce or remove the mucus coating inside your mouth, increasing the feeling of dryness.

- **Lip balm.** You can soothe dry, cracked lips by using oil- or petroleum-based lip balm or lipstick. If your mouth hurts, your doctor may give you medicine in a mouth rinse, ointment, or gel to apply to the sore areas to control pain and inflammation.

- **Other therapies.** Other therapies such as saliva substitutes or medications that stimulate the salivary glands to produce saliva are sometimes indicated.

Treatments for Symptoms in Other Parts of the Body

If you have extraglandular involvement, that is, a problem that extends beyond the moisture-producing glands of your eyes and mouth, your doctor—or the appropriate specialist—may also treat those problems using nonsteroidal anti-inflammatory drugs (NSAIDs), or immune-modifying drugs.

Chapter 71

Thyroid Disease

Chapter Contents

Section 71.1

Graves Disease

This section includes text excerpted from "Graves' Disease,"
National Institute of Diabetes and Digestive and Kidney
Diseases (NIDDK), August 2012. Reviewed October 2016.

What Is Graves Disease?

Graves disease, also known as toxic diffuse goiter, is the most common cause of hyperthyroidism in the United States. Hyperthyroidism is a disorder that occurs when the thyroid gland makes more thyroid hormone than the body needs.

The Thyroid

The thyroid is a 2-inch-long, butterfly-shaped gland in the front of the neck below the larynx, or voice box. The thyroid makes two thyroid hormones, triiodothyronine (T3) and thyroxine (T4). T3 is made from T4 and is the more active hormone, directly affecting the tissues. Thyroid hormones circulate throughout the body in the bloodstream and act on virtually every tissue and cell in the body.

Thyroid hormones affect metabolism, brain development, breathing, heart and nervous system functions, body temperature, muscle strength, skin dryness, menstrual cycles, weight, and cholesterol levels. Hyperthyroidism causes many of the body's functions to speed up.

Thyroid hormone production is regulated by another hormone called thyroid-stimulating hormone (TSH), which is made by the pituitary gland in the brain. When thyroid hormone levels in the blood are low, the pituitary releases more TSH. When thyroid hormone levels are high, the pituitary responds by decreasing TSH production.

Autoimmune Disorder

Graves disease is an autoimmune disorder. Normally, the immune system protects the body from infection by identifying and destroying bacteria, viruses, and other potentially harmful foreign substances.

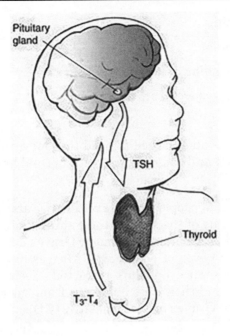

Figure 71.1. *Thyroid Gland*

The thyroid's production of thyroid hormones—T3 and T4—is regulated by thyroid-stimulating hormone (TSH), which is made by the pituitary gland.

But in autoimmune diseases, the immune system attacks the body's own cells and organs.

With Graves disease, the immune system makes an antibody called thyroid-stimulating immunoglobulin (TSI)—sometimes called TSH receptor antibody—that attaches to thyroid cells. TSI mimics TSH and stimulates the thyroid to make too much thyroid hormone. Sometimes the TSI antibody instead blocks thyroid hormone production, leading to conflicting symptoms that may make correct diagnosis more difficult.

What Are the Symptoms of Graves Disease?

People with Graves disease may have common symptoms of hyperthyroidism such as

- nervousness or irritability
- fatigue or muscle weakness
- heat intolerance

415

- trouble sleeping

- hand tremors

- rapid and irregular heartbeat

- frequent bowel movements or diarrhea

- weight loss

- goiter, which is an enlarged thyroid that may cause the neck to look swollen and can interfere with normal breathing and swallowing

A small number of people with Graves disease also experience thickening and reddening of the skin on their shins. This usually painless problem is called pretibial myxedema or Graves dermopathy.

In addition, the eyes of people with Graves disease may appear enlarged because their eyelids are retracted—seem pulled back into the eye sockets—and their eyes bulge out from the eye sockets. This condition is called Graves ophthalmopathy (GO).

What Is Graves Ophthalmopathy?

Go is a condition associated with Graves disease that occurs when cells from the immune system attack the muscles and other tissues around the eyes.

The result is inflammation and a buildup of tissue and fat behind the eye socket, causing the eyeballs to bulge out. Rarely, inflammation is severe enough to compress the optic nerve that leads to the eye, causing vision loss.

Other GO symptoms are

- dry, gritty, and irritated eyes

- puffy eyelids

- double vision

- light sensitivity

- pressure or pain in the eyes

- trouble moving the eyes

About 25 to 30 percent of people with Graves disease develop mild GO, and 2 to 5 percent develop severe GO. This eye condition usually lasts 1 to 2 years and often improves on its own.

GO can occur before, at the same time as, or after other symptoms of hyperthyroidism develop and may even occur in people whose thyroid function is normal. Smoking makes GO worse.

Who Is Likely to Develop Graves Disease?

Scientists cannot predict who will develop Graves disease. However, factors such as age, sex, heredity, and emotional and environmental stress are likely involved.

Graves disease usually occurs in people younger than age 40 and is seven to eight times more common in women than men. Women are most often affected between ages 30 and 60. And a person's chance of developing Graves disease increases if other family members have the disease.

Researchers have not been able to find a specific gene that causes the disease to be passed from parent to child. While scientists know some people inherit an immune system that can make antibodies against healthy cells, predicting who will be affected is difficult.

People with other autoimmune diseases have an increased chance of developing Graves disease. Conditions associated with Graves disease include type 1 diabetes, rheumatoid arthritis, and vitiligo—a disorder in which some parts of the skin are not pigmented.

How Is Graves Disease Diagnosed?

Healthcare providers can sometimes diagnose Graves disease based only on a physical examination and a medical history. Blood tests and other diagnostic tests, such as the following, then confirm the diagnosis.

TSH test. The ultrasensitive TSH test is usually the first test performed. This test detects even tiny amounts of TSH in the blood and is the most accurate measure of thyroid activity available.

T3 and T4 test. Another blood test used to diagnose Graves disease measures T3 and T4 levels. In making a diagnosis, healthcare providers look for below-normal levels of TSH, normal to elevated levels of T4, and elevated levels of T3.

Because the combination of low TSH and high T3 and T4 can occur with other thyroid problems, healthcare providers may order other tests to finalize the diagnosis. The following two tests use small, safe doses of radioactive iodine because the thyroid uses iodine to make thyroid hormone.

Radioactive iodine uptake test. This test measures the amount of iodine the thyroid collects from the bloodstream. High levels of iodine uptake can indicate Graves disease.

Thyroid scan. This scan shows how and where iodine is distributed in the thyroid. With Graves disease the entire thyroid is involved, so the iodine shows up throughout the gland. Other causes of hyperthyroidism such as nodules—small lumps in the gland—show a different pattern of iodine distribution.

TSI test. Healthcare providers may also recommend the TSI test, although this test usually isn't necessary to diagnose Graves disease. This test, also called a TSH antibody test, measures the level of TSI in the blood. Most people with Graves disease have this antibody, but people whose hyperthyroidism is caused by other conditions do not.

How Is Graves Disease Treated?

People with Graves disease have three treatment options: radioiodine therapy, medications, and thyroid surgery. Radioiodine therapy is the most common treatment for Graves disease in the United States. Graves disease is often diagnosed and treated by an endocrinologist—a doctor who specializes in the body's hormone- secreting glands.

Can Treatment for Graves Disease Affect Pregnancy?

Treatment for Graves disease can sometimes affect pregnancy. After treatment with surgery or radioactive iodine, TSI antibodies can still be present in the blood, even when thyroid levels are normal. If a pregnant woman has received either of these treatments prior to becoming pregnant, the antibodies she produces may travel across the placenta to the baby's bloodstream and stimulate the fetal thyroid.

A pregnant woman who has been treated with surgery or radioactive iodine should inform her healthcare provider so her baby can be monitored for thyroid-related problems later in the pregnancy. Pregnant women may safely be treated with anti-thyroid medications.

Eating, Diet, and Nutrition

Experts recommend that people eat a balanced diet to obtain most nutrients.

Iodine is an essential mineral for the thyroid. However, people with autoimmune thyroid disease may be sensitive to harmful side effects from iodine. Taking iodine drops or eating foods containing large amounts of iodine—such as seaweed, dulse, or kelp—may cause or worsen hyperthyroidism.

Women need more iodine when they are pregnant—about 250 micrograms a day—because the baby gets iodine from the mother's diet. In the United States, about 7 percent of pregnant women may not get enough iodine in their diet or through prenatal vitamins. Choosing iodized salt—salt supplemented with iodine—over plain salt and prenatal vitamins containing iodine will ensure this need is met.

To help ensure coordinated and safe care, people should discuss their use of dietary supplements, such as iodine, with their healthcare provider.

Section 71.2

Hashimoto Disease

This section includes text excerpted from "Hashimoto's Disease," National Institute of Diabetes and Digestive and Kidney Diseases (NIDDK), May 2014.

What Is Hashimoto Disease?

Hashimoto disease, also called chronic lymphocytic thyroiditis or autoimmune thyroiditis, is an autoimmune disease. An autoimmune disease is a disorder in which the body's immune system attacks the body's own cells and organs. Normally, the immune system protects the body from infection by identifying and destroying bacteria, viruses, and other potentially harmful foreign substances.

In Hashimoto disease, the immune system attacks the thyroid gland, causing inflammation and interfering with its ability to produce thyroid hormones. Large numbers of white blood cells called lymphocytes accumulate in the thyroid. Lymphocytes make the antibodies that start the autoimmune process.

Hashimoto disease often leads to reduced thyroid function, or hypothyroidism. Hypothyroidism is a disorder that occurs when the thyroid doesn't make enough thyroid hormone for the body's needs. Thyroid hormones regulate metabolism—the way the body uses energy—and affect nearly every organ in the body. Without enough thyroid hormone, many of the body's functions slow down. Hashimoto disease is the most common cause of hypothyroidism in the United States.

What Are the Symptoms of Hashimoto Disease?

Many people with Hashimoto disease have no symptoms at first. As the disease slowly progresses, the thyroid usually enlarges and may cause the front of the neck to look swollen. The enlarged thyroid, called a goiter, may create a feeling of fullness in the throat, though it is usually not painful. After many years, or even decades, damage to the thyroid causes it to shrink and the goiter to disappear.

Not everyone with Hashimoto disease develops hypothyroidism. For those who do, the hypothyroidism may be subclinical—mild and without symptoms, especially early in its course. With progression to hypothyroidism, people may have one or more of the following symptoms:

- fatigue

- weight gain

- cold intolerance

- joint and muscle pain

- constipation, or fewer than three bowel movements a week

- dry, thinning hair

- heavy or irregular menstrual periods and problems becoming pregnant

- depression

- memory problems

- a slowed heart rate

Who Is More Likely to Develop Hashimoto Disease?

Hashimoto disease is much more common in women than men. Although the disease often occurs in adolescent or young women, it more commonly appears between 30 and 50 years of age.

Hashimoto disease tends to run in families. Researchers are working to identify the gene or genes that cause the disease to be passed from one generation to the next.

Possible environmental factors are also being studied. For example, researchers have found that consuming too much iodine may inhibit thyroid hormone production in susceptible individuals. Chemicals released into the environment, such as pesticides, along with certain medications or viral infections may also contribute to autoimmune thyroid diseases.

People with other autoimmune diseases are more likely to develop Hashimoto disease. The opposite is also true—people with Hashimoto disease are more likely to develop other autoimmune diseases. These diseases include

- **vitiligo,** a condition in which some areas of the skin lose their natural color.

- **rheumatoid arthritis,** a disease that causes pain, swelling, stiffness, and loss of function in the joints when the immune system attacks the membrane lining the joints.

- **Addison disease,** in which the adrenal glands are damaged and cannot produce enough of certain critical hormones.

- **type 1 diabetes,** in which the pancreas is damaged and can no longer produce insulin, causing high blood glucose, also called blood sugar.

- **pernicious anemia,** a type of anemia caused by not having enough vitamin B12 in the body. In anemia, the number of red blood cells is less than normal, resulting in less oxygen carried to the body's cells and extreme fatigue.

- **celiac disease,** a form of gastrointestinal gluten sensitivity, an autoimmune disorder in which people cannot tolerate gluten because it will damage the lining of the small intestine and prevent adsorption of nutrients. Gluten is a protein found in wheat, rye, and barley and in some products.

- **autoimmune hepatitis,** or nonviral liver inflammation, a disease in which the immune system attacks liver cells.

How Is Hashimoto Disease Diagnosed?

Diagnosis begins with a physical exam and medical history. A goiter, nodules, or growths may be found during a physical exam, and symptoms may suggest hypothyroidism. Healthcare providers will then perform blood tests to confirm the diagnosis. A blood test involves drawing blood at a healthcare provider's office or a commercial facility and sending the sample to a lab for analysis. Diagnostic blood tests may include the

- TSH test
- T4 test
- Antithyroid antibody test
- Ultrasound
- CT scan

How Is Hashimoto Disease Treated?

Treatment generally depends on whether the thyroid is damaged enough to cause hypothyroidism. In the absence of hypothyroidism, some healthcare providers treat Hashimoto disease to reduce the size of the goiter. Others choose not to treat the disease and simply monitor their patients for disease progression.

Hashimoto disease, with or without hypothyroidism, is treated with synthetic thyroxine, which is man-made T4. Healthcare providers prefer to use synthetic T4, such as Synthroid, rather than synthetic T3, because T4 stays in the body longer, ensuring a steady supply of thyroid hormone throughout the day. The thyroid preparations made with animal thyroid are not considered as consistent as synthetic thyroid (Levothyroxine) and rarely prescribed today.

Healthcare providers routinely test the blood of patients taking synthetic thyroid hormone and adjust the dose as necessary, typically based on the result of the TSH test. Hypothyroidism can almost always be completely controlled with synthetic thyroxine, as long as the recommended dose is taken every day as instructed.

How Does Hashimoto Disease Affect Pregnant Women?

During pregnancy, hypothyroidism is usually caused by Hashimoto disease and occurs in three to five out of every 1,000 pregnancies. Uncontrolled hypothyroidism raises the chance of miscarriage, premature birth, stillbirth, and preeclampsia—a dangerous rise in blood pressure in late pregnancy.

Untreated hypothyroidism during pregnancy may also affect the baby's growth and brain development. Thyroid medications can help prevent these problems and are safe to take during pregnancy. Women with Hashimoto disease should discuss their condition with their healthcare provider before becoming pregnant.

Eating, Diet, and Nutrition

Iodine is an essential mineral for the thyroid. However, people with Hashimoto's disease may be sensitive to harmful side effects from iodine. Taking iodine drops or eating foods containing large amounts of iodine—such as seaweed, dulse, or kelp—may cause or worsen hypothyroidism.

Women need more iodine when they are pregnant—about 220 micrograms a day—because the baby gets iodine from the mother's diet. Women who are breastfeeding need about 290 micrograms a day. In the United States, about 7 percent of pregnant women may not get enough iodine in their diet or through prenatal vitamins. Pregnant women should choose iodized salt—salt supplemented with iodine— over plain salt and take prenatal vitamins containing iodine to ensure this need is met.

To help ensure coordinated and safe care, people should discuss their use of complementary and alternative medical practices, including their use of dietary supplements such as iodine, with their health-care provider.

Chapter 72

Uveitis

What Is Uveitis?

Uveitis is a general term describing a group of inflammatory diseases that produces swelling and destroys eye tissues. These diseases can slightly reduce vision or lead to severe vision loss.

The term "uveitis" is used because the diseases often affect a part of the eye called the uvea. Nevertheless, uveitis is not limited to the uvea. These diseases also affect the lens, retina, optic nerve, and vitreous, producing reduced vision or blindness.

Uveitis may be caused by problems or diseases occurring in the eye or it can be part of an inflammatory disease affecting other parts of the body.

It can happen at all ages and primarily affects people between 20 and 60 years old.

Uveitis can last for a short (acute) or a long (chronic) time. The severest forms of uveitis reoccur many times.

Eye care professionals may describe the disease more specifically as:

- Anterior uveitis

- Intermediate uveitis

- Posterior uveitis

- Panuveitis uveitis

This chapter includes text excerpted from "Uveitis," National Eye Institute (NEI), National Institutes of Health (NIH), August 2011. Reviewed October 2016.

Eye care professionals may also describe the disease as infectious or noninfectious uveitis.

What Is the Uvea and What Parts of the Eye Are Most Affected by Uveitis?

The uvea is the middle layer of the eye which contains much of the eye's blood vessels. This is one way that inflammatory cells can enter the eye. Located between the sclera, the eye's white outer coat, and the inner layer of the eye, called the retina, the uvea consists of the iris, ciliary body, and choroid:

Iris: The colored circle at the front of the eye. It defines eye color, secretes nutrients to keep the lens healthy, and controls the amount of light that enters the eye by adjusting the size of the pupil.

Ciliary Body: It is located between the iris and the choroid. It helps the eye focus by controlling the shape of the lens and it provides nutrients to keep the lens healthy.

Choroid: A thin, spongy network of blood vessels, which primarily provides nutrients to the retina.

Uveitis disrupts vision by primarily causing problems with the lens, retina, optic nerve, and vitreous:

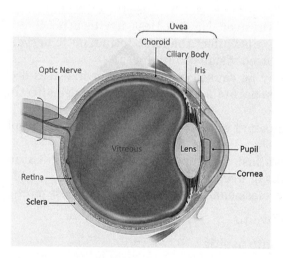

Figure 72.1. *Cross Section of the Eye*

Lens: Transparent tissue that allows light into the eye.

Retina: The layer of cells on the back, inside part of the eye that converts light into electrical signals sent to the brain.

426

Optic Nerve: A bundle of nerve fibers that transmits electrical signals from the retina to the brain.

Vitreous: The fluid filled space inside the eye.

Causes and Risk Factors of Uveitis

Uveitis is caused by inflammatory responses inside the eye.

Inflammation is the body's natural response to tissue damage, germs, or toxins. It produces swelling, redness, heat, and destroys tissues as certain white blood cells rush to the affected part of the body to contain or eliminate the insult.

Uveitis may be caused by:

- An attack from the body's own immune system (autoimmunity).

- Infections or tumors occurring within the eye or in other parts of the body.

- Bruises to the eye.

- Toxins that may penetrate the eye.

The disease will cause symptoms, such as decreased vision, pain, light sensitivity, and increased floaters. In many cases the cause is unknown.

Uveitis is usually classified by where it occurs in the eye.

What Is Anterior Uveitis?

Anterior uveitis occurs in the front of the eye. It is the most common form of uveitis, predominantly occurring in young and middle-aged people. Many cases occur in healthy people and may only affect one eye but some are associated with rheumatologic, skin, gastrointestinal, lung and infectious diseases.

What Is Intermediate Uveitis?

Intermediate uveitis is commonly seen in young adults. The center of the inflammation often appears in the vitreous. It has been linked to several disorders including, sarcoidosis and multiple sclerosis.

What Is Posterior Uveitis?

Posterior uveitis is the least common form of uveitis. It primarily occurs in the back of the eye, often involving both the retina and the choroid. It is often called choroditis or chorioretinitis. There are many infectious and non-infectious causes to posterior uveitis.

What Is Pan-Uveitis?

Pan-uveitis is a term used when all three major parts of the eye are affected by inflammation. Behcet disease is one of the most well-known forms of pan-uveitis and it greatly damages the retina.

Intermediate, posterior, and pan-uveitis are the most severe and highly recurrent forms of uveitis. They often cause blindness if left untreated.

Diseases Associated with Uveitis

Uveitis can be associated with many diseases including:

- AIDS
- Ankylosing spondylitis
- Behcet syndrome
- CMV retinitis
- Herpes zoster infection
- Histoplasmosis
- Kawasaki disease
- Multiple sclerosis
- Psoriasis
- Reactive arthritis
- Rheumatoid arthritis
- Sarcoidosis
- Syphilis
- Toxoplasmosis
- Tuberculosis
- Ulcerative colitis
- Vogt Koyanagi Harada disease

Symptoms and Detection of Uveitis

Uveitis can affect one or both eyes. Symptoms may develop rapidly and can include:

- blurred vision
- dark, floating spots in the vision (floaters)
- eye pain
- redness of the eye
- sensitivity to light (photophobia)

Anyone suffering eye pain, severe light sensitivity, and any change in vision should immediately be examined by an ophthalmologist.

The signs and symptoms of uveitis depend on the type of inflammation.

Acute anterior uveitis may occur in one or both eyes and in adults is characterized by eye pain, blurred vision, sensitivity to light, a small pupil, and redness.

Intermediate uveitis causes blurred vision and floaters. Usually it is not associated with pain.

Posterior uveitis can produce vision loss. This type of uveitis can only be detected during an eye examination.

How Is Uveitis Detected?

Diagnosis of uveitis includes a thorough examination and the recording of the patient's complete medical history. Laboratory tests may be done to rule out an infection or an autoimmune disorder.

A central nervous system evaluation will often be performed on patients with a subgroup of intermediate uveitis, called pars planitis, to determine whether they have multiple sclerosis which is often associated with pars planitis.

The eye exams used, include:

- *An Eye Chart or Visual Acuity Test:* This test measures whether a patient's vision has decreased.

- *A Funduscopic Exam:* The pupil is widened (dilated) with eye drops and then a light is shown through with an instrument called an ophthalmoscope to noninvasively inspect the back, inside part of the eye.

- Ocular Pressure: An instrument, such a tonometer or a tonopen, measures the pressure inside the eye. Drops that numb the eye may be used for this test.

- *A Slit Lamp Exam:* A slit lamp noninvasively inspects much of the eye. It can inspect the front and back parts of the eye and some lamps may be equipped with a tonometer to measure eye pressure. A dye called fluorescein, which makes blood vessels easier to see, may be added to the eye during the examination. The dye only temporarily stains the eye.

How Is Uveitis Treated?

Uveitis treatments primarily try to eliminate inflammation, alleviate pain, prevent further tissue damage, and restore any loss of vision. Treatments depend on the type of uveitis a patient displays. Some, such as using corticosteroid eye drops and injections around the eye or inside the eye, may exclusively target the eye whereas other treatments, such immunosuppressive agents taken by mouth, may be used when the disease is occurring in both eyes, particularly in the back of both eyes.

An eye care professional will usually prescribe steroidal anti-inflammatory medication that can be taken as eye drops, swallowed as a pill, injected around or into the eye, infused into the blood intravenously, or, released into the eye via a capsule that is surgically implanted inside the eye. Long-term steroid use may produce side effects such as stomach ulcers, osteoporosis (bone thinning), diabetes, cataracts, glaucoma, cardiovascular disease, weight gain, fluid retention, and Cushing syndrome. Usually other agents are started if it appears that patients need moderate or high doses of oral steroids for more than 3 months.

Other immunosuppressive agents that are commonly used include medications such as methotrexate, mycophenolate, azathioprine, and cyclosporine. These treatments require regular blood tests to monitor for possible side effects. In some cases, biologic response modifiers (BRM), or biologics, such as, adalimumab, infliximab, daclizumab, abatacept, and rituximab are used. These drugs target specific elements of the immune system. Some of these drugs may increase the risk of having cancer.

Chapter 73

Vitiligo

What Is Vitiligo?

Vitiligo is a disorder in which white patches of skin appear on different parts of the body. This happens because the cells that make pigment (color) in the skin are destroyed. These cells are called melanocytes. Vitiligo can also affect the mucous membranes (such as the tissue inside the mouth and nose) and the eye.

What Causes Vitiligo?

The cause is not known. Vitiligo may be an autoimmune disease. These diseases happen when your immune system mistakenly attacks some part of your own body. In vitiligo, the immune system may destroy the melanocytes in the skin. It is also possible that one or more genes may make a person more likely to get the disorder.

Some researchers think that the melanocytes destroy themselves. Others think that a single event such as sunburn or emotional distress can cause vitiligo. But these events have not been proven to cause vitiligo.

Who Is Affected by Vitiligo?

Many people develop it in their twenties, but it can occur at any age. The disorder affects all races and both sexes equally, however, it is more noticeable in people with dark skin.

This chapter includes text excerpted from "Vitiligo," National Institute of Arthritis and Musculoskeletal and Skin Diseases (NIAMS), November 2014.

People with certain autoimmune diseases (such as hyperthyroidism) are more likely to get vitiligo than people who don't have any autoimmune diseases. Scientists do not know why vitiligo is connected with these diseases. However, most people with vitiligo have no other autoimmune disease.

Vitiligo may also run in families. Children whose parents have the disorder are more likely to develop vitiligo. However, most children will not get vitiligo even if a parent has it.

What Are the Symptoms of Vitiligo?

White patches on the skin are the main sign of vitiligo. These patches are more common in areas where the skin is exposed to the sun. The patches may be on the hands, feet, arms, face, and lips. Other common areas for white patches are:

- the armpits and groin (where the leg meets the body)
- around the mouth
- eyes
- nostrils
- navel
- genitals
- rectal areas.

People with vitiligo often have hair that turns gray early. Those with dark skin may notice a loss of color inside their mouths.

Will the White Patches Spread?

There is no way to tell if vitiligo will spread. For some people, the white patches do not spread. But often the white patches will spread to other areas of the body. For some people, vitiligo spreads slowly, over many years. For other people, spreading occurs quickly. Some people have reported more white patches after physical or emotional stress.

How Is Vitiligo Diagnosed?

The doctor will use a family and medical history, physical exam, and tests to diagnose vitiligo. The doctor may ask questions such as:

- Do you have family members with vitiligo?
- Do you or family members have any autoimmune diseases?

- Did you have a rash, sunburn, or other skin problem before the white patches appeared?
- Did you have some type of stress or physical illness?
- Did your hair turn gray before age 35?
- Are you sensitive to the sun?

The doctor will do a physical exam to rule out other medical problems.

Tests might include:

- taking a small sample (biopsy) of the affected skin to be examined
- blood tests
- an eye exam.

How Is Vitiligo Treated?

Treatment may help make the skin look more even. The choice of treatment depends on:

- The number of white patches
- How widespread the patches are
- The treatment the person prefers to use.

Some treatments are not right for everyone. Many treatments can have unwanted side effects. Treatments can take a long time, and sometimes they don't work.

Current treatment options for vitiligo include medical, surgical, and other treatments. Most treatments are aimed at restoring color to the white patches of skin.

Medical treatments include:

- Medicines (such as creams) that you put on the skin
- Medicines that you take by mouth
- A treatment that uses medicine plus ultraviolet A (UVA) light (PUVA)
- Removing the color from other areas so they match the white patches.

Surgical treatments include:

- skin grafts from a person's own tissues. The doctor takes skin from one area of a patient's body and attaches it to another area. This is sometimes used for people with small patches of vitiligo.

- tattooing small areas of skin.

Other treatments include:

- sunscreens

- cosmetics, such as makeup or dye, to cover the white patches

- counseling and support.

What Can People Do to Cope with Vitiligo?

When you have vitiligo, you may be upset or depressed about the change in your appearance. There are several things you can do to cope with the disorder:

- Find a doctor who knows how to treat vitiligo. The doctor should also be a good listener and be able to provide emotional support.

- Learn about the disorder and treatment choices. This can help you make decisions about your treatment.

- Talk with other people who have vitiligo. A vitiligo group can help you find a support group (check your local listings). Family and friends are another source of support.

Some people with vitiligo have found that cosmetics that cover the white patches improve their appearance and help them feel better about themselves. A person may need to try several brands of concealing cosmetics before finding the product that works best.

Part Six

Other Altered Immune Responses

Chapter 74

Allergies and Asthma

Allergy Basics

Allergies are the 6th leading cause of chronic illness in the United States with an annual cost in excess of $18 billion. More than 50 million Americans suffer from allergies each year.

Allergies are an overreaction of the immune system to substances that generally do not affect other individuals. These substances, or allergens, can cause sneezing, coughing, and itching. Allergic reactions range from merely bothersome to life-threatening. Some allergies are seasonal, like hay fever. Allergies have also been associated with chronic conditions like sinusitis and asthma.

Who's at Risk?

Anyone may have or develop an allergy—from a baby born with an allergy to cow's milk, to a child who gets poison ivy, to a senior citizen who develops hives after taking a new medication.

This chapter contains text excerpted from the following sources: Text beginning with the heading "Allergy Basics" is excerpted from "Allergies," Centers for Disease Control and Prevention (CDC), February 2, 2011. Reviewed October 2016; Text under the heading "Asthma Basics" is excerpted from "Asthma," National Heart, Lung, and Blood Institute (NHLBI), August 4, 2014; Text under the heading "Allergens and Asthma" is excerpted from "Asthma Triggers: Gain Control," U.S. Environmental Protection Agency (EPA), October 26, 2015.

Can It Be Prevented?

Allergies can generally not be prevented but allergic reactions can be. Once a person knows they are allergic to a certain substance, they can avoid contact with the allergen. Strategies for doing this include being in an air-conditioned environment during peak hay-fever season, avoiding certain foods, and eliminating dust mites and animal dander from the home. They can also control the allergy by reducing or eliminating the symptoms. Strategies include taking medication to counteract reactions or minimize symptoms and being immunized with allergy injection therapy.

The Bottom Line

- The most common allergic diseases include: hay fever, asthma, conjunctivitis, hives, eczema, dermatitis and sinusitis.

- Food allergies are most prevalent in young children and are frequently outgrown.

- Latex allergies are a reaction to the proteins in latex rubber, a substance used in gloves, condoms and other products.

- Bees, hornets, wasps, yellow jackets, and fire ants can cause insect sting allergies.

- Allergies to drugs, like penicillin, can affect any tissue or organ in the body.

Anaphylaxis is the most severe allergic reaction. Symptoms include flush; tingling of the palms of the hands, soles of the feet or lips; light-headedness, and chest-tightness. If not treated, these can progress into seizures, cardiac arrhythmia, shock, and respiratory distress. Anaphylaxis can result in death. Food, latex, insect sting, and drug allergies can all result in anaphylaxis.

Asthma Basics

Asthma is a chronic (long-term) lung disease that inflames and narrows the airways. Asthma causes recurring periods of wheezing (a whistling sound when you breathe), chest tightness, shortness of breath, and coughing. The coughing often occurs at night or early in the morning.

Asthma affects people of all ages, but it most often starts during childhood. In the United States, more than 25 million people are known to have asthma. About 7 million of these people are children.

Overview

To understand asthma, it helps to know how the airways work. The airways are tubes that carry air into and out of your lungs. People who have asthma have inflamed airways. The inflammation makes the airways swollen and very sensitive. The airways tend to react strongly to certain inhaled substances.

When the airways react, the muscles around them tighten. This narrows the airways, causing less air to flow into the lungs. The swelling also can worsen, making the airways even narrower. Cells in the airways might make more mucus than usual. Mucus is a sticky, thick liquid that can further narrow the airways.

This chain reaction can result in asthma symptoms. Symptoms can happen each time the airways are inflamed. Sometimes asthma symptoms are mild and go away on their own or after minimal treatment with asthma medicine. Other times, symptoms continue to get worse.

When symptoms get more intense and/or more symptoms occur, you're having an asthma attack. Asthma attacks also are called flareups or exacerbations.

Treating symptoms when you first notice them is important. This will help prevent the symptoms from worsening and causing a severe asthma attack. Severe asthma attacks may require emergency care, and they can be fatal.

Outlook

Asthma has no cure. Even when you feel fine, you still have the disease and it can flare up at any time.

However, with today's knowledge and treatments, most people who have asthma are able to manage the disease. They have few, if any, symptoms. They can live normal, active lives and sleep through the night without interruption from asthma.

If you have asthma, you can take an active role in managing the disease. For successful, thorough, and ongoing treatment, build strong partnerships with your doctor and other health care providers.

Allergens and Asthma

Dust Mites and Asthma

Dust mites are tiny bugs that are too small to see. Every home has dust mites. They feed on human skin flakes and are found in mattresses, pillows, carpets, upholstered furniture, bedcovers, clothes, stuffed toys and fabric and fabric-covered items.

Body parts and droppings from dust mites can trigger asthma in individuals with allergies to dust mites. Exposure to dust mites can cause asthma in children who have not previously exhibited asthma symptoms.

Actions You Can Take

Common house dust may also contain asthma triggers. These simple steps can help:

- Wash bedding in hot water once a week. Dry completely.
- Use dust proof covers on pillows and mattresses.
- Vacuum carpets and furniture every week.
- Choose stuffed toys that you can wash. Wash stuffed toys in hot water. Dry completely before your child plays with the toy.
- Dust often with a damp cloth.
- Use a vacuum with a high-efficiency particulate air (HEPA) filter on carpet and fabric-covered furniture to reduce dust build-up. People with asthma or allergies should leave the area being vacuumed.

Molds and Asthma

Molds create tiny spores to reproduce, just as plants produce seeds. Mold spores float through the indoor and outdoor air continually. When mold spores land on damp places indoors, they may begin growing. Molds are microscopic fungi that live on plant and animal matter. Molds can be found almost anywhere when moisture is present.

For people sensitive to molds, inhaling mold spores can trigger an asthma attack.

Actions You Can Take

- If mold is a problem in your home, you need to clean up the mold and eliminate sources of moisture.
- If you see mold on hard surfaces, clean it up with soap and water. Let the area dry completely.
- Use exhaust fans or open a window in the bathroom and kitchen when showering, cooking or washing dishes.

- Fix water leaks as soon as possible to keep mold from growing.

- Dry damp or wet things completely within one to two days to keep mold from growing.

- Maintain low indoor humidity, ideally between 30–50 percent relative humidity. Humidity levels can be measured by hygrometers, which are available at local hardware stores.

Cockroaches, Other Pests, and Asthma

Droppings or body parts of cockroaches and other pests can trigger asthma. Certain proteins are found in cockroach feces and saliva and can cause allergic reactions or trigger asthma symptoms in some individuals.

Cockroaches are commonly found in crowded cities and the southern regions of the United States. Cockroach allergens likely play a significant role in asthma in many urban areas.

Actions You Can Take

- Insecticides and pesticides are not only toxic to pests—they can harm people too. Try to use pest management methods that pose less of a risk. Keep counters, sinks, tables, and floors clean and free of clutter.

- Clean dishes, crumbs and spills right away.

- Store food in airtight containers.

- Seal cracks or openings around or inside cabinets.

Pets and Asthma

Proteins in your pet's skin flakes, urine, feces, saliva, and hair can trigger asthma. Dogs, cats, rodents (including hamsters and guinea pigs), and other warm-blooded mammals can trigger asthma in individuals with an allergy to animal dander.

The most effective method to control animal allergens in the home is to not allow animals in the home. If you remove an animal from the home, it is important to thoroughly clean the floors, walls, carpets and upholstered furniture.

Some individuals may find isolation measures to be sufficiently effective. Isolation measures that have been suggested include keeping pets out of the sleeping areas, keeping pets away from upholstered furniture, carpets and stuffed toys, keeping the pet outdoors as much as possible and isolating sensitive individuals from the pet as much as possible.

Actions You Can Take

- Find another home for your cat or dog.
- Keep pets outside if possible.
- If you have to have a pet inside, keep it out of the bedroom of the person with asthma.
- Keep pets off of your furniture.
- Vacuum carpets and furniture when the person with asthma is not around.

Nitrogen Dioxide NO$_2$ and Asthma

Nitrogen dioxide (NO$_2$) is an odorless gas that can irritate your eyes, nose and throat and cause shortness of breath. NO$_2$ can come from appliances inside your home that burn fuels such as gas, kerosene and wood. NO2 forms quickly from emissions from cars, trucks and buses, power plants and off-road equipment. Smoke from your stove or fireplace can trigger asthma.

In people with asthma, exposure to low levels of NO$_2$ may cause increased bronchial reactivity and make young children more susceptible to respiratory infections. Long-term exposure to high levels of NO$_2$ can lead to chronic bronchitis. Studies show a connection between breathing elevated short-term NO$_2$ concentrations, and increased visits to emergency departments and hospital admissions for respiratory issues, especially asthma.

Actions You Can Take

If possible, use fuel-burning appliances that are vented to the outside. Always follow the manufacturer's instructions on how to use these appliances.

- Gas cooking stoves: If you have an exhaust fan in the kitchen, use it when you cook. Never use the stove to keep you warm or heat your house.
- Unvented kerosene or gas space heaters: Use the proper fuel and keep the heater adjusted the right way. Open a window slightly or use an exhaust fan when you are using the heater.

Outdoor Air Pollution and Asthma

Outdoor air pollution is caused by small particles and ground level ozone that comes from car exhaust, smoke, road dust, and factory emissions. Outdoor air quality is also affected by pollen from plants, crops and weeds. Particle pollution can be high any time of year and are higher near busy roads and where people burn wood.

When inhaled, outdoor pollutants and pollen can aggravate the lungs, and can lead to:

- Chest pain
- Coughing
- Digestive problems
- Dizziness
- Fever
- Lethargy
- Sneezing
- Shortness of breath
- Throat irritation
- Watery eyes

Outdoor air pollution and pollen may also worsen chronic respiratory diseases, such as asthma.

Actions You Can Take

- Monitor the Air Quality Index (AQI) on your local weather report.

- Know when and where air pollution may be bad.

- Regular exercise is healthy. Check your local air quality to know when to play and when to take it a little easier.

- Schedule outdoor activities at times when the air quality is better.

- In the summer, this may be in the morning.

- Stay inside with the windows closed on high pollen days and when pollutants are high.

- Use your air conditioner to help filter the air coming into the home. Central air systems are the best.

- Remove indoor plants if they irritate or produce symptoms for you or your family.

- Pay attention to asthma warning signs. If you start to see signs, limit outdoor activity. Be sure to talk about this with your child's doctor.

Chemical Irritants and Asthma

Chemical irritants are found in some products in your house and may trigger asthma. Your asthma or your child's asthma may be worse around products such as cleaners, paints, adhesives, pesticides, cosmetics or air fresheners. Chemical irritants are also present in schools and can be found in commonly used cleaning supplies and educational kits.

Chemical irritants may exacerbate asthma. At sufficient concentrations in the air, many products can trigger a reaction.

Actions You Can Take

If you find that your asthma or your child's asthma gets worse when you use a certain product, consider trying different products. If you must use a product, then you should:

- Make sure your child is not around.

- Open windows or doors, or use an exhaust fan.

- Always follow the instructions on the product label.

Wood Smoke and Asthma

Smoke from wood-burning stoves and fireplaces contain a mixture of harmful gases and small particles. Breathing these small particles can cause asthma attacks and severe bronchitis, aggravate heart and lung disease and may increase the likelihood of respiratory illnesses. If you're using a wood stove or fireplace and smell smoke in your home, it probably isn't working as it should.

Actions You Can Take

- To help reduce smoke, make sure to burn dry wood that has been split, stacked, covered, and stored for at least 6 months.

- Have your stove and chimney inspected every year by a certified professional to make sure there are no gaps, cracks, unwanted drafts or to remove dangerous creosote build-up.

- If possible, replace your old wood stove with a new, cleaner heating appliance. Newer wood stoves are at least 50 percent more efficient and pollute 70 percent less than older models.

- This can help make your home healthier and safer and help cut fuel costs.

Secondhand Smoke and Asthma

Secondhand smoke is the smoke from a cigarette, cigar or pipe, and the smoke exhaled by a smoker. Secondhand smoke contains more than 4,000 substances, including several compounds that cause cancer.

Secondhand smoke can trigger asthma episodes and increase the severity of attacks. Secondhand smoke is also a risk factor for new cases of asthma in preschool-aged children. Children's developing bodies make them more susceptible to the effects of secondhand smoke and, due to their small size, they breathe more rapidly than adults, thereby taking in more secondhand smoke. Children receiving high doses of secondhand smoke, such as those with smoking parents, run the greatest relative risk of experiencing damaging health effects.

Actions You Can Take

- Don't let anyone smoke near your child.

- If you smoke—until you can quit, don't smoke in your home or car.

Chapter 75

Serum Sickness

Similar to an allergic reaction, serum sickness is a delayed response to certain medications or to foreign proteins, particularly the substances found in antiserums. Serum is the clear portion of blood that does not contain red or white blood cells but does contain proteins, electrolytes, antibodies, antigens, hormones, and other substances. An antiserum is a preparation of plasma (the liquid portion of blood) that has been removed from an animal or person who has already developed an immunity to a particular disease and is then used to treat that condition in other animals or people.

While vaccines may also be prepared from serum in a similar fashion, they are intended to prevent illness by "teaching" the body to develop an immunity to a particular disease, while antiserums are primarily used to stimulate the immune system to combat an existing infection or disease. Antiserums have commonly been made from the plasma of animals, such as horses, sheep, oxen, and rabbits, which have been exposed to a disease and have produced antibodies in response to it. The animal's blood is then withdrawn and purified, and the antibodies are used in the production of antiserum.

In serum sickness, as with an allergy, the body erroneously identifies the medicine or foreign protein as a threat, and the immune system responds by attacking it with its own antibodies. These combine with the antigens (foreign substances) to form immune complexes that can

"Serum Sickness," © 2017 Omnigraphics. Reviewed October 2016.

collect on the blood vessels, heart, and other body parts to cause the illness.

Serum sickness resulting from animal-based antiserums is becoming less common because of the decrease in the use of foreign serum proteins in the treatment of human diseases. However, the condition still occurs with some regularity and is most prevalent as a reaction to various medications.

Causes

Penicillin reaction is one of the most common causes of serum sickness, affecting an estimated 10 percent of patients treated with this it. Other medications that can trigger the response include various other antibiotics, thiazides (used to treat hypertension and edema), aspirin, fluoxetine (used in the treatment of depression), and, occasionally, vaccines. Serum sickness can also be caused by bee or wasp stings, by antivenoms made to treat bites from venomous snakes, spiders, insects, or fish, and by antiserums used in the treatment of such conditions as tetanus and rabies.

Symptoms

Symptoms of serum sickness typically appear seven to ten days after exposure to a medication or foreign protein, primarily because it takes time for the immune system to produce the antibodies needed to fight the introduced substance. However, re-exposure can accelerate the process, with symptoms developing in as little as a day.

Symptoms of serum sickness include:

- fever
- skin rash
- joint pain
- itching
- swollen lymph nodes
- diarrhea
- nausea
- low blood pressure
- general malaise

Diagnosis

To diagnose serum sickness, a doctor will generally begin by taking the patient's history, in particular asking about medications taken, as well as any recent insect bites or stings. A physical exam will reveal lymph nodes that are enlarged and sore, skin rashes, or reactions at an injection site. Laboratory tests may include blood work to detect antibodies that have developed to counter foreign proteins, a urine test to see if it contains blood or proteins, and biopsies of rashes or skin eruptions.

Treatment

The first treatment for serum sickness is to discontinue the use of the medicine, antiserum, or antivenom that caused the condition. A corticosteroid cream or ointment applied to the skin may relieve discomfort from a rash and itching. In most instances, serum sickness resolves in a relatively short time, but more serious cases may require high doses of IV corticosteroids followed by reduced doses of oral steroids.

Antihistamines can help shorten the length of serum sickness and relieve symptoms such as itching and rash, while nonsteroidal anti-inflammatory drugs (NSAIDs), like ibuprofen and naproxen, may be prescribed to reduce joint pain.

In some very severe cases, plasmapheresis has been used to treat serum sickness. This procedure involves circulating the patient's blood through a centrifuge or filter to remove antibodies, immune complexes, and proteins, and then returning it to the body.

Complications

With proper treatment, the symptoms of serum sickness generally improve in seven to ten days, and a full recovery can be expected within 30 days. Although the condition is usually not life-threatening, it is important to consult a physician when symptoms appear, since serum sickness can on occasion lead to very serious disorders.

Some possible complications include:

- recurrence from future exposure to the causative substance

- inflammation of the blood vessels

- angioedema (swelling of the face, arms, and legs)

- nervous-system disorders, such as Guillain-Barre syndrome and peripheral neuritis

- anaphylaxis (a potentially fatal allergic reaction)

- kidney disorders

- heart inflammation

Prevention

Obviously, anyone who has experienced serum sickness as a reaction to a certain medication or antiserum injection should avoid that treatment in the future. But for those who have no known sensitivity to a given substance, it is very difficult to predict a reaction until one takes place. However, there are a couple ways in which a physician may be able to prevent the condition from occurring or recurring.

In some cases, a doctor may be able to test for sensitivity to a particular antiserum before administering it. For example, prior to injecting the antiserum, he or she could try a skin-prick test using a diluted version of the substance to see if a minor reaction occurs.

And when a patient has experienced serum sickness in the past, it might be possible for the physician to administer a desensitization treatment, which will temporarily prevent a reaction. This is done by injecting small amounts of the antiserum before administering the full dose. However, this method is only used in specific cases and is not always successful.

References

1. Dyall-Smith, Dewlyn, MD, FACD. "Serum Sickness," Dermnet New Zealand, n.d.

2. Alissa, Hassan M., MD. "Serum Sickness," Medscape.com, February 15, 2016.

3. Henochowicz, Stuart I.,MD, FACP. "Serum Sickness," Medline Plus, March 14, 2016.

4. Ronis, Tova, MD. "Pediatric Serum Sickness," MedScape.com, April 25, 2016.

5. "Serum Sickness," University of Maryland Medical Center, March 24, 2015.

6. Wener, Mark H., MD. "Serum Sickness and Serum Sickness-Like Reactions," UpToDate.com, October 19, 2015.

Chapter 76

Blood Transfusion Reaction

Blood transfusions save lives every day. Hospitals use blood trans-fusions to help people who are injured, having surgery, getting cancer treatments, or being treated for other diseases that affect the blood, like sickle cell anemia. In fact, about 5 million people each year in the United States get blood transfusions.

A Bit about Blood

As blood moves throughout the body, it carries oxygen and nutrients to all the places they're needed. Blood also collects waste products, like carbon dioxide, and takes them to the organs responsible for making sure wastes leave the body.

Blood is a mixture of cells and liquid. Each has a specific job:

- **Red blood cells** carry oxygen to the body's tissues and remove carbon dioxide. Red blood cells make up about 40 percent–45 percent of a person's blood and live for 120 days.

This chapter contains text excerpted from the following sources: Text in this chapter begins with excerpts from "Blood Transfusion," © 1995–2016. The Nemours Foundation/KidsHealth®. Reprinted with permission; Text under the heading "What Are the Risks of a Blood Transfusion?" is excerpted from "Blood Transfusion," National Heart, Lung, and Blood Institute (NHLBI), January 30, 2012. Reviewed October 2016; Text under the heading "Adverse Reactions Asso-ciated with Blood Transfusions" is excerpted from "Blood Safety," Centers for Disease Control and Prevention (CDC), August 1, 2011. Reviewed October 2016.

- **White blood cells** are part of the immune system, and its main defense against infection. White blood cells make up less than 1 percent of a person's blood.

- **Platelets** are cell fragments that help blood clot, which helps to prevent and control bleeding. A person's blood has about 1 platelet for every 20 red blood cells.

- **Plasma** is a pale yellow liquid mixture of water, proteins, electrolytes, carbohydrates, cholesterol, hormones, and vitamins. About 55 percent of our blood is plasma.

Blood cells are made in the bone marrow (a spongy material inside many of the bones in the body). A full-grown adult has about 10 pints of blood (almost 5 liters) in his or her body.

What Is a Blood Transfusion?

A transfusion is a simple medical procedure that doctors use to make up for a loss of blood—or for any part of the blood, such as red blood cells or platelets.

A person usually gets a blood transfusion through an intravenous line, a tiny tube that is inserted into a vein with a small needle. The whole process takes about 1 to 4 hours, depending on how much blood is needed.

Blood from a donor needs to match the blood type of the person receiving it. There are eight main blood types:

1. O positive

2. O negative

3. A positive

4. A negative

5. B positive

6. B negative

7. AB positive

8. AB negative

In emergencies, there are exceptions to the rule that the donor's blood type must match the recipient's exactly. Blood type O negative is the only type of blood that people of all other blood types can receive. Medical teams use it in situations when patients need a transfusion but their blood type is unknown. Because of this, O negative donors are called "universal donors." People who have type AB blood are called "universal recipients" because they can safely receive any type of blood.

A blood transfusion usually isn't whole blood—it could be any one of the blood's components. For example, chemotherapy can affect how bone marrow makes new blood cells. So some people getting treatment for cancer might need a transfusion of red blood cells or platelets.

Other people might need plasma or only certain parts of plasma. People who have hemophilia, a disease that affects the blood's ability to clot, need plasma or the clotting factors contained in plasma to help their blood clot and prevent internal bleeding.

Where Does the Blood Come From?

In the United States, the blood supply for transfusions comes from people who volunteer to donate their blood. Donors give blood at local blood banks, at community centers during blood drives, or through the American Red Cross.

When people know they are going to have an operation that might include a blood transfusion, they may choose to receive blood from one of several different places. Most patients choose to receive blood from the donated supply, but some decide to use their own blood. Providing your own blood before surgery is called **autologous** blood donation.

Another option for blood transfusions is called **directed donation**. This is when a family member or friend donates blood specifically to be used by a designated patient. For directed donation, the donor must have a blood type that is compatible with the recipient's. He or she must also meet all the requirements of a regular volunteer blood donor. There is no medical or scientific evidence that blood from directed donors is safer or better than blood from volunteer donors.

How Safe Is Donated Blood?

Some people worry about getting diseases from infected blood, but the United States has one of the safest blood supplies in the world. Many organizations, including community blood banks and the federal government, work hard to ensure that the blood supply is safe.

All blood donors must provide a detailed history, including recent travel, infections, medicines, and health problems. In addition, the American Red Cross and other donation groups test donated blood for viruses like HIV (the virus that causes AIDS), hepatitis B, hepatitis C, syphilis, and West Nile virus. Since blood can also be infected with bacteria or parasites, some blood components also get tested for these. If any of these things are found, the blood is destroyed.

The U.S. Food and Drug Administration (FDA) regulates U.S. blood banks. All blood centers must pass regular inspections in order to continue their operations.

What Are the Risks of a Blood Transfusion?

Most blood transfusions go very smoothly. However, mild problems and, very rarely, serious problems can occur.

Allergic Reactions

Some people have allergic reactions to the blood given during transfusions. This can happen even when the blood given is the right blood type.

Allergic reactions can be mild or severe. Symptoms can include:

- anxiety
- chest and/or back pain
- trouble breathing
- fever, chills, flushing, and clammy skin
- a quick pulse or low blood pressure
- nausea (feeling sick to the stomach)

A nurse or doctor will stop the transfusion at the first signs of an allergic reaction. The health care team determines how mild or severe the reaction is, what treatments are needed, and whether the transfusion can safely be restarted.

Viruses and Infectious Diseases

Some infectious agents, such as HIV, can survive in blood and infect the person receiving the blood transfusion. To keep blood safe, blood banks carefully screen donated blood.

The risk of catching a virus from a blood transfusion is very low.

- HIV. Your risk of getting HIV from a blood transfusion is lower than your risk of getting killed by lightning. Only about 1 in 2 million donations might carry HIV and transmit HIV if given to a patient.

- Hepatitis B and C. The risk of having a donation that carries hepatitis B is about 1 in 205,000. The risk for hepatitis C is 1 in 2 million. If you receive blood during a transfusion that contains hepatitis, you'll likely develop the virus.

- Variant Creutzfeldt-Jakob disease (vCJD). This disease is the human version of Mad Cow Disease. It's a very rare, yet fatal brain disorder. There is a possible risk of getting vCJD from a blood transfusion, although the risk is very low. Because of this, people who may have been exposed to vCJD aren't eligible blood donors.

Fever

You may get a sudden fever during or within a day of your blood transfusion. This is usually your body's normal response to white blood cells in the donated blood. Over-the-counter fever medicine usually will treat the fever.

Some blood banks remove white blood cells from whole blood or different parts of the blood. This makes it less likely that you will have a reaction after the transfusion.

Iron Overload

Getting many blood transfusions can cause too much iron to build up in your blood (iron overload). People who have a blood disorder like thalassemia, which requires multiple transfusions, are at risk for iron overload. Iron overload can damage your liver, heart, and other parts of your body.

If you have iron overload, you may need iron chelation. For this therapy, medicine is given through an injection or as a pill to remove the extra iron from your body.

Lung Injury

Although it's unlikely, blood transfusions can damage your lungs, making it hard to breathe. This usually occurs within about 6 hours of the procedure.

Most patients recover. However, 5 to 25 percent of patients who develop lung injuries die from the injuries. These people usually were very ill before the transfusion.

Doctors aren't completely sure why blood transfusions damage the lungs. Antibodies (proteins) that are more likely to be found in the plasma of women who have been pregnant may disrupt the normal way that lung cells work. Because of this risk, hospitals are starting to use men's and women's plasma differently.

Graft-Versus-Host Disease

Graft-versus-host disease (GVHD) is a condition in which white blood cells in the new blood attack your tissues. GVHD usually is fatal. People who have weakened immune systems are the most likely to get GVHD.

Symptoms start within a month of the blood transfusion. They include fever, rash, and diarrhea. To protect against GVHD, people who have weakened immune systems should receive blood that has been treated so the white blood cells can't cause GVHD.

Adverse Reactions Associated with Blood Transfusions

The chance of having a reaction to a blood transfusion is very small. The most common adverse reactions from blood transfusions are allergic and febrile (fever–associated) reactions, which make up over half of all adverse reactions reported. Rare but serious adverse reactions include infection caused by bacterial contamination of blood products and immune reactions due to problems in blood type matching between donor and recipient.

The following is a list of blood transfusion-associated adverse reactions that are tracked through the National Healthcare Safety Network (NHSN) Hemovigilance Module. These adverse reactions are not common following blood transfusions but are tracked so that the Centers for Disease Control and Prevention (CDC) can better understand them and develop interventions to prevent them.

- **Acute hemolytic transfusion reaction (AHTR)**

  An acute hemolytic transfusion reaction is the rapid destruction of red blood cells that occurs during, immediately after, or within 24 hours of a transfusion when a patient is given an incompatible blood type. The recipient's body immediately begins to destroy the donated red blood cells resulting in fever, pain, and sometimes severe complications such as kidney failure.

- **Delayed hemolytic transfusion reaction (DHTR)**

  A delayed hemolytic transfusion reaction occurs when the recipient develops antibodies to red blood cell antigen(s) between 24 hours and 28 days after a transfusion. Symptoms are usually milder than in acute hemolytic transfusion reactions and may even be absent. DHTR is diagnosed with laboratory testing.

- **Delayed serologic transfusion reaction (DSTR)**

  A delayed serologic transfusion reaction occurs when a recipient develops new antibodies against red blood cells between 24 hours and 28 days after a transfusion without clinical symptoms or laboratory evidence of hemolysis. Clinical symptoms are rarely associated with DSTR

- **Febrile non-hemolytic transfusion reaction (FNHTR)**

  Febrile non-hemolytic transfusion reactions are the most common reaction reported after a transfusion. FNHTR is characterized by fever and/or chills in the absence of hemolysis (breakdown of red blood cells) occurring in the patient during or up to 4 hours after a transfusion. These reactions are generally mild and respond quickly to treatment. Fever can be a symptom of a more severe reaction with more serious causes, and should be fully investigated.

- **Hypotensive transfusion reaction**

  A hypotensive transfusion reaction is a drop in systolic blood pressure occurring soon after a transfusion begins that responds quickly to cessation of the transfusion and supportive treatment. Hypotension also can be a symptom of a more severe reaction and should be fully investigated.

- **Post-transfusion purpura (PTP)**

  Post-transfusion purpura is a rare but potentially fatal condition that occurs when a transfusion recipient develops antibodies against platelets, resulting in rapid destruction of both transfused and the patient's own platelets and a severe decline in the platelet count. PTP usually occurs 5-12 days after a transfusion and is more common in women than in men.

- **Transfusion-associated circulatory overload (TACO)**

  Transfusion-associated circulatory overload occurs when the volume of blood or blood components are transfused cannot be effectively processed by the recipient. TACO can occur due to an excessively high infusion rate and/or volume or due to an underlying heart or kidney condition. Symptoms may include difficulty breathing, cough, and fluid in the lungs.

- **Transfusion-related acute lung injury (TRALI)**

  Transfusion-related acute lung injury is a serious but rare reaction that occurs when fluid builds up in the lungs, but is not related to excessive volume of blood or blood products transfused. Symptoms include acute respiratory distress with no other explanation for lung injury such as pneumonia or trauma occurring within 6 hours of transfusion. TRALI is a leading cause of transfusion-related death reported to the FDA. The mechanism of TRALI is not well understood, but is thought to be associated with the presence of antibodies in donor blood.

- **Transfusion-associated dyspnea (TAD)**

  Transfusion associated dyspnea is the onset of respiratory distress within 24 hours of transfusion that cannot be defined as TACO, TRALI, or an allergic reaction.

- **Transfusion-associated graft vs. host disease (TAGVHD)**

  Transfusion-associated graft vs. host disease is a rare complication of transfusion that occurs when donor T-lymphocytes (the "graft") introduced by the blood transfusion rapidly increase in number in the recipient (the "host") and then attack the recipient's own cells. Symptoms include fever, a characteristic rash, enlargement of the liver, and diarrhea that occur between 2 days and 6 weeks post transfusion. Though very rare, this inflammatory response is difficult to treat and often results in death.

- **Transfusion-transmitted infection (TTI)**

  A transfusion-transmitted infection occurs when a bacterium, parasite, virus, or other potential pathogen is transmitted in donated blood to the transfusion recipient.

Chapter 77

Transplant Rejection

Understanding Transplantation

A transplant replaces a failed or damaged organ or tissue with a healthy one. People may need transplants because disease, injury, or an inherited defect causes organ failure. Despite tremendous progress over the years, several major barriers remain to the overall success of transplantation. While survival rates after transplantation surgery have improved markedly, there has been little improvement in reversing long-term declines in the function of transplanted organs. Transplant recipients have a shorter life expectancy compared to the general population due, in part, to the accelerated cardiovascular disease, kidney disease, infection, and cancer associated with the use of immunosuppressive drugs.

Immune System in Transplantation

The immune system is a network of organs, cells, and tissues found throughout the body that protects the body from diseases of infectious and non-infectious origin. There are numerous types of immune cells that play unique roles, with different ways of recognizing problems and responding to eliminate or limit the disease. Research resulting in a better understanding of how the immune system functions has allowed clinicians to modulate immune responses to improve outcomes in many conditions including organ transplantation.

This chapter includes text excerpted from "Transplantation," National Institute of Allergy and Infectious Alcoholism (NIAAA), January 21, 2015.

A primary function of the immune system is to distinguish cells and tissues that belong to the body ("self") from those that do not ("non-self"), enabling it to swiftly respond to an infection or other foreign presence. Immune cells interact with a set of proteins called human leukocyte antigens (HLAs), which are expressed on the surface of most cells, to determine if a cell is self or non-self. When non-self HLAs are encountered, the immune system reacts by attacking and eliminating the foreign cells. However, in transplantation, these immune responses are unfavorable and can damage or destroy a transplanted tissue or organ—a process known as rejection.

The HLA system is the most diverse and variable region in the human genome, and it is rare that unrelated people will have the same set of HLA markers. Closely matched HLAs help reduce the risk of an adverse outcome following transplantation. The number of HLA variants is quite large, and it is very rare to get an exact match between two people. The chance of two unrelated people having identical transplant markers is about one in 100,000. Similarities are more common among family members.

How Are Transplants Matched?

There are many considerations in matching a transplant donor and recipient. When the donor and recipient are closely matched, a transplant is more likely to be successful. This matching process is organ-specific and may include HLA, gender, height, weight, blood type, the geographical distance between the donor and the recipient, the recipient's medical condition and infection status, and genetic matching.

The requirements for a compatible match vary depending on the organ needed. For example, body size is a major factor for heart and lung transplants—especially in pediatric transplantation. In some cases, an urgent, life-sustaining transplant is required despite the lack of an ideal match. Transplant physicians must assess these factors to determine the best decision available for a patient. National Institute of Allergy and Infectious Diseases (NIAID) supports research to help inform these decisions, better predict which transplants will have favorable outcomes, and address the unique needs of special and/or vulnerable populations of transplant recipients, such as children or HIV-infected people.

In bone marrow transplantation, detailed genetic testing and matching of the HLA system of the donor and recipient is critical to avoid rejection. Without HLA matching, the risk that the transplanted cells will be detected as foreign by the recipient's immune system is greatly increased. The immune system will respond by attacking the transplanted organ or cells as if they were an infection or tumor, and the transplant will undergo rejection. Transplanted immune cells from a mismatched donor can also attack recipient cells, resulting in graft-versus-host disease. NIAID supports research to better understand how transplantation outcome is linked to HLA matching and how some mismatches may be more harmful than others.

An accurate understanding of the immune system is critical for understanding why a transplant is accepted or rejected, minimizing complications, and improving transplantation outcomes. The criteria used for donor and recipient matching, as well as the drugs prescribed to prevent transplant rejection, are based on decades of research identifying how the immune system distinguishes between self and non-self. Expansion of such knowledge promises to offer better therapies and more effective transplants.

Transplant Rejection and Treatment

Transplant rejection occurs as a consequence of normal, but undesired actions of the immune system. While matching donors and recipients helps reduce the chances of rejection, anti-rejection drugs are also given to suppress the immune system, thereby preventing it from attacking the transplanted organ or cells. Currently, these drugs are required for successful organ transplantation.

The prevention and treatment of rejection requires a fine balance: insufficient anti-rejection drugs may not suppress the immune system enough to protect the transplanted organ, resulting in rejection. On the other hand, anti-rejection drugs may lead to complications from side effects such as infection, high blood pressure, kidney damage, diabetes, and cancer. Knowing if or when these drugs can be reduced or discontinued has significant health and quality-of-life implications for transplant recipients. NIAID-supported researchers are working to better understand the effects of these drugs, how to optimize their use, and develop new anti-rejection or immunosuppressive therapies.

Researchers also are studying ways to modify the immune system so that it accepts a transplanted organ without needing immunosuppressive drugs. This state is called immune tolerance. NIAID supports a wide range of research activities in pursuit of this goal. For example, the Immune Tolerance Network is an international consortium of investigators dedicated to the clinical evaluation of novel, tolerance-inducing strategies in three disease areas: autoimmunity, asthma and allergy, and transplantation.

Chapter 78

Anaphylaxis

Anaphylaxis is a serious allergic reaction that involves more than one organ system (for example, skin, respiratory tract, and/or gastrointestinal tract). It can begin very rapidly, and symptoms may be severe or life-threatening.

Causes

The most common causes of anaphylaxis are reactions to foods (especially peanuts), medications, and stinging insects. Other potential triggers include exercise and exposure to latex. Sometimes, anaphylaxis occurs without an identifiable trigger. This is called idiopathic anaphylaxis.

Symptoms

Anaphylaxis includes a wide range of symptoms that can occur in many combinations and may be difficult to recognize. Some symptoms are not life-threatening, but the most severe ones restrict breathing and blood circulation.

Many of the body's organs can be affected:

- Skin—itching, hives, redness, swelling

- Nose—sneezing, stuffy nose, runny nose

This chapter includes text excerpted from "Anaphylaxis," National Institute of Allergy and Infectious Diseases (NIAID), April 23, 2015.

- Mouth—itching, swelling of the lips or tongue
- Throat—itching, tightness, difficulty swallowing, swelling of the back of the throat
- Chest—shortness of breath, cough, wheeze, chest pain, tightness
- Heart—weak pulse, passing out, shock
- Gastrointestinal (GI) tract—vomiting, diarrhea, cramps
- Nervous system—dizziness or fainting

How Soon after Exposure Will Symptoms Occur?

Symptoms can begin within minutes to hours after exposure to the allergen. Sometimes the symptoms go away, only to return anywhere from 8 to 72 hours later. When you begin to experience symptoms, seek immediate medical attention because anaphylaxis can be life-threatening.

How Do You Know If a Person Is Having an Anaphylactic Reaction?

Anaphylaxis is likely if a person experiences two or more of the following symptoms within minutes to several hours after exposure to an allergen:

- Hives, itchiness, or redness all over the body and swelling of the lips, tongue, or back of the throat
- Trouble breathing
- Severe GI symptoms such as abdominal cramps, diarrhea, or vomiting
- Dizziness or fainting (signs of a drop in blood pressure)

If you are experiencing symptoms of anaphylaxis, seek immediate treatment and tell your healthcare professional if you have a history of allergic reactions.

Can Anaphylaxis Be Predicted?

Anaphylaxis caused by an allergic reaction is highly unpredictable. The severity of a one attack does not predict the severity of subsequent attacks. Any anaphylactic reaction can become dangerous quickly and must be evaluated immediately by a health-care professional.

Timing

An anaphylactic reaction can occur as any of the following:

- A single reaction that occurs immediately after exposure to the allergen and gets better with or without treatment within minutes to hours. Symptoms do not recur later in relation to that episode.

- A double reaction. The first reaction occurs within minutes or hours. The initial symptoms seem to go away but later reappear in a second reaction, which typically occurs 8 to 72 hours after the first reaction.

- A single, long-lasting reaction that continues for hours or days.

Treatment

If you or someone you know is having an anaphylactic episode, health experts advise using an auto-injector, if available, to inject epinephrine into the thigh muscle, and calling 9-1-1 if you are not in a hospital. (Epinephrine is a hormone that increases heart rate, constricts the blood vessels, and opens the airways.) If you are in a hospital, summon a resuscitation team.

If epinephrine is not given promptly, rapid decline and death could occur within 30 to 60 minutes. Epinephrine acts immediately but does not last long in the body, so it may be necessary to give repeat doses.

After epinephrine has been given, the patient can be placed in a reclining position with feet elevated to help restore normal blood flow.

A healthcare professional also may give the patient any of the following secondary treatments:

- Medicines to open the airways

- Antihistamines to relieve itching and hives

- Corticosteroids (a class of drugs used to treat inflammatory diseases) to prevent prolonged inflammation and long-lasting reactions

- Additional medicines to constrict blood vessels and increase heart rate

- Supplemental oxygen therapy

- Intravenous fluids

Conditions such as asthma, chronic lung disease, and cardiovascular disease may increase the risk of death from anaphylaxis. Medicines such as those that treat high blood pressure also may worsen symptom severity and limit response to treatment.

Antihistamines should be used only as a secondary treatment. Giving antihistamines instead of epinephrine may increase the risk of a life-threatening allergic reaction.

Management

Before leaving emergency medical care, your healthcare professional should provide the following:

- An epinephrine auto-injector or a prescription for two doses and training on how to use the auto-injector

- A follow-up appointment or an appointment with a clinical specialist such as an allergist or immunologist

- Information on where to get medical identification jewelry or an anaphylaxis wallet card that alerts others of the allergy

- Education about allergen avoidance, recognizing the symptoms of anaphylaxis, and giving epinephrine

- An anaphylaxis emergency action plan

If you or someone you know has a history of severe allergic reactions or anaphylaxis, your healthcare professional should remember to keep you S.A.F.E.

- **Seek support:** Your healthcare professional should tell you the following:

  - Anaphylaxis is a life-threatening condition.

  - The symptoms of the current episode may occur again (sometimes up to three days later).

  - You are at risk for anaphylaxis in the future.

  - At the first sign of symptoms, give yourself epinephrine and then immediately call an ambulance or have someone else take you to the nearest emergency facility.

- **Allergen identification and avoidance:** Before you leave the hospital, your healthcare professional should have done the following:

  - Made efforts to identify the allergen by taking your medical history

  - Explained the importance of getting additional testing to confirm what triggered the reaction, so you can successfully avoid it in the future

- **Follow-up with specialty care:** Your healthcare professional should encourage you to consult a specialist for an allergy evaluation.

- **Epinephrine for emergencies:** Your healthcare professional should give you the following:

  - An epinephrine auto-injector or a prescription and training on how to use an auto-injector

  - Advice to routinely check the expiration date of the auto-injector

Part Seven

Treatments for Immune Deficiencies and Diseases

Chapter 79

Immune Globulin
Intravenous Injection (IGIV)

Immune globulin intravenous (IGIV) is a sterilized, highly purified medication made from human plasma that contains antibodies
to help fight infections and other diseases. Its principal use is in the
treatment of primary immunodeficiency (PI), a group of hundreds of
mostly genetic disorders in which the body's immune system is unable
to produce enough antibodies on its own, as well as some secondary
immunodeficiencies, those caused by other conditions.

Primary immunodeficiency disorders include X-linked agammaglobulinemia, common variable immunodeficiency, Wiskott-Aldrich
syndrome, DiGeorge Syndrome, chronic mucocutaneous candidiasis,
chronic granulomatous disease, and C2 deficiency. Secondary immunodeficiencies (sometimes called acquired immunodeficiencies) include
such disorders as human immunodeficiency virus (HIV), lymphocytic
leukemia, and severe malnutrition, as well as chronic diseases, like
diabetes. It can also be caused by certain immunosuppressive medications or by chemotherapy.

In addition, IGIV may be used to increase the platelet count in
individuals with blood disorders, like idiopathic thrombocytopenia
purpura, and to treat certain muscle and nerve conditions, as well
as blood-vessel diseases, such as Kawasaki syndrome, and nerve

disorders, like chronic inflammatory demyelinating polyneuropathy (CIDP).

How It Is Made

IGIV is made from plasma collected from large numbers of donors who have been carefully screened to ensure that they are healthy, free of disease, have not traveled to high-risk areas, and have not engaged in behaviors that might increase their risk of contracting an infectious disease. Donation centers are carefully monitored by the U.S. Food and Drug Administration (FDA) and the American Association of Blood Banks (AABB) to be sure that proper safety procedures are followed.

The plasma from many donors is pooled together, purified to remove any viruses or other pathogens, and treated to extract the immune globulins. Depending on the particular type of IGIV being prepared, sugars, amino acids, or other substances may be added to help preserve the solution for storage and transportation. The product is then packaged, stored, and finally shipped to healthcare providers.

Administering IGIV

IGIV is known as a replacement therapy, because it is replenishing a substance (such as antibodies) that the body is incapable of producing—or producing in sufficient quantities—on its own. Since it does not prompt the immune system to begin making antibodies, but rather provides the necessary antibodies from an outside source, and since the supply of antibodies constantly becomes depleted, IGIV is a temporary treatment that must be repeated on a regular basis.

IGIV treatments are usually given by infusion but in some cases may also be administered by intramuscular or subcutaneous injection. With infusion, the medication is introduced directly into a vein through a needle or catheter over a two-to-four-hour period in sessions that are repeated approximately every three to four weeks. Prior to the introduction of infusion therapy, intramuscular injections were the norm, but this method fell out of favor because it is less effective and causes pain in many patients. A better alternative for some types of immunoglobulins is subcutaneous (under skin) injection, which is more convenient but may need to be repeated more often, depending on the condition.

IGIV can be administered at a medical facility or at home. If self-administered, it is important that the patient fully understand proper storage of the medication, exact dosages required, and the cleaning, use, and disposal of needles and other equipment. Some types of IGIV need to be kept in a refrigerator, while others may be stored at room temperature. Medication that has changed color or contains particles is not safe to use. The prescribing healthcare provider will explain the proper storage and use of IGIV to the patient, and his or her instructions must be followed carefully to ensure the safe and effective use of the medication.

Risks Associated with IGIV

Even though multiple precautions are taken in screening donors, treating fluids, and testing the product, because IGIV is made from human plasma there is a risk—however slight—that the medication could transmit viruses or other diseases. But with modern screening and processing methods, this risk is so low that it is far outweighed by the benefits of treatment.

In the very unlikely event that transmission of infection via IGIV is suspected, it is important to consult a physician as soon as possible. Signs of infection include:

- high fever
- flu symptoms
- mouth sores
- severe headache
- neck stiffness
- increased sensitivity to light
- nausea and vomiting

IGIV has been associated with kidney failure and other serious renal disorders. It is important that the physician be informed if the patient has ever had kidney disease, diabetes, sepsis, plasma cell disease, paraproteinemia, or fluid volume depletion. Many other drugs, including over-the-counter medications, can increase the chance of kidney disease. So patients taking medicines like antivirals, chemotherapy, certain antibiotics, or drugs for pain, osteoporosis, bowel disorders, or to prevent rejection of organ transplants may be at even greater risk when undergoing IGIV treatment.

Most IGIV solutions contain additives like amino acids or sugars, which help preserve them and also reduce the incidence of side effects. These substances are harmless for most patients, however some of them may cause adverse reactions in a small percentage of individuals. The administering physician will monitor for such reactions and recommend a different type of IGIV is necessary.

Side Effects

IGIV is a well-established form of treatment that has proven to be safe and effective for most patients. However, as with any medication, some individuals may experience side effects, which can commonly include:

- headache
- dizziness
- low-grade fever
- chills
- muscle cramps
- vomiting
- diarrhea
- muscle or back pain
- pain, swelling, or redness at the injection site
- flushing or rash
- fatigue

Some reactions to IGIV require the immediate attention of a medical professional. These uncommon but more serious side effects may include:

- blood clots
- severe allergic reactions
- chest pain
- difficulty breathing
- sudden cough
- fainting
- hives
- severe headaches
- slurred speech
- liver problems (characterized by jaundice or dark urine)
- signs of infection (including fever, neck stiffness, or flu-like symptoms)
- pulmonary embolism
- aseptic meningitis

- kidney problems (indicated by rapid weight gain, swelling, or low urine output)

To reduce the risk of side effects, it is important to be well hydrated before each IGIV treatment. It is also vital to give the physician a complete medical history prior to beginning treatment. This includes conditions like allergies, high blood pressure, lung disease, and any prescription or over-the-counter medications being taken. IGIV can interfere with the effectiveness of certain vaccines, so it is wise to inform the doctor of any recent or planned immunizations. The physician should also be told if the patient is pregnant, plans to be become pregnant, or is currently breast feeding.

References

1. "Immune globulin (Injection)," University of Maryland Medical Center, December 4, 2015.

2. "Immune Globulin Intravenous," Web MD, n.d.

3. "Immune Globulin (Intravenous) (IGIV)," Drugs.com, November 14, 2013.

4. "Immunoglobulin Therapy and Other Medical Therapies for Antibody Deficiencies," Immune Deficiency Foundation, n.d.

5. "The Immune System and Primary Immunodeficiency," Immune Deficiency Foundation, n.d.

6. Scheinfeld, Noah S., JD, MD, FAAD. "Intravenous Immunoglobulin," Medscape.com, February 3, 2016.

7. "What Is Immune Globulin?" BDI Pharma, n.d.

Chapter 80

Plasmapheresis for Autoimmune Disease

What Is Plasmapheresis?

Plasmapheresis, also called plasma exchange, is a procedure in which blood is removed from the body and the liquid part, called plasma, is separated from the red and white blood cells. The plasma is then typically discarded, and the blood cells are returned to the body, along with fresh plasma or other fluids. This procedure is a successful method of treating some autoimmune diseases, such as multiple sclerosis, Guillain-Barre syndrome, Miller Fisher syndrome, chronic inflammatory demyelinating polyneuropathy, Goodpasture syndrome, and Lambert-Eaton syndrome.

An autoimmune disease causes the body's immune system to attack healthy cells or its own tissues. The immune system produces antibodies to protect the body from infections, bacteria, viruses, and other invaders, but when the antibodies, which are proteins in blood plasma, attack their own body, they became autoantibodies. Plasma exchange helps remove autoantibodies from the blood. An alternative treatment for some disorders is to use medication to suppress the immune system, but this approach can lead to serious side effects, and in some case, the body may no longer be able to fight infection. So plasmapheresis

---

"Plasmapheresis for Autoimmune Disease," © 2017 Omnigraphics. Reviewed October 2016.

is often the preferred method of fighting a number of autoimmune disorders.

Procedure for Plasmapheresis

Anesthesia is generally not necessary for the plasmapheresis treatment itself, but it is sometimes used for the placement of the two relatively large needles that must be used. Once the needles are positioned, patients may feel some discomfort, but no pain, for the remainder of the procedure.

Before the start of plasmapheresis, the patient is asked to lie down or sit in a reclining chair. A needle or catheter tube is placed in a large vein in the crook of the arm, and another needle or tube is placed in the opposite arm or foot. In some cases, the needle or catheter is placed in the shoulder or groin area. Blood is removed through one of the tubes and passed into an apheresis machine, or cell separator. This device separates the plasma from the blood cells, either by spinning at high speed, or by passing the blood through a membrane with tiny pores, which allow only the plasma to pass through, but not the blood cells.

The removed plasma is then discarded, along with the autoantibodies it contains. The replacement plasma, or a plasma substitute, is blended with the blood cells, and the mixture is returned to the body through the other tube. The amount of blood that is outside the body at any given time during the procedure is generally less than the amount a donor would contribute at a blood bank.

Plasmapheresis is usually done on an outpatient basis, and the procedure can take from one to three hours. For an average patient, treatments are repeated six to ten times over span of two to ten weeks. The length and number of treatments depends on the diagnosis and the general condition of the patient.

Before the Procedure

Prior to plasmapheresis, the patient will be examined by his or her physician. A thorough medical history will be taken, and all medication will be reviewed by the doctor in order to determine whether the patient will need to stop taking certain medicines for a given amount of time before and after the treatment.

A few other things to keep in mind:

- Drink plenty of fluids for several days before the procedure to stay hydrated.

- Eat a well-balanced meal prior to treatment.

- Wear comfortable clothing with sleeves that can be easily pulled above the elbows.

- Bring something to read or a portable music device with head-phones to help pass the time.

After the Procedure

Following the procedure, the patient will be allowed to leave the hospital or medical center after resting for a short time. Since many people feel tired or weak after plasmapheresis, the patient will need someone to drive him or her home. After the procedure, care must be taken to follow the doctor's instructions regarding medication dosages, which may need to be adjusted, and preventing infection. The patient can show improvement within days or, at most, a few weeks, and the positive effects of the course of treatment can be expected to last for several months. But since plasmapheresis is a temporary treatment, the procedure may have to be repeated on a regular basis.

Risks and Complications

Although plasmapheresis is a safe form of treatment, and complications don't occur often, like most medical procedures, it does carry some risks. Awareness of these risks can help the patient to be better prepared.

A few of the possible risks and complications include:

- Bleeding, which can occur because of the medication given to prevent clotting during the procedure.

- A drop in blood pressure, which can be helped by lowering the patient's head, raising his or her legs, and giving an intravenous fluid.

- Dizziness, blurred vision, sweating, and abdominal cramps.

- Allergic reaction resulting in fever, chills, or rashes.

- Reactions to medication, such as tingling in the mouth or limbs or metallic taste in the mouth.

- Swelling, bruises, or rashes where needles or tubes were inserted.

- Infection.

- Anaphylaxis, a potentially dangerous reaction to the solutions used in plasma replacement. The procedure needs to be stopped if this complication occurs.

- Severe bleeding, which can lead to irregular heartbeats or seizures; this needs immediate attention.

- Fatigue, weakness, or joint pain.

- Excessive suppression of the immune system can occur during the plasma exchange, however this generally resolves in a short time as the body produces more antibodies.

- Patients can occasionally develop an allergy to the solutions and equipment used in the procedure. If so, the medical technician or doctor would administer intravenous medication.

A doctor should be contacted immediately if any of the following serious complications develop:

- seizures

- signs of infection, such as chills or fever

- severe bleeding or swelling where the needle or tube was inserted

- persistent itching or rashes

- severe pain

- dizziness, shortness of breath, chest pain, or wheezing

References

1. "Plasmapheresis," Mount Sinai Hospital, 2016.

2. Heitz, David. "Plasmapheresis," Healthline, January 6, 2014.

3. Winkler, Sarah. "Plasmapheresis Procedure," How Stuff Works Health, October 10, 2011.

4. "Facts About Plasmapheresis," Muscular Dystrophy Association, July, 2005.

5. "What is Plasmapheresis?" PMWO Life Saving Organization, n.d.

Chapter 81

Gene Therapy

What Is Gene Therapy?

Gene therapy is an experimental technique that uses genes to treat or prevent disease. In the future, this technique may allow doctors to treat a disorder by inserting a gene into a patient's cells instead of using drugs or surgery. Researchers are testing several approaches to gene therapy, including:

- Replacing a mutated gene that causes disease with a healthy copy of the gene.

- Inactivating, or "knocking out," a mutated gene that is functioning improperly.

- Introducing a new gene into the body to help fight a disease.

Although gene therapy is a promising treatment option for a number of diseases (including inherited disorders, some types of cancer, and certain viral infections), the technique remains risky and is still under study to make sure that it will be safe and effective. Gene therapy is currently only being tested for the treatment of diseases that have no other cures.

This chapter includes text excerpted from "Gene Therapy," Genetics Home Reference (GHR), National Institutes of Health (NIH), October 4, 2016.

481

How Does Gene Therapy Work?

Gene therapy is designed to introduce genetic material into cells to compensate for abnormal genes or to make a beneficial protein. If a mutated gene causes a necessary protein to be faulty or missing, gene therapy may be able to introduce a normal copy of the gene to restore the function of the protein.

A gene that is inserted directly into a cell usually does not function. Instead, a carrier called a vector is genetically engineered to deliver the gene. Certain viruses are often used as vectors because they can deliver the new gene by infecting the cell. The viruses are modified so they can't cause disease when used in people. Some types of virus, such as retroviruses, integrate their genetic material (including the new gene) into a chromosome in the human cell. Other viruses, such as adenoviruses, introduce their deoxyribonucleic acid (DNA) into the nucleus of the cell, but the DNA is not integrated into a chromosome.

The vector can be injected or given intravenously (by IV) directly into a specific tissue in the body, where it is taken up by individual cells. Alternately, a sample of the patient's cells can be removed and exposed to the vector in a laboratory setting. The cells containing the vector are then returned to the patient. If the treatment is successful, the new gene delivered by the vector will make a functioning protein.

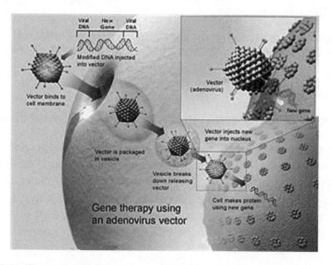

Figure 81.1. *Therapy Vector*

A new gene is injected into an adenovirus vector, which is used to introduce the modified DNA into a human cell. If the treatment is successful, the new gene will make a functional protein.

Researchers must overcome many technical challenges before gene therapy will be a practical approach to treating disease. For example, scientists must find better ways to deliver genes and target them to particular cells. They must also ensure that new genes are precisely controlled by the body.

Is Gene Therapy Safe?

Gene therapy is under study to determine whether it could be used to treat disease. Current research is evaluating the safety of gene therapy; future studies will test whether it is an effective treatment option. Several studies have already shown that this approach can have very serious health risks, such as toxicity, inflammation, and cancer. Because the techniques are relatively new, some of the risks may be unpredictable; however, medical researchers, institutions, and regulatory agencies are working to ensure that gene therapy research is as safe as possible.

Comprehensive federal laws, regulations, and guidelines help protect people who participate in research studies. The U.S. Food and Drug Administration (FDA) regulates all gene therapy products in the United States and oversees research in this area. Researchers who wish to test an approach in a clinical trial must first obtain permission from the FDA. The FDA has the authority to reject or suspend clinical trials that are suspected of being unsafe for participants.

The National Institutes of Health (NIH) also plays an important role in ensuring the safety of gene therapy research. NIH provides guidelines for investigators and institutions (such as universities and hospitals) to follow when conducting clinical trials with gene therapy. These guidelines state that clinical trials at institutions receiving NIH funding for this type of research must be registered with the NIH Office of Biotechnology Activities. The protocol, or plan, for each clinical trial is then reviewed by the NIH Recombinant DNA Advisory Committee (RAC) to determine whether it raises medical, ethical, or safety issues that warrant further discussion at one of the RAC's public meetings.

An Institutional Review Board (IRB) and an Institutional Biosafety Committee (IBC) must approve each gene therapy clinical trial before it can be carried out. An IRB is a committee of scientific and medical advisors and consumers that reviews all research within an institution. An IBC is a group that reviews and approves an institution's potentially hazardous research studies. Multiple levels of evaluation and oversight ensure that safety concerns are a top priority in the planning and carrying out of gene therapy research.

What Are the Ethical Issues Surrounding Gene Therapy?

Because gene therapy involves making changes to the body's set of basic instructions, it raises many unique ethical concerns. The ethical questions surrounding gene therapy include:

- How can "good" and "bad" uses of gene therapy be distinguished?

- Who decides which traits are normal and which constitute a disability or disorder?

- Will the high costs of gene therapy make it available only to the wealthy?

- Could the widespread use of gene therapy make society less accepting of people who are different?

- Should people be allowed to use gene therapy to enhance basic human traits such as height, intelligence, or athletic ability?

Current gene therapy research has focused on treating individuals by targeting the therapy to body cells such as bone marrow or blood cells. This type of gene therapy cannot be passed on to a person's children. Gene therapy could be targeted to egg and sperm cells (germ cells), however, which would allow the inserted gene to be passed on to future generations. This approach is known as germline gene therapy.

The idea of germline gene therapy is controversial. While it could spare future generations in a family from having a particular genetic disorder, it might affect the development of a fetus in unexpected ways or have long-term side effects that are not yet known. Because people who would be affected by germline gene therapy are not yet born, they can't choose whether to have the treatment. Because of these ethical concerns, the U.S. Government does not allow federal funds to be used for research on germline gene therapy in people.

Chapter 82

Stem Cell Transplantation

Clearing the Way for New Stem Cells

Stem cell transplantation can be a lifesaving treatment for patients with some types of cancer, primarily blood cancers like leukemia and lymphoma.

However, the procedure is sometimes grueling for patients and potentially dangerous. Prior to the transplant, patients are often treated with radiation and chemotherapy to kill existing stem cells in the bone marrow so the transplanted donor stem cells have a safe harbor in which to grow and repopulate the body with healthy blood cells (a process called engraftment). And, in the case of hematopoietic (blood) stem cells (HSCs) from a genetically similar but not identical donor (an allogeneic transplant), these conditioning treatments help to suppress an immune response against the transplanted cells.

But the conditioning regimen can damage a patient's healthy cells and tissues as well as their HSCs, resulting in side effects, including infections, respiratory problems, and organ damage that can be fatal in a small percentage of patients.

If the preparation for transplantation could be made less toxic to healthy cells, explained Judith Shizuru, M.D., Ph.D., the study's senior author, the procedure could potentially be used not just for cancer but for other indications. These include treating diseases caused by

This chapter includes text excerpted from "Approach May Allow for Stem Cell Transplant without Radiation, Chemotherapy," National Cancer Institute (NCI), September 7, 2016.

485

malfunctioning blood and immune cells, including autoimmune diseases and blood disorders marked by abnormal hemoglobin (such as sickle cell anemia or thalassemia), as well as improving gene therapy and organ transplantation.

Previous research, by the Stanford team and others, has shown that biological agents that target c-kit, a protein that HSCs use for many of their normal cellular functions, can deplete HSCs in mice lacking a functioning immune system. However, in earlier studies, targeting this single protein did not deplete the HSCs in mice with a functioning immune system.

So the Stanford researchers tested whether targeting a second protein, called CD47, in addition to c-kit could eliminate HSCs in mice with a healthy immune system. CD47 serves as a "marker of self" for HSCs and some other types of cells, telling the immune system not to attack them. By blocking CD47 with a specially designed molecule, the researchers hoped to make HSCs vulnerable to treatment with an agent targeting c-kit.

The combination worked. In mice with healthy immune systems that were treated with both agents, the researchers saw a 10,000-fold reduction in the targeted HSCs, to the point where "we could no longer measure them," said the study's lead author, Akanksha Chhabra, Ph.D.

In further experiments, mice with healthy immune systems were treated with both agents or with a c-kit-targeting agent alone and then underwent a modified form of anautologous stem cell transplant. The mice that received both agents showed 100 times more engraftment of the donor stem cells in their bone marrow than mice treated with the anti-c-kit agent alone, and healthy cells derived from the transplanted HSCs were found in the blood, spleen, bone marrow, and thymus.

The researchers also tested in mice whether the general approach would work in a type of allogeneic transplant. They treated mice with the two-agent conditioning regimen and with additional biological agents to deplete immune cells (T cells) to prevent the immune system from attacking the transplanted cells. The transplant was successful, with the donor cells successfully establishing themselves in the recipient's bone marrow and producing healthy blood and immune cells.

Toward Human Trials

Agents that target c-kit and CD47 have already been tested in human studies in healthy volunteers and cancer patients, respectively, explained Dr. Shizuru, and no major side effect have been observed. The team has also recently begun enrolling patients in a clinical trial using an agent that targets c-kit for children with severe combined immunodeficiency disease. In mice, added Dr. Chhabra, researchers have seen some graying of the fur and drops in sperm counts due to the c-kit antibody, but "when the treatment stopped, the sperm counts did go [back] up," she said. The current study did not look at long-term effects on fertility.

The next step is to test the drug combination as a conditioning regimen for HSC transplantation in nonhuman primates, said Dr. Shizuru. Since the drugs have already begun human safety studies as single agents, she thinks early human trials of the combination for HSC transplantation could begin in the next 3 to 5 years.

"The goal of this study, and what we're hoping we've shown, is that we're going to change the way that blood and marrow transplants will be done in the near future," Dr. Shizuru said. "We foresee that transplants will be safer to perform and that many more patients can be treated with this potentially curative cellular therapy."

Chapter 83

Treatment of Human Immunodeficiency Virus (HIV) Infection

What Is Antiretroviral Therapy?

Antiretroviral therapy (ART) is the use of human immunodeficiency virus (HIV) medicines to treat HIV infection. People on ART take a combination of HIV medicines (called an HIV regimen) every day.

ART is recommended for everyone infected with HIV. ART can't cure HIV, but HIV medicines help people with HIV live longer, healthier lives. ART also reduces the risk of HIV transmission.

How Do HIV Medicines Work?

HIV attacks and destroys the infection-fighting CD4 cells of the immune system. Loss of CD4 cells makes it hard for the body to fight off infections and certain HIV-related cancers.

HIV medicines prevent HIV from multiplying (making copies of itself), which reduces the amount of HIV in the body. Having less HIV in the body gives the immune system a chance to recover.

This chapter includes text excerpted from "HIV Treatment: The Basics," AIDS *info*, National Institutes of Health (NIH), March 1, 2016.

Even though there is still some HIV in the body, the immune system is strong enough to fight off infections and certain HIV-related cancers.

By reducing the amount of HIV in the body, HIV medicines also reduce the risk of HIV transmission.

When Is It Time to Start Taking HIV Medicine?

People infected with HIV should start ART as soon as possible. In people with the following conditions, it's especially important to start ART right away: pregnancy, AIDS, certain HIV-related illnesses and coinfections, and early HIV infection. (Early HIV infection is the period up to 6 months after infection with HIV.)

What HIV Medicines Are Included in an HIV Regimen?

There are many HIV medicines available to make up an HIV regimen. The HIV medicines are grouped into six drug classes according to how they fight HIV. A person's initial HIV regimen usually includes three or more HIV medicines from at least two different HIV drug classes.

Selection of an HIV regimen depends on several factors, including possible side effects of HIV medicines and potential drug interactions between medicines. Because the needs of people with HIV vary, there are several HIV regimens to choose from.

What Are Risks of Taking HIV Medicines?

Potential risks of ART include side effects from HIV medicines and drug interactions between HIV medicines or between HIV medicines and other medicines a person is taking. Poor adherence—not taking HIV medicines every day and exactly as prescribed—increases the risk of drug resistance and treatment failure.

Side Effects

Side effects from HIV medicines can vary depending on the medicine and the person taking the medicine. People taking the same HIV medicine can have very different side effects. Some side effects, for example, headache or occasional dizziness, may not be serious. Other side effects, such as swelling of the mouth and tongue or liver damage, can be life-threatening.

Drug Interactions

HIV medicines can interact with other HIV medicines in an HIV regimen. They can also interact with other medicines that a person with HIV is taking. A drug interaction can reduce or increase a medicine's effect on the body. Drug interactions can also cause unwanted side effects.

Drug Resistance

When HIV multiplies in the body, the virus sometimes mutates (changes form) and makes variations of itself. Variations of HIV that develop while a person is taking HIV medicines can lead to drug-resistant strains of HIV. HIV medicines that previously controlled a person's HIV are not effective against the new, drug-resistant HIV. In other words, the person's HIV continues to multiply.

Poor adherence to an HIV regimen increases the risk of drug resistance and treatment failure.

Chapter 84

Treatments for Rheumatic Conditions

What Is Arthritis?

"Arthritis" literally means joint inflammation. Although joint inflammation is a symptom or sign rather than a specific diagnosis, the term arthritis is often used to refer to any disorder that affects the joints. These disorders fall within the broader category of rheumatic diseases. These are diseases characterized by inflammation (signs include redness or heat, swelling, and symptoms such as pain) and loss of function of one or more connecting or supporting structures of the body. They especially affect joints, tendons, ligaments, bones, and muscles. Common signs and symptoms are pain, swelling, and stiffness. Some rheumatic diseases also can involve internal organs. There are more than 100 rheumatic diseases that collectively affect more than 46 million Americans.

Examples of Rheumatic Diseases

The most common type of arthritis, osteoarthritis, damages both the cartilage, which is the tissue that cushions the ends of bones within the joint and the underlying bone. Osteoarthritis can cause joint pain and

This chapter includes text excerpted from "Arthritis and Rheumatic Diseases," National Institute of Arthritis and Musculoskeletal and Skin Diseases (NIAMS), October 2014.

stiffness. Disability results most often when the disease affects the spine and the weight-bearing joints (the knees and hips). Rheumatoid arthritis, which is less common, is an inflammatory disease of the immune system that attacks the lining of the joint, called the "synovium," resulting in pain and swelling and loss of function in the joints. The most commonly affected joints are those in the hands and feet.

Finding Effective Treatments

Treatments for arthritis and rheumatic diseases vary depending on the specific disease or condition; however, treatment generally includes the following:

Exercise. Physical activity can reduce joint pain and stiffness and increase flexibility, muscle strength, and endurance. Exercise also can result in weight loss, which in turn reduces stress on painful joints. The best exercises for people with arthritis are those that place the least stress on the joints, such as walking, stretching, using weight machines, stationary cycling, exercising in water, and swimming. A doctor or physical therapist can recommend a safe, wellrounded exercise program. People with arthritis should speak with their doctor before beginning any new exercise program.

Diet. Although there is not a specific diet that helps arthritis, a well-balanced diet, along with exercise, helps people manage their body weight and stay healthy. Diet is especially important for people who have gout. People with gout should avoid alcohol and foods that are high in purines, such as organ meats (liver, kidney), sardines, anchovies, and gravy.

Medications. A variety of medications are used to treat rheumatic diseases. The type of medication depends on the specific disease and the individual patient. The medications used to treat most rheumatic diseases do not provide a cure, but rather limit the symptoms of the disease. In some cases, especially when a person has rheumatoid arthritis or another type of inflammatory arthritis, the medication may slow the course of the disease and prevent further damage to joints or other parts of the body.

Following are some of the types of medications commonly used in the treatment of rheumatic diseases.

- **Oral analgesics.** Medications that are designed purely for pain relief. These include over-the-counter analgesics such as

494

acetaminophen and stronger narcotic medications such as oxyco-
done or hydrocodone, which are usually reserved for severe pain
or pain following surgery or a fracture.

- **Topical analgesics.** Creams or ointments that are rubbed into
  the skin over sore muscles or joints and relieve pain through one
  or more active ingredients.

- **Nonsteroidal anti-inflammatory drugs (NSAIDs).** A large
  class of medications useful against both pain and inflammation.
  Two NSAIDs, ibuprofen and naproxen sodium, are available
  over the counter. More than two dozen others, including a sub-
  class of NSAIDs called COX-2 inhibitors, are available only with
  a prescription.

- **Disease-modifying antirheumatic drugs (DMARDs).** A
  family of medicines that is used to slow or stop the immune
  system from attacking the joints and causing damage in inflammatory arthritis like rheumatoid arthritis and ankylosing
  spondylitis.

- **Biologic response modifiers.** A relatively new family of genetically engineered drugs that block specific molecular pathways
  of the immune system that are involved in the inflammatory
  process.

- **Janus kinase inhibitors.** A new class of medications that work
  by blocking Janus-associated kinase, or JAK, pathways that are
  involved in the body's immune response.

- **Corticosteroids.** Strong inflammation-fighting drugs that are
  similar to the cortisone made by our bodies. Corticosteroids can
  be given by mouth, in creams applied to the skin, intravenously,
  or by injection directly into the affected joint(s).

Although all of these drugs have the potential to help arthritis and
rheumatic diseases, all have the potential for dangerous side effects.
When prescribing medications, doctors and patients must weigh the
potential risks against the expected benefits.

Heat and cold therapies. Heat and cold can both be used to
reduce the pain and inflammation of arthritis. Heat therapy increases
blood flow, tolerance for pain, and flexibility. Cold therapy numbs the
nerves around the joint to reduce pain and may relieve inflammation
and muscle spasms. Heat therapy can involve placing warm towels or
hot packs on the inflamed joint or taking a warm bath or shower. Cold

therapy can involve cold packs, ice massage, soaking in cold water, or over-the-counter sprays and ointments that cool the skin and joints.

Relaxation therapy. Relaxation therapy helps reduce pain by teaching people various ways to release muscle tension throughout the body. In one method of relaxation therapy, known as progressive relaxation, the patient tightens a muscle group and then slowly releases the tension. Doctors and physical therapists can teach patients a variety of relaxation techniques.

Splints and braces. Splints and braces are used to support weakened joints or allow them to rest. Some prevent the joint from moving; others allow some movement. A splint or brace should be used only when recommended by a doctor or therapist, who will ensure a proper fit and provide instructions for its use.

The incorrect use of a splint or brace can cause joint damage, stiffness, and pain.

Assistive devices. A person with arthritis can use many kinds of devices to ease the pain. For example, using a cane when walking can reduce some of the weight placed on a knee or hip affected by arthritis. A shoe insert (orthotic) can ease the pain of walking caused by arthritis of the foot or knee. Other devices can help with activities such as opening jars, closing zippers, and holding pencils.

Surgery. Surgery may be required to repair damage to a joint after an injury or to restore function or relieve pain in a joint damaged by arthritis. Many types of surgery are performed for arthritis. They range from outpatient procedures performed arthroscopically (through small incisions over the joints) to the surgical removal and replacement of a damaged joint with an artificial joint, known as total joint replacement.

Chapter 85

Immunotherapy for Allergies

Most people manage their allergies by avoiding allergy-triggering substances (allergens) and taking medications to provide temporary relief from symptoms. For some types of allergies, allergen immunotherapy is an additional and often useful approach that involves introducing increasing amounts of allergens to the immune system. Immunotherapy is a long-term treatment that may help prevent or reduce the severity of allergic reactions and can change the course of allergic disease by modifying the body's immune response to allergens. Immunotherapy can be used to treat environmental allergies and is particularly effective at reducing the risk of severe allergic reactions to stings from some insects, such as bees and yellow jackets. Improvements in allergy symptoms may last for several years after stopping immunotherapy. Scientists are attempting to use immunotherapy to prevent and treat food allergy. However, the balance between the benefits and risks of immunotherapy for food allergy has not yet been

This chapter contains text excerpted from the following sources: Text in this chapter begins with excerpts from "Allergen Immunotherapy," National Institute of Allergy and Infectious Diseases (NIAID), April 22, 2015; Text under the heading "Immunotherapy for Environmental Allergies" is excerpted from "Immunotherapy for Environmental Allergies," National Institute of Allergy and Infectious Diseases (NIAID), May 12, 2015; and text under the heading "Immunotherapy for Food Allergy" is excerpted from "Immunotherapy for Food Allergy," National Institute of Allergy and Infectious Diseases (NIAID), May 12, 2015.

well-studied, and it currently is not recommended except as an experimental approach.

National Institute of Allergy and Infectious Diseases (NIAID) research efforts on allergen immunotherapy focus on the prevention and treatment of asthma, allergic rhinitis (hay fever), and food allergy.

NIAID-supported research aims to increase the effectiveness and safety of immunotherapy, reduce the duration of treatment, advance the development of safe and effective immunotherapy for food allergy, and improve understanding of how immunotherapy helps reduce allergic symptoms in these diseases.

Types of Allergen Immunotherapies

1. Immunotherapy for environmental allergies

2. Immunotherapy for food allergies

Immunotherapy for Environmental Allergies

Allergic rhinitis, commonly known as hay fever, occurs when the immune system overreacts to airborne allergens, such as those from pollens, animal dander, dust mites, cockroaches, and molds. These environmental allergies can cause symptoms such as sneezing, a runny and stuffy nose, and itchy or watery eyes. Reactions to allergens often also play an important role in asthma. Surveys performed at clinical practices suggest that many patients do not get complete relief from medications and may be candidates for immunotherapy.

Allergy shots, or subcutaneous immunotherapy (SCIT), have been used for more than 100 years and can provide long-lasting symptom relief. In 2014, the Food and Drug Administration approved three types of under-the-tongue tablets for allergies to grass and ragweed. The treatments, called sublingual immunotherapy (SLIT), offer a potential alternative to allergy shots for people with these allergies.

Subcutaneous Immunotherapy (SCIT)

SCIT involves a series of shots containing small amounts of allergen into the fat under the skin.

SCIT includes two phases: a buildup phase and a maintenance phase. During the buildup phase, doctors administer injections containing gradually increasing amounts of allergen once or twice per week. This phase generally lasts from three to six months, depending on how often the shots are given and the body's response. The aim is to reach a target dose that has been shown to be effective. Once the target dose is reached, the maintenance phase begins. Shots are given less frequently during the maintenance phase, typically every two to four weeks. Some people begin experiencing a decrease in symptoms during the buildup phase, but others may not notice an improvement until the maintenance phase.

Maintenance therapy generally lasts three to five years. The decision about how long to continue SCIT is based on how well it is working and how well a person tolerates the shots. For example, if after one year of maintenance therapy there is no evidence of improvement, it is hard to justify continuing immunotherapy for another two to four years. On the other hand, if a person is entirely symptom-free, he or she may choose to stop after three years rather than complete five years of treatment. Many people continue to experience benefits for several years after the shots are stopped, and the theoretical potential of "curing" allergy makes the concept of immunotherapy very attractive.

Side-effects from SCIT are usually minor and may include swelling or redness at the injection site. However, there is a small risk of serious allergic reactions such as anaphylaxis. Because most severe reactions occur shortly after injection, it is recommended that patients remain under medical supervision for at least half an hour after receiving a shot. Patients whose asthma is not under control are recommended to postpone their shot until their asthma is stable.

An estimated 5 percent of people with environmental allergies receive SCIT for allergic rhinitis and asthma, and less than 20 percent of people who begin SCIT finish the entire treatment course. The time and cost commitments that SCIT requires likely discourage some people from starting or completing treatment. Development of new forms of immunotherapy that require shorter treatment duration may result in more patients being interested in receiving allergen immunotherapy.

NIAID funds research to investigate several approaches to improve the effectiveness and safety of SCIT and decrease the duration of treatment. Scientists are exploring the use of modified allergens that may elicit the same or better effects with fewer shots, while decreasing the risk of side effects. Scientists also are developing treatment approaches that combine SCIT with other medications. For example, researchers from the NIAID-sponsored Immune Tolerance Network are testing a combination of SCIT and an investigational allergy drug as a potential treatment for cat allergy.

Sublingual Immunotherapy (SLIT)

People taking SLIT place a tablet containing allergen under the tongue. SLIT tablets are taken daily and kept under the tongue for one to two minutes, then swallowed. The allergen doses used in SLIT typically are higher than those used in SCIT. For example, a daily SLIT dose for grass pollen is roughly equivalent to a monthly SCIT dose.

- SLIT has been widely used in Europe for several years and is available in the United States for treatment of grass and ragweed allergies. Studies show that there are fewer allergic reactions to SLIT compared to SCIT. After the first SLIT dose is given at the doctor's office, patients can take subsequent doses at home. However, even though therapy is taken at home, many people do not complete the recommended three years of treatment.

- Side effects of SLIT are usually minor and may include itching of the mouth, lips, or throat. Severe allergic reactions (anaphylaxis) are extremely rare, and this represents a clear advantage over allergy shots. Nevertheless, because treatment takes place at home, doctors may prescribe an epinephrine autoinjector (EpiPen) to people receiving SLIT for use in the event of a severe allergic reaction. The NIAID-funded Immune Tolerance Network is conducting a side-by-side evaluation of SLIT or SCIT for grass allergy. This will help determine whether there are any differences in the effectiveness of these two types of immunotherapy.

How Does Immunotherapy Work?

Scientists have developed a general understanding of how SCIT and SLIT may work to prevent and treat allergies, although many of the details of this process have yet to be unraveled. An allergic response begins when an allergen is taken up by cells known as antigen-presenting cells (APCs). The APCs break down the allergen and display fragments of it on their surfaces, alerting other cells to become active and starting a chain of events that leads to allergy symptoms. The amount of allergen given in an allergy shot or as an under-the-tongue tablet is much larger than the amount that would be encountered during a natural exposure. This difference in quantity may be responsible for the change in the kind of immune response that is started by the APCs. Instead of activating type 2 T helper (Th2) cells, which play a key role in promoting an allergic response, APCs activate specialized immune cells called regulatory T cells (Tregs). Tregs begin to release a variety of chemical messengers that lead to the suppression, change in function, or elimination of the Th2 cells. Tregs can also influence B cells, the cells that develop into antibody-producing plasma cells. As a result, plasma cells produce less IgE, the main type of antibody involved in allergic reactions and also may make more of other types of allergen-specific antibodies known as "blocking" antibodies. Blocking antibodies recognize and bind to the allergen, preventing it from binding to IgE and triggering an allergic reaction.

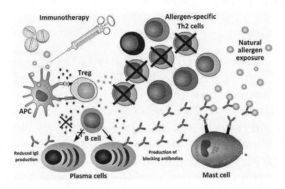

Figure 85.1. *Immunotherapy*

Allergen introduced to the body by allergy shots or under-the-tongue tablets is processed by antigen-presenting cells (APCs), which activate regulatory cells (Tregs). Signals sent by the APCs and Tregs lead to changes in production of chemical messengers, increasing those that are anti-allergic and decreasing those that are pro-allergic. In addition, allergy-promoting type 2 T helper (Th2) cells that specifically recognize the allergen are suppressed or deleted. However, other Th2 cells that do not contribute to the allergic response are not affected. Tregs can also influence B cells, which develop into antibody-producing plasma cells. Plasma cells are driven to produce less IgE and more blocking antibodies. Blocking antibodies bind to allergen and do not allow it to reach the mast cells and start an allergic reaction.

Immunotherapy for Food Allergy

Current strategies to manage food allergy involve avoiding foods that may cause an allergic reaction and treating severe reactions as they arise. However, avoiding food allergens can be difficult because they are often "hidden" in unexpected foods. For example, the coating of a fruit-flavored jelly bean may contain peanut allergen. Therefore, scientists are working to develop immunotherapy approaches to prevent and treat food allergy. These experimental therapies include oral immunotherapy, therapy with baked milk or egg, sublingual (under-the-tongue) immunotherapy, and epicutaneous (skin patch) immunotherapy. Initial attempts to use allergy shots, or subcutaneous immunotherapy, to treat food allergy have been stopped because too many people experienced severe allergic reactions after receiving the injections.

All forms of immunotherapy for food allergy are experimental, and although some trained clinicians offer them, these therapies are not approved by the U.S. Food and Drug Administration (FDA). People should not try immunotherapy on their own because of the risk of severe reactions. The therapy should be administered only under the guidance of trained clinicians.

Oral Immunotherapy

Oral immunotherapy (OIT) currently is being tested in several NIAID-funded and other clinical trials. It involves eating small but gradually increasing doses of the food that causes the allergy every day, usually in the form of a powder mixed with a harmless food. The most common side effects associated with OIT are mouth itching and swelling and stomach aches. However, severe allergic reactions requiring treatment with epinephrine, an emergency rescue medication that is given by injection, have occurred in some cases. Some people who have participated in OIT studies discontinued OIT due to side effects. The gastrointestinal side effects of OIT sometimes can be severe and may be due to the development of a condition called eosinophilic esophagitis, which often is associated with food allergy.

OIT has shown some benefits in small clinical trials for treatment of milk, egg, and peanut allergies. However, there are still many issues that need to be addressed, including the safety of the treatment, the number of people who will benefit, the duration of improvement, and the effectiveness of OIT for a wider variety of foods. NIAID supports research to evaluate the role of OIT in treating and managing food allergy. A study from the NIAID-funded Consortium of Food Allergy Research suggested that egg OIT can benefit children with egg allergy. Most of the study participants could be safely exposed to egg while on egg OIT, and some were able to safely eat egg after stopping OIT for four to six weeks.

NIAID also is funding peanut OIT trials in older children and adults, as well as another trial to evaluate OIT for multiple food allergies at the same time.

Baked Milk and Egg Therapy

Consumption of baked milk and egg is a potential alternative to OIT for treatment of milk and egg allergies. Temperature-associated changes in certain milk and egg proteins may render baked versions of these foods less allergenic. However, the same does not hold true for all allergy-triggering foods. Roasting peanuts, for example, can make them more likely to cause allergic reactions.

Studies have suggested that some children who are allergic to uncooked egg and milk can tolerate small amounts of these foods in fully cooked products such as muffins. An NIAID-funded study found that more than half of baked-milk-tolerant children who followed specific instructions to include baked milk products into their diets eventually were able to tolerate foods containing uncooked milk. The results also suggested that children who ate baked milk outgrew their milk allergies more quickly than children who did not eat baked milk. However, many children treated with baked products may never be able to eat unheated milk without allergic reactions. More studies need to be done to determine whether the baked food approach benefits some people with food allergy.

Sublingual Immunotherapy

SLIT involves holding drops containing food allergen extract under the tongue, then swallowing or spitting them out. Currently, very little information is available regarding food allergen SLIT. More work is needed to determine the potential role of this therapy in treating food allergy, including appropriate dosing and length of treatment, before SLIT can be considered a safe or effective option.

Epicutaneous Immunotherapy

In epicutaneous immunotherapy (EPIT), another experimental form of immunotherapy, allergen is delivered to the skin surface by a patch. The NIAID-funded Consortium of Food Allergy Research currently is conducting a clinical trial evaluating EPIT for the treatment of peanut allergy in children and young adults.

Prevention of Food Allergy

For many years, parents of children at high risk of developing food allergies were advised to wait to put common food allergens into their children's diet. For example, it was recommended that eggs be avoided until 2 years of age and peanuts until 3 years. However, food allergy continued to become more common, suggesting that delayed introduction was not helping, and in 2008, this practice was no longer recommended by the American Academy of Pediatrics. In fact, by 2008, there was some evidence to suggest that early introduction might decrease the likelihood of developing food allergy.

In February 2015, scientists reported results from the Learning Early About Peanut Allergy (LEAP) study, a large clinical trial conducted by the NIAID-funded Immune Tolerance Network. The goal of this trial was to determine whether early exposure to peanut-containing foods can prevent the development of peanut allergy. The study enrolled 640 children under a year of age thought to be at high risk of peanut allergy because they had severe eczema, an allergy to egg, or both. These children were divided into a group that avoided peanuts until they were 5 years old and a group that immediately started eating peanut-containing foods at least three times per week. When the children reached 5 years of age, the rate of peanut allergy was 80 percent lower in the group that had eaten peanut products compared to the group that had avoided them. These results suggest that the early introduction of peanut into the diet may prevent the development of peanut allergy. Medical experts currently are discussing how the LEAP findings will change recommendations about introducing peanuts into the diet of infants and young children.

Chapter 86

Immunotherapy for Cancer

Immunotherapy: Using the Immune System to Treat Cancer

The immune system's natural capacity to detect and destroy abnormal cells may prevent the development of many cancers. However, cancer cells are sometimes able to avoid detection and destruction by the immune system. Cancer cells may:

- reduce the expression of tumor antigens on their surface, making it harder for the immune system to detect them

- express proteins on their surface that induce immune cell inactivation

- induce cells in the surrounding environment (microenvironment) to release substances that suppress immune responses and promote tumor cell proliferation and survival

In the past few years, the rapidly advancing field of cancer immunology has produced several new methods of treating cancer, called immunotherapies, that increase the strength of immune responses against tumors. Immunotherapies either stimulate the activities of specific components of the immune system or counteract signals produced by cancer cells that suppress immune responses.

This chapter includes text excerpted from "Immunotherapy: Using the Immune System to Treat Cancer," National Cancer Institute (NCI), September 14, 2015.

These advances in cancer immunotherapy are the result of long-term investments in basic research on the immune system—research that continues today. Additional research is currently under way to:

- understand why immunotherapy is effective in some patients but not in others who have the same cancer

- expand the use of immunotherapy to more types of cancer

- increase the effectiveness of immunotherapy by combining it with other types of cancer treatment, such as targeted therapy, chemotherapy, and radiation therapy

Immune Checkpoint Modulators

One immunotherapy approach is to block the ability of certain proteins, called immune checkpoint proteins, to limit the strength and duration of immune responses. These proteins normally keep immune responses in check by preventing overly intense responses that might damage normal cells as well as abnormal cells. But, researchers have learned that tumors can commandeer these proteins and use them to suppress immune responses.

Blocking the activity of immune checkpoint proteins releases the "brakes" on the immune system, increasing its ability to destroy cancer cells. Several immune checkpoint inhibitors have been approved by the U.S. Food and Drug Administration (FDA). The first such drug to receive approval, ipilimumab (Yervoy®), for the treatment of advanced melanoma, blocks the activity of a checkpoint protein known as CTLA4, which is expressed on the surface of activated immune cells called cytotoxic T lymphocytes. CTLA4 acts as a "switch" to inactivate these T cells, thereby reducing the strength of immune responses; ipilimumab binds to CTLA4 and prevents it from sending its inhibitory signal.

Two other FDA-approved checkpoint inhibitors, nivolumab (Opdivo®) and pembrolizumab (Keytruda®), work in a similar way, but they target a different checkpoint protein on activated T cells known as PD-1. Nivolumab is approved to treat some patients with advanced melanoma or advanced lung cancer, and pembrolizumab is approved to treat some patients with advanced melanoma.

Researchers have also developed checkpoint inhibitors that disrupt the interaction of PD-1 and proteins on the surface of tumor cells known as PD-L1 and PD-L2. Agents that target other checkpoint proteins are also being developed, and additional research is aimed at understanding why checkpoint inhibitors are effective in some patients but not in others and identifying ways to expand the use of checkpoint inhibitors to other cancer types.

Immune Cell Therapy

Progress is also being made with an experimental form of immunotherapy called adoptive cell transfer (ACT). In several small clinical trials testing ACT, some patients with very advanced cancer—primarily blood cancers—have had their disease completely eradicated. In some cases, these treatment responses have lasted for years.

In one form of ACT, T cells that have infiltrated a patient's tumor, called tumor-infiltrating lymphocytes (TILs), are collected from samples of the tumor. TILs that show the greatest recognition of the patient's tumor cells in laboratory tests are selected, and large populations of these cells are grown in the laboratory. The cells are then activated by treatment with immune system signaling proteins called cytokines and infused into the patient's bloodstream.

The idea behind this approach is that the TILs have already shown the ability to target tumor cells, but there may not be enough of them within the tumor microenvironment to eradicate the tumor or overcome the immune suppressive signals that are being released there. Introducing massive amounts of activated TILs can help to overcome these barriers and shrink or destroy tumors.

Another form of ACT that is being actively studied is CAR T-cell therapy. In this treatment approach, a patient's T cells are collected from the blood and genetically modified to express a protein known as a chimeric antigen receptor, or CAR. Next, the modified cells are grown in the laboratory to produce large populations of the cells, which are then infused into the patient.

CARs are modified forms of a protein called a T-cell receptor, which is expressed on the surface of T cells. These receptors allow the modified T cells to attach to specific proteins on the surface of cancer cells. Once bound to the cancer cells, the modified T cells become activated and attack the cancer cells.

Therapeutic Antibodies

Therapeutic antibodies are antibodies made in the laboratory that are designed to cause the destruction of cancer cells.

One class of therapeutic antibodies, called antibody-drug conjugates (ADCs), has proven to be particularly effective, with several ADCs having been approved by the FDA for the treatment of different cancers.

ADCs are created by chemically linking antibodies, or fragments of antibodies, to a toxic substance. The antibody portion of the ADC allows it to bind to a target molecule that is expressed on the surface of cancer cells. The toxic substance can be a poison, such as a bacterial toxin; a small-molecule drug; or a radioactive compound. Once an ADC binds to a cancer cell, it is taken up by the cell and the toxic substance kills the cell.

The FDA has approved several ADCs for the treatment of patients with cancer, including:

• ado-trastuzumab emtansine (Kadcyla®) for the treatment of some types of breast cancer

• brentuximab vedotin (Adcetris®) for Hodgkin lymphoma and a type of non-Hodgkin T-cell lymphoma

• ibritumomab tiuxetan (Zevalin®) for a type of non-Hodgkin B-cell lymphoma

Other therapeutic antibodies do not carry toxic payloads. Some of these antibodies cause cancer cells to commit suicide (apoptosis) when they bind to them. In other cases, antibody binding to cancer cells is recognized by certain immune cells or proteins known collectively as "complement," which are produced by immune cells, and these cells and proteins mediate cancer cell death (via antibody-dependent cell-mediated cytotoxicity or complement-dependent cytotoxicity, respectively). Sometimes all three mechanisms of inducing cancer cell death can be involved.

One example of this type of therapeutic antibody is rituximab (Rituxan®), which targets a protein on the surface of B lymphocytes called CD20. Rituximab has become a mainstay in the treatment of some B-cell lymphomas and B-cell chronic lymphocytic leukemia. When CD20-expressing cells become coated with rituximab, the drug kills the cells by inducing apoptosis, as well as by antibody-dependent cell-mediated cytotoxicity and complement-dependent cytotoxicity.

Other therapies combine non-antibody immune system molecules and cancer-killing agents. For example, denileukin diftitox (ONTAK®), which is approved for the treatment of cutaneous T-cell lymphoma, consists of the cytokine interleukin-2 (IL-2) attached to a toxin produced by the bacterium *Corynebacterium diphtheria*, which causes diphtheria. Some leukemia and lymphoma cells express receptors for IL-2 on their surface. Denileukin diftitox uses its IL-2 portion to target these cancer cells and the diphtheria toxin to kill them.

Cancer Treatment Vaccines

The use of cancer treatment (or therapeutic) vaccines is another approach to immunotherapy. These vaccines are usually made from a patient's own tumor cells or from substances produced by tumor cells. They are designed to treat cancers that have already developed by strengthening the body's natural defenses against the cancer.

In 2010, the FDA approved the first cancer treatment vaccine, sipuleucel-T (Provenge®), for use in some men with metastatic prostate cancer. Other therapeutic vaccines are being tested in clinical trials to treat a range of cancers, including brain, breast, and lung cancer.

Immune System Modulators

Yet another type of immunotherapy uses proteins that normally help regulate, or modulate, immune system activity to enhance the body's immune response against cancer. These proteins include cytokines and certain growth factors. Two types of cytokines are used to treat patients with cancer: interleukins and interferons.

Immune-modulating agents may work through different mechanisms. One type of interferon, for example, enhances a patient's immune response to cancer cells by activating certain white blood cells, such as natural killer cells and dendritic cells. Recent advances in understanding how cytokines stimulate immune cells could enable the development of more effective immunotherapies and combinations of these agents.

Chapter 87

Asthma Treatment

What Is Asthma?

Asthma is a chronic (long-term) lung disease that inflames and narrows the airways. Asthma causes recurring periods of wheezing (a whistling sound when you breathe), chest tightness, shortness of breath, and coughing. The coughing often occurs at night or early in the morning.

Asthma affects people of all ages, but it most often starts during childhood. In the United States, more than 25 million people are known to have asthma. About 7 million of these people are children.

Sometimes asthma symptoms are mild and go away on their own or after minimal treatment with asthma medicine. Other times, symptoms continue to get worse.

When symptoms get more intense and/or more symptoms occur, you're having an asthma attack. Asthma attacks also are called flareups or exacerbations.

Treating symptoms when you first notice them is important. This will help prevent the symptoms from worsening and causing a severe asthma attack. Severe asthma attacks may require emergency care, and they can be fatal.

This chapter includes text excerpted from "Asthma," National Heart, Lung, and Blood Institute (NHLBI), August 4, 2014.

How Is Asthma Treated and Controlled?

Asthma is a long-term disease that has no cure. The goal of asthma treatment is to control the disease. Good asthma control will:

- prevent chronic and troublesome symptoms, such as coughing and shortness of breath

- reduce your need for quick-relief medicines

- help you maintain good lung function

- let you maintain your normal activity level and sleep through the night

- prevent asthma attacks that could result in an emergency room visit or hospital stay

To control asthma, partner with your doctor to manage your asthma or your child's asthma. Children aged 10 or older—and younger children who are able—should take an active role in their asthma care.

Taking an active role to control your asthma involves:

- Working with your doctor to treat other conditions that can interfere with asthma management.

- Avoiding things that worsen your asthma (asthma triggers). However, one trigger you should not avoid is physical activity. Physical activity is an important part of a healthy lifestyle. Talk with your doctor about medicines that can help you stay active.

- Working with your doctor and other healthcare providers to create and follow an asthma action plan.

An asthma action plan gives guidance on taking your medicines properly, avoiding asthma triggers (except physical activity), tracking your level of asthma control, responding to worsening symptoms, and seeking emergency care when needed.

Asthma is treated with two types of medicines: long-term control and quick-relief medicines. Long-term control medicines help reduce airway inflammation and prevent asthma symptoms. Quick-relief, or "rescue," medicines relieve asthma symptoms that may flare up.

Your initial treatment will depend on the severity of your asthma. Followup asthma treatment will depend on how well your asthma action plan is controlling your symptoms and preventing asthma attacks.

Your level of asthma control can vary over time and with changes in your home, school, or work environments. These changes can alter how often you're exposed to the factors that can worsen your asthma.

Your doctor may need to increase your medicine if your asthma doesn't stay under control. On the other hand, if your asthma is well controlled for several months, your doctor may decrease your medicine. These adjustments to your medicine will help you maintain the best control possible with the least amount of medicine necessary.

Asthma treatment for certain groups of people—such as children, pregnant women, or those for whom exercise brings on asthma symptoms—will be adjusted to meet their special needs.

Follow an Asthma Action Plan

You can work with your doctor to create a personal asthma action plan. The plan will describe your daily treatments, such as which medicines to take and when to take them. The plan also will explain when to call your doctor or go to the emergency room.

If your child has asthma, all of the people who care for him or her should know about the child's asthma action plan. This includes babysitters and workers at daycare centers, schools, and camps. These caretakers can help your child follow his or her action plan.

Avoid Things That Can Worsen Your Asthma

Many common things (called asthma triggers) can set off or worsen your asthma symptoms. Once you know what these things are, you can take steps to control many of them.

For example, exposure to pollens or air pollution might make your asthma worse. If so, try to limit time outdoors when the levels of these substances in the outdoor air are high. If animal fur triggers your asthma symptoms, keep pets with fur out of your home or bedroom.

One possible asthma trigger you shouldn't avoid is physical activity. Physical activity is an important part of a healthy lifestyle. Talk with your doctor about medicines that can help you stay active.

If your asthma symptoms are clearly related to allergens, and you can't avoid exposure to those allergens, your doctor may advise you to get allergy shots.

You may need to see a specialist if you're thinking about getting allergy shots. These shots can lessen or prevent your asthma symptoms, but they can't cure your asthma.

Several health conditions can make asthma harder to manage. These conditions include runny nose, sinus infections, reflux disease, psychological stress, and sleep apnea. Your doctor will treat these conditions as well.

Medicines

Your doctor will consider many things when deciding which asthma medicines are best for you. He or she will check to see how well a medicine works for you. Then, he or she will adjust the dose or medicine as needed.

Asthma medicines can be taken in pill form, but most are taken using a device called an inhaler. An inhaler allows the medicine to go directly to your lungs.

Not all inhalers are used the same way. Ask your doctor or another healthcare provider to show you the right way to use your inhaler. Review the way you use your inhaler at every medical visit.

Long-Term Control Medicines

Most people who have asthma need to take long-term control medicines daily to help prevent symptoms. The most effective long-term medicines reduce airway inflammation, which helps prevent symptoms from starting. These medicines don't give you quick relief from symptoms.

Inhaled corticosteroids. Inhaled corticosteroids are the preferred medicine for long-term control of asthma. They're the most effective option for long-term relief of the inflammation and swelling that makes your airways sensitive to certain inhaled substances.

Reducing inflammation helps prevent the chain reaction that causes asthma symptoms. Most people who take these medicines daily find they greatly reduce the severity of symptoms and how often they occur.

Inhaled corticosteroids generally are safe when taken as prescribed. These medicines are different from the illegal anabolic steroids taken by some athletes. Inhaled corticosteroids aren't habit-forming, even if you take them every day for many years.

Like many other medicines, though, inhaled corticosteroids can have side effects. Most doctors agree that the benefits of taking inhaled corticosteroids and preventing asthma attacks far outweigh the risk of side effects.

One common side effect from inhaled corticosteroids is a mouth infection called thrush. You might be able to use a spacer or holding chamber on your inhaler to avoid thrush. These devices attach to your inhaler. They help prevent the medicine from landing in your mouth or on the back of your throat.

Check with your doctor to see whether a spacer or holding chamber should be used with the inhaler you have. Also, work with your healthcare team if you have any questions about how to use a spacer or holding chamber. Rinsing your mouth out with water after taking inhaled corticosteroids also can lower your risk for thrush.

If you have severe asthma, you may have to take corticosteroid pills or liquid for short periods to get your asthma under control.

If taken for long periods, these medicines raise your risk for cataracts and osteoporosis. A cataract is the clouding of the lens in your eye. Osteoporosis is a disorder that makes your bones weak and more likely to break.

Your doctor may have you add another long-term asthma control medicine so he or she can lower your dose of corticosteroids. Or, your doctor may suggest you take calcium and vitamin D pills to protect your bones.

Other long-term control medicines. Other long-term control medicines include:

- Cromolyn. This medicine is taken using a device called a nebulizer. As you breathe in, the nebulizer sends a fine mist of medicine to your lungs. Cromolyn helps prevent airway inflammation.

- Omalizumab (anti-IgE). This medicine is given as a shot (injection) one or two times a month. It helps prevent your body from reacting to asthma triggers, such as pollen and dust mites. Anti-IgE might be used if other asthma medicines have not worked well.

A rare, but possibly life-threatening allergic reaction called anaphylaxis might occur when the Omalizumab injection is given. If you take this medication, work with your doctor to make sure you understand the signs and symptoms of anaphylaxis and what actions you should take.

- Inhaled long-acting beta$_2$-agonists. These medicines open the airways. They might be added to inhaled corticosteroids to improve asthma control. Inhaled long-acting beta$_2$-agonists should never be used on their own for long-term asthma control. They must used with inhaled corticosteroids.

515

- Leukotriene modifiers. These medicines are taken by mouth. They help block the chain reaction that increases inflammation in your airways.

- Theophylline. This medicine is taken by mouth. Theophylline helps open the airways.

If your doctor prescribes a long-term control medicine, take it every day to control your asthma. Your asthma symptoms will likely return or get worse if you stop taking your medicine.

Long-term control medicines can have side effects. Talk with your doctor about these side effects and ways to reduce or avoid them.

With some medicines, like theophylline, your doctor will check the level of medicine in your blood. This helps ensure that you're getting enough medicine to relieve your asthma symptoms, but not so much that it causes dangerous side effects.

Quick-Relief Medicines

All people who have asthma need quick-relief medicines to help relieve asthma symptoms that may flare up. Inhaled short-acting beta$_2$-agonists are the first choice for quick relief.

These medicines act quickly to relax tight muscles around your airways when you're having a flareup. This allows the airways to open up so air can flow through them.

You should take your quick-relief medicine when you first notice asthma symptoms. If you use this medicine more than 2 days a week, talk with your doctor about your asthma control. You may need to make changes to your asthma action plan.

Carry your quick-relief inhaler with you at all times in case you need it. If your child has asthma, make sure that anyone caring for him or her has the child's quick-relief medicines, including staff at the child's school. They should understand when and how to use these medicines and when to seek medical care for your child.

You shouldn't use quick-relief medicines in place of prescribed long-term control medicines. Quick-relief medicines don't reduce inflammation.

Track Your Asthma

To track your asthma, keep records of your symptoms, check your peak flow number using a peak flow meter, and get regular asthma checkups.

Record Your Symptoms

You can record your asthma symptoms in a diary to see how well your treatments are controlling your asthma.

Asthma is well controlled if:

- You have symptoms no more than 2 days a week, and these symptoms don't wake you from sleep more than 1 or 2 nights a month.

- You can do all your normal activities.

- You take quick-relief medicines no more than 2 days a week.

- You have no more than one asthma attack a year that requires you to take corticosteroids by mouth.

- Your peak flow doesn't drop below 80 percent of your personal best number.

If your asthma isn't well controlled, contact your doctor. He or she may need to change your asthma action plan.

Use a Peak Flow Meter

This small, hand-held device shows how well air moves out of your lungs. You blow into the device and it gives you a score, or peak flow number. Your score shows how well your lungs are working at the time of the test.

Your doctor will tell you how and when to use your peak flow meter. He or she also will teach you how to take your medicines based on your score.

Your doctor and other healthcare providers may ask you to use your peak flow meter each morning and keep a record of your results. You may find it very useful to record peak flow scores for a couple of weeks before each medical visit and take the results with you.

When you're first diagnosed with asthma, it's important to find your "personal best" peak flow number. To do this, you record your score each day for a 2- to 3-week period when your asthma is well-controlled. The highest number you get during that time is your personal best. You can compare this number to future numbers to make sure your asthma is controlled.

Your peak flow meter can help warn you of an asthma attack, even before you notice symptoms. If your score shows that your breathing is getting worse, you should take your quick-relief medicines the way your asthma action plan directs. Then you can use the peak flow meter to check how well the medicine worked.

Get Asthma Checkups

When you first begin treatment, you'll see your doctor about every 2 to 6 weeks. Once your asthma is controlled, your doctor may want to see you from once a month to twice a year.

During these checkups, your doctor may ask whether you've had an asthma attack since the last visit or any changes in symptoms or peak flow measurements. He or she also may ask about your daily activities. This information will help your doctor assess your level of asthma control.

Your doctor also may ask whether you have any problems or concerns with taking your medicines or following your asthma action plan. Based on your answers to these questions, your doctor may change the dose of your medicine or give you a new medicine.

If your control is very good, you might be able to take less medicine. The goal is to use the least amount of medicine needed to control your asthma.

Emergency Care

Most people who have asthma, including many children, can safely manage their symptoms by following their asthma action plans. However, you might need medical attention at times.

Call your doctor for advice if:

- Your medicines don't relieve an asthma attack.
- Your peak flow is less than half of your personal best peak flow number.

Call 9–1–1 for emergency care if:

- You have trouble walking and talking because you're out of breath.
- You have blue lips or fingernails.

At the hospital, you'll be closely watched and given oxygen and more medicines, as well as medicines at higher doses than you take at home. Such treatment can save your life.

Asthma Treatment for Special Groups

The treatments described above generally apply to all people who have asthma. However, some aspects of treatment differ for people in certain age groups and those who have special needs.

Children

It's hard to diagnose asthma in children younger than 5 years. Thus, it's hard to know whether young children who wheeze or have other asthma symptoms will benefit from long-term control medicines. (Quick-relief medicines tend to relieve wheezing in young children whether they have asthma or not.)

Doctors will treat infants and young children who have asthma symptoms with long-term control medicines if, after assessing a child, they feel that the symptoms are persistent and likely to continue after 6 years of age.

Inhaled corticosteroids are the preferred treatment for young children. Montelukast and cromolyn are other options. Treatment might be given for a trial period of 1 month to 6 weeks. Treatment usually is stopped if benefits aren't seen during that time and the doctor and parents are confident the medicine was used properly.

Inhaled corticosteroids can possibly slow the growth of children of all ages. Slowed growth usually is apparent in the first several months of treatment, is generally small, and doesn't get worse over time. Poorly controlled asthma also may reduce a child's growth rate.

Many experts think the benefits of inhaled corticosteroids for children who need them to control their asthma far outweigh the risk of slowed growth.

Older Adults

Doctors may need to adjust asthma treatment for older adults who take certain other medicines, such as beta blockers, aspirin and other pain relievers, and anti-inflammatory medicines. These medicines can prevent asthma medicines from working well and may worsen asthma symptoms.

Be sure to tell your doctor about all of the medicines you take, including over-the-counter medicines.

Older adults may develop weak bones from using inhaled corticosteroids, especially at high doses. Talk with your doctor about taking calcium and vitamin D pills, as well as other ways to help keep your bones strong.

Pregnant Women

Pregnant women who have asthma need to control the disease to ensure a good supply of oxygen to their babies. Poor asthma control increases the risk of preeclampsia, a condition in which a pregnant woman develops high blood pressure and protein in the urine. Poor asthma control also increases the risk that a baby will be born early and have a low birth weight.

Studies show that it's safer to take asthma medicines while pregnant than to risk having an asthma attack.

Talk with your doctor if you have asthma and are pregnant or planning a pregnancy. Your level of asthma control may get better or it may get worse while you're pregnant. Your healthcare team will check your asthma control often and adjust your treatment as needed.

People Whose Asthma Symptoms Occur with Physical Activity

Physical activity is an important part of a healthy lifestyle. Adults need physical activity to maintain good health. Children need it for growth and development.

In some people, however, physical activity can trigger asthma symptoms. If this happens to you or your child, talk with your doctor about the best ways to control asthma so you can stay active.

The following medicines may help prevent asthma symptoms caused by physical activity:

- Short-acting beta$_2$-agonists (quick-relief medicine) taken shortly before physical activity can last 2 to 3 hours and prevent exercise-related symptoms in most people who take them.

- Long-acting beta$_2$-agonists can be protective for up to 12 hours. However, with daily use, they'll no longer give up to 12 hours of protection. Also, frequent use of these medicines for physical activity might be a sign that asthma is poorly controlled.

- Leukotriene modifiers. These pills are taken several hours before physical activity. They can help relieve asthma symptoms brought on by physical activity.

- Long-term control medicines. Frequent or severe symptoms due to physical activity may suggest poorly controlled asthma and the need to either start or increase long-term control medicines that reduce inflammation. This will help prevent exercise-related symptoms.

Easing into physical activity with a warmup period may be helpful. You also may want to wear a mask or scarf over your mouth when exercising in cold weather.

If you use your asthma medicines as your doctor directs, you should be able to take part in any physical activity or sport you choose.

People Having Surgery

Asthma may add to the risk of having problems during and after surgery. For instance, having a tube put into your throat may cause an asthma attack.

Tell your surgeon about your asthma when you first talk with him or her. The surgeon can take steps to lower your risk, such as giving you asthma medicines before or during surgery.

Part Eight

Coping with Immune Disease

Chapter 88

Coping with Autoimmunity

What Are Autoimmune Diseases?

Our bodies have an immune system, which is a complex network of special cells and organs that defends the body from germs and other foreign invaders. At the core of the immune system is the ability to tell the difference between self and nonself: what's you and what's foreign. A flaw can make the body unable to tell the difference between self and nonself. When this happens, the body makes autoantibodies that attack normal cells by mistake. At the same time special cells called regulatory T cells fail to do their job of keeping the immune system in line. The result is a misguided attack on your own body. This causes the damage we know as autoimmune disease. The body parts that are affected depend on the type of autoimmune disease. There are more than 80 known types.

How Can I Manage My Life Now That I Have an Autoimmune Disease?

Although most autoimmune diseases don't go away, you can treat your symptoms and learn to manage your disease, so you can enjoy life! Women with autoimmune diseases lead full, active lives. Your life goals should not have to change. It is important, though, to see a

This chapter includes text excerpted from "Autoimmune Diseases Fact Sheet," Office on Women's Health (OWH), U.S. Department of Health and Human Services (HHS), July 16, 2012. Reviewed October 2016.

doctor who specializes in these types of diseases, follow your treatment plan, and adopt a healthy lifestyle.

How Can I Deal with Flares?

Flares are the sudden and severe onset of symptoms. You might notice that certain triggers, such as stress or being out in the sun, cause your symptoms to flare. Knowing your triggers, following your treatment plan, and seeing your doctor regularly can help you to prevent flares or keep them from becoming severe. If you suspect a flare is coming, call your doctor. Don't try a "cure" you heard about from a friend or relative.

What Are Some Things I Can Do to Feel Better?

If you are living with an autoimmune disease, there are things you can do each day to feel better:

- **Eat healthy, well-balanced meals.** Make sure to include fruits and vegetables, whole grains, fat-free or low-fat milk products, and lean sources of protein. Limit saturated fat, *trans* fat, cholesterol, salt, and added sugars. If you follow a healthy eating plan, you will get the nutrients you need from food.

- **Get regular physical activity. But be careful not to overdo it.** Talk with your doctor about what types of physical activity you can do. A gradual and gentle exercise program often works well for people with long-lasting muscle and joint pain. Some types of yoga or tai chi exercises may be helpful.

- **Get enough rest.** Rest allows your body tissues and joints the time they need to repair. Sleeping is a great way you can help both your body and mind. If you don't get enough sleep, your stress level and your symptoms could get worse. You also can't fight off sickness as well when you sleep poorly. When you are well-rested, you can tackle your problems better and lower your risk for illness. Most people need at least 7 to 9 hours of sleep each day to feel well-rested.

- **Reduce stress.** Stress and anxiety can trigger symptoms to flare up with some autoimmune diseases. So finding ways to simplify your life and cope with daily stressors will help you to feel your best. Meditation, self-hypnosis, and guided imagery, are simple relaxation techniques that might help you to reduce stress, lessen your pain, and deal with other aspects of living with your disease. You can learn to do these through self-help books, tapes, or with the help of an instructor. Joining a support group or talking with a counselor might also help you to manage your stress and cope with your disease.

You Have Some Power to Lessen Your Pain! Try Using Imagery for 15 Minutes, Two or Three Times Each Day.

1. Put on your favorite calming music.

2. Lie back on your favorite chair or sofa. Or if you are at work, sit back and relax in your chair.

3. Close your eyes.

4. Imagine your pain or discomfort.

5. Imagine something that confronts this pain and watch it "destroy" the pain.

Chapter 89

Students with Chronic Illnesses: Guidance for Families, Schools, and Students

Chronic illnesses affect at least 10 to 15 percent of American children. Responding to the needs of students with chronic conditions, such as asthma, allergies, diabetes, and epilepsy (also known as seizure disorders), in the school setting requires a comprehensive, coordinated, and systematic approach. Students with chronic health conditions can function to their maximum potential if their needs are met. The benefits to students can include better attendance, improved alertness and physical stamina, fewer symptoms, fewer restrictions on participation in physical activities and special activities, such as field trips, and fewer medical emergencies. Schools can work together with parents, students, healthcare providers, and the community to provide a safe and supportive educational environment for students with chronic illnesses and to ensure that students with chronic illnesses have the same educational opportunities as do other students.

This chapter includes text excerpted from "Students with Chronic Illnesses: Guidance for Families, Schools, and Students," National Heart, Lung, and Blood Institute (NHLBI), September 6, 2015.

Family's Responsibilities

- Notify the school of the student's health management needs and diagnosis when appropriate. Notify schools as early as possible and whenever the student's health needs change.

- Provide a written description of the student's health needs at school, including authorizations for medication administration and emergency treatment, signed by the student's healthcare provider.

- Participate in the development of a school plan to implement the student's health needs:

  - Meet with the school team to develop a plan to accommodate the student's needs in all school settings.

  - Authorize appropriate exchange of information between school health program staff and the student's personal healthcare providers.

  - Communicate significant changes in the student's needs or health status promptly to appropriate school staff.

- Provide an adequate supply of student's medication, in pharmacy-labeled containers, and other supplies to the designated school staff, and replace medications and supplies as needed. This supply should remain at school.

- Provide the school a means of contacting you or another responsible person at all times in case of an emergency or medical problem.

- Educate the student to develop age-appropriate self-care skills.

- Promote good general health, personal care, nutrition, and physical activity.

School District's Responsibilities

- Develop and implement districtwide guidelines and protocols applicable to chronic illnesses generally and specific protocols for asthma, allergies, diabetes, epilepsy (seizure disorders), and other common chronic illnesses of students.

- Guidelines should include safe, coordinated practices (as age and skill level appropriate) that enable the student to successfully manage his or her health in the classroom and at all school-related activities.

- Protocols should be consistent with established standards of care for students with chronic illnesses and Federal laws that provide protection to students with disabilities, including ensuring confidentiality of student healthcare information and appropriate information sharing.

- Protocols should address education of all members of the school environment about chronic illnesses, including a component addressing the promotion of acceptance and the elimination of stigma surrounding chronic illnesses.

- Develop, coordinate, and implement necessary training programs for staff that will be responsible for chronic illness care tasks at school and school-related activities.

- Monitor schools for compliance with chronic illness care protocols.

- Meet with parents, school personnel, and healthcare providers to address issues of concern about the provision of care to students with chronic illnesses by school district staff.

School's Responsibilities

- Identify students with chronic conditions, and review their health records as submitted by families and healthcare providers.

- Arrange a meeting to discuss health accommodations and educational aids and services that the student may need and to develop a 504 Plan, Individualized Education Program (IEP), or other school plan, as appropriate. The participants should include the family, student (if appropriate), school health staff, 504/IEP coordinator (as applicable), individuals trained to assist the student, and the teacher who has primary responsibility for the student. Healthcare provider input may be provided in person or in writing.

- Provide nondiscriminatory opportunities to students with disabilities. Be knowledgeable about and ensure compliance with applicable Federal laws, including Americans With Disabilities Act (ADA), Individuals With Disabilities Education Act (IDEA), Section 504, and Family Educational Rights and Privacy Act of 1974 (FERPA). Be knowledgeable about any State or local laws or district policies that affect the implementation of students' rights under Federal law.

- Clarify the roles and obligations of specific school staff, and provide education and communication systems necessary to ensure that students' health and educational needs are met in a safe and coordinated manner.

- Implement strategies that reduce disruption in the student's school activities, including physical education, recess, offsite events, extracurricular activities, and field trips.

- Communicate with families regularly and as authorized with the student's healthcare providers.

- Ensure that the student receives prescribed medications in a safe, reliable, and effective manner and has access to needed medication at all times during the school day and at school-related activities.

- Be prepared to handle health needs and emergencies and to ensure that there is a staff member available who is properly trained to administer medications or other immediate care during the school day and at all school-related activities, regardless of time or location.

- Ensure that all staff who interact with the student on a regular basis receive appropriate guidance and training on routine needs, precautions, and emergency actions.

- Provide appropriate health education to students and staff.

- Provide a safe and healthy school environment.

- Ensure that case management is provided as needed. Ensure proper record keeping, including appropriate measures to both protect confidentiality and to share information.

- Promote a supportive learning environment that views students with chronic illnesses the same as other students except to respond to health needs.

- Promote good general health, personal care, nutrition, and physical activity.

Student's Responsibilities

- Notify an adult about concerns and needs in managing his or her symptoms or the school environment.

- Participate in the care and management of his or her health as appropriate to his or her developmental level.

Chapter 90

Immunization Recommendations for People with a Weakened Immune System

Weakened Immune System and Adult Vaccinations

Vaccines are especially critical for people with health conditions such as a weakened immune system.

If you have cancer or other immunocompromising conditions, talk with your doctor about:

- Influenza vaccine each year to protect against seasonal flu

- Tdap vaccine to protect against whooping cough and tetanus

- Pneumococcal vaccine (both types) to protect against pneumonia and other pneumococcal diseases

- HPV vaccine series to protect against human papillomavirus if you are a man or woman up to age 26 years

This chapter includes text excerpted from "Vaccine Information for Adults," Centers for Disease Control and Prevention (CDC), January 25, 2013.

Asplenia and Adult Vaccination

Vaccines are especially critical for people with chronic health conditions such as asplenia.

If your spleen has been surgically removed (by a procedure called splenectomy), or your spleen does not work well, talk with your doctor about:

- Influenza vaccine each year to protect against seasonal flu
- Tdap vaccine to protect against whooping cough and tetanus
- Hib vaccine to protect against *Haemophilus influenzae* type b (Hib) if you were not previously vaccinated with the vaccine
- Pneumococcal vaccines (both types) to protect against pneumonia and other pneumococcal disease
- Meningococcal vaccines (both types) to protect against meningitis and other meningococcal disease
- Zoster vaccine to protect against shingles if you are 60 years and older
- HPV vaccine series to protect against human papillomavirus if you are a man up to age 21 or woman up to age 26
- MMR vaccine to protect against measles, mumps, and rubella if you were born in 1957 or after and have not gotten this vaccine or have immunity to these diseases
- Varicella vaccine to protect against chickenpox if you were born in 1980 or after and have not gotten two doses of this vaccine or have immunity to this disease

Diabetes Type 1 and Type 2 and Adult Vaccination

Each year thousands of adults in the United States get sick from diseases that could be prevented by vaccines—some people are hospitalized, and some even die. People with diabetes (both type 1 and type 2) are at higher risk for serious problems from certain vaccine-preventable diseases. Getting vaccinated is an important step in staying healthy. **If you have diabetes, talk with your doctor about getting your vaccinations up-to-date.**

Why Vaccines are Important for You

- Diabetes, even if well managed, can make it harder for your immune system to fight infections, so you may be at risk for more serious complications from an illness compared to people without diabetes.

- Some illnesses, like influenza, can raise your blood glucose to dangerously high levels.
- People with diabetes have higher rates of hepatitis B than the rest of the population. Outbreaks of hepatitis B associated with blood glucose monitoring procedures have happened among people with diabetes.
- People with diabetes are at increased risk for death from pneumonia (lung infection), bacteremia (blood infection) and meningitis (infection of the lining of the brain and spinal cord).

- Immunization provides the best protection against vaccine-preventable diseases.
- Vaccines are one of the safest ways for you to protect your health, even if you are taking prescription medications. Vaccine side effects are usually mild and go away on their own. Severe side effects are very rare.

Vaccines You Need

- Influenze vaccine: to protect against seasonal flu every year
- Pnemococcal vaccine: to protect against pneumonia
- Tdap vaccine: to protect against whooping cough and tetanus
- Hep B vaccine: to protect against hepatitis B
- Zoster vaccine: to protect against shingles

Getting Vaccinated

You regularly see your provider for diabetes care, and that is a great place to start!

Heart Disease, Stroke, or Other Cardiovascular Disease and Adult Vaccination

People with heart disease and those who have suffered stroke are at higher risk for serious problems from certain diseases. Getting vaccinated is an important step in staying healthy. If you have cardiovascular disease, talk with your doctor about getting your vaccinations up-to-date.

Why Vaccines are Important for You

- Heart disease can make it harder for you to fight off certain diseases or make it more likely that you will have serious complications from certain diseases.

- Immunization provides the best protection against vaccine-preventable diseases.

- Vaccines are one of the safest ways for you to protect your health, even if you are taking prescription medications. Vaccine side effects are usually mild and go away on their own. Severe side effects are very rare.

- Some vaccine-preventable diseases, like the flu, can increase the risk of another heart attack.

Vaccines You Need

- Influenze vaccine: to protect against seasonal flu every year

- Pneumococcal vaccine: to protect against pneumonia

- Tdap vaccine: to protect against whooping cough and tetanus

- Zoster vaccine: to protect against shingles

Getting Vaccinated

You may regularly see a cardiologist, or your primary care provider. Either is a great place to start!

HIV Infection and Adult Vaccination

Vaccines are especially critical for people with chronic health conditions such as HIV infection.

If you have HIV infection and your CD4 count is 200 or greater, talk with your doctor about:

- Influenza vaccine each year to protect against seasonal flu

- Tdap vaccine to protect against whooping cough and tetanus

- Pneumococcal vaccine to protect against pneumonia and other pneumococcal diseases

- Hepatitis B vaccine series to protect against hepatitis B

- HPV vaccine series to protect against human papillomavirus if you are a man or woman up to age 26 years

- MMR vaccine to protect against measles, mumps, and rubella if you were born in 1957 or after and have not gotten this vaccine or have immunity to these diseases

- Varicella vaccine to protect against chickenpox if you were born in 1980 or after and have not gotten two doses of this vaccine or have immunity to this disease

If you have HIV infection and your CD4 count is less than 200, talk with your doctor about:

- Influenza vaccine each year to protect against seasonal flu

- Tdap vaccine to protect against whooping cough and tetanus

- Pneumococcal vaccine to protect against pneumonia and other pneumococcal diseases

- Hepatitis B vaccine series to protect against hepatitis B

- HPV vaccine series to protect against human papillomavirus if you are a man or woman up to age 26 years

Liver Disease and Adult Vaccination

Vaccines are especially critical for people with health conditions such as liver disease.

If you have chronic liver disease, talk with your doctor about:

- Influenza vaccine each year to protect against seasonal flu

- Tdap vaccine to protect against whooping cough and tetanus

- Pneumococcal polysaccharide vaccine to protect against pneumonia and other pneumococcal diseases

- Hepatitis B vaccine series to protect against hepatitis B

- Hepatitis A vaccine series to protect against hepatitis A

- Zoster vaccine to protect against shingles if you are 60 years and older

- HPV vaccine to protect against human papillomavirus if you are a woman up to age 26 and a man up to age 21

537

- MMR vaccine to protect against measles, mumps, and rubella if you were born in 1957 or after and have not gotten this vaccine or have immunity to these diseases

- Varicella vaccine to protect against chickenpox if you were born in 1980 or after and have not gotten two doses of this vaccine or have immunity to this disease

Lung Disease Including Asthma and Adult Vaccination

People with asthma or chronic obstructive pulmonary disease (COPD) are at higher risk for serious problems from certain vaccine-preventable diseases. Getting vaccinated is an important step in staying healthy. If you have lung disease, talk with your doctor about getting your vaccinations up-to-date.

Why Vaccines are Important for You

- Adults with COPD or asthma are more likely to get complications from the flu.

- COPD and asthma cause your airways to swell and become blocked with mucus, which can make it hard to breathe. Certain vaccine preventable diseases can also increase swelling of your airways and lungs. The combination of the two can lead to pneumonia and other serious respiratory illnesses.

- Vaccines are one of the safest ways for you to protect your health, even if you are taking prescription medications. Vaccine side effects are usually mild and go away on their own. Severe side effects are very rare.

- Immunization provides the best protection against vaccine-preventable diseases.

Vaccines You Need

- Influenze vaccine: to protect against seasonal flu every year

- Pnemococcal vaccine: to protect against pneumonia

- Tdap vaccine: to protect against whooping cough and tetanus

- Zoster vaccine: to protect against shingles

Getting Vaccinated

You may regularly see your COPD or asthma specialist, or maybe your primary care provider. Either is a great place to start!

Renal Disease and Adult Vaccination

Vaccines are especially critical for people with health conditions such as renal disease.

If you have renal disease or kidney failure, talk with your doctor about:

- Influenza vaccine each year to protect against seasonal flu

- Tdap vaccine to protect against whooping cough and tetanus

- Pneumococcal polysaccharide vaccine to protect against pneumonia and other pneumococcal diseases

- Hepatitis B vaccine series to protect against hepatitis B

- Zoster vaccine to protect against shingles if you are 60 years and older

- HPV vaccine to protect against human papillomavirus if you are a woman up to age 26 and a man up to age 21

- MMR vaccine to protect against measles, mumps, and rubella if you were born in 1957 or after and have not gotten this vaccine or have immunity to these diseases

- Varicella vaccine to protect against chickenpox if you were born in 1980 or after and have not gotten two doses of this vaccine or have immunity to this disease

Chapter 91

Recommendations for Travelers with Immune System Disorders

Travelers with Weakened Immune Systems

Many illnesses can weaken the immune system, including HIV/AIDS, different kinds of cancer, liver disease, kidney disease, and multiple sclerosis. In addition, many medicines can weaken the immune system, including steroids, cancer chemotherapy, and drugs to treat rheumatoid arthritis or psoriasis. Regardless of the cause, if you have a weakened immune system and are planning a trip overseas, make an appointment with a travel medicine specialist to talk about what you should do to prepare for safe and healthy travel.

Vaccines

Check the Centers for Disease Control and Prevention (CDC) Travelers' Health website (wwwnc.cdc.gov/travel) to see what vaccines might be recommended for your destination, and talk to your doctor about which of them are right for you. Most travel vaccines are made from killed bacteria or viruses and can be given safely to people with

This chapter includes text excerpted from "Travelers with Weakened Immune Systems," Centers for Disease Control and Prevention (CDC), May 3, 2013.

weakened immune systems. However, they may be less effective than in people with normal immune systems, and you may not be fully protected. Your doctor may recommend blood tests to confirm that a vaccine was effective, or he or she may recommend additional precautions to keep you safe.

Some vaccines, such as MMR (measles, mumps, and rubella) and varicella, are made from live viruses. Many people with weakened immune systems should not receive these vaccines. Talk to your doctor what your options are for protecting yourself against these diseases.

Yellow fever vaccine is made from a live virus, and it cannot be safely given to people whose immune systems are very weak, such as people with HIV infection and low T-cell counts or people receiving cancer chemotherapy. If there is a risk of yellow fever at your destination, CDC recommends delaying your trip until your immune system is strong enough for you to have the vaccine. Some countries may require the vaccine, even if there is no risk of yellow fever. If that's the case, ask your doctor about a medical waiver for the vaccine.

Medicines

If there is a risk of malaria at your destination, you may need to take medicine to prevent it. People who have weakened immune systems can get seriously ill from malaria, so it's important to closely follow your doctor's instructions for taking the medicine, which may include taking it for several weeks before and after the trip. You should also take steps to avoid mosquito bites: wear insect repellent, wear long pants and sleeves, and sleep under a net if your rooms are exposed to the outdoors.

Depending on where you are going and your planned activities, your doctor may also prescribe medicine to prevent altitude illness or to treat travelers' diarrhea. These drugs, as well as any you are prescribed to prevent malaria, can interact with medicines you usually take. Make sure your travel doctor knows about all the medicines you take regularly, including vitamin supplements, so that he or she can anticipate potential interactions.

Other Precautions

Not all illnesses can be prevented with vaccines or medicines, and people with weakened immune systems are especially prone to travelers' diarrhea. Make sure you follow CDC's advice for eating and drinking safely. You should also wash your hands often and try to avoid touching surfaces that other people have touched, such as doorknobs and stair rails, with your bare hands.

With a little advance preparation and a few precautions, people who have weakened immune systems can safely travel almost anywhere in the world.

Food and Water Safety

Contaminated food or drinks can cause travelers' diarrhea and other diseases. Travelers to developing countries are especially at risk. Reduce your risk by sticking to safe eating and drinking habits.

Food

Usually Safe

Hot food

High heat kills the germs that cause travelers' diarrhea, so food that is cooked thoroughly is usually safe as long as it is served steaming hot. Be careful of food that is cooked and allowed to sit at warm or room temperatures, such as on a buffet. It could become contaminated again.

Dry or packaged food

Most germs require moisture to grow, so food that is dry, such as bread or potato chips, is usually safe. Additionally, food from factory-sealed containers, such as canned tuna or packaged crackers, is safe as long as it was not opened and handled by another person.

Can Be Risky

Raw food

Raw food should generally be avoided. Raw fruits or vegetables may be safe if you can peel them yourself or wash them in safe (bottled or disinfected) water. Steer clear of platters of cut-up fruit or vegetables. (Did you see the hands that cut them? Can you be sure those hands were clean?) Salads are especially problematic because shredded or finely cut vegetables offer a lot of surface area for germs to grow on. Also avoid fresh salsas or other condiments made from raw fruits or vegetables. Raw meat or seafood may contain germs; this includes raw meat that is "cooked" with citrus juice, vinegar, or other acidic liquid (such as ceviche, a dish of raw seafood marinated in citrus juice).

Street food

Street vendors in developing countries may not be held to the same hygiene standards as restaurants (which may be low to begin with), so eat food from street vendors with caution. If you choose to eat street food, apply the same rules as to other food; for example, if you watch something come straight off the grill (cooked and steaming hot), it's more likely to be safe.

Bushmeat

Bushmeat refers to local wild game, generally animals not typically eaten in the United States, such as bats, monkeys, or rodents. Bushmeat can be a source of animal-origin diseases, such as Ebola or severe acute respiratory syndrome (SARS), and is best avoided.

Drinks

Usually Safe

Bottled or canned drinks

Drinks from factory-sealed bottles or cans are safe; however, dishonest vendors in some countries may sell tap water in bottles that are "sealed" with a drop of glue to mimic the factory seal. Carbonated drinks, such as sodas or sparkling water, are safest since the bubbles indicate that the bottle was sealed at the factory. If drinking directly from a can, wipe off the lip of the can before your mouth comes into contact with it.

Hot drinks

Hot coffee or tea should be safe if it is served steaming hot. It's okay to let it cool before you drink it, but be wary of coffee or tea that is served only warm or at room temperature. Be careful about adding things that may be contaminated (cream, lemon) to your hot drinks (sugar should be fine; see "Dry food" above).

Milk

Pasteurized milk from a sealed bottle should be okay, but watch out for milk in open containers (such as pitchers) that may have been sitting at room temperature. This includes the cream you put in your coffee or tea. People who are pregnant or have weakened immune systems should stay away from unpasteurized milk or other dairy products (cheese, yogurt).

Alcohol

The alcohol content of most liquors is sufficient to kill germs; however, stick to the guidelines above when choosing mixers and avoid drinks "on the rocks" (see "Ice" below). The alcohol content of beer and wine is probably not high enough to kill germs, but if it came from a sealed bottle or can, it should be okay.

Can Be Risky

Tap water

In most developing countries, tap water should probably not be drunk, even in cities. This includes swallowing water when showering or brushing your teeth. In some areas, it may be advisable to brush your teeth with bottled water. Tap water can be disinfected by boiling, filtering, or chemically treating it, for example with chlorine.

Fountain drinks

Sodas from a fountain are made by carbonating water and mixing it with flavored syrup. Since the water most likely came from the tap, these sodas are best avoided. Similarly, juice from a fountain is most likely juice concentrate mixed with tap water and should be avoided.

Ice

Avoid ice in developing countries; it was likely made with tap water.

Freshly squeezed juice

If you washed the fruit in safe water and squeezed the juice yourself, drink up. Juice that was squeezed by unknown hands may be risky. The same goes for ice pops and other treats that are made from freshly squeezed juice.

Part Nine

Additional Help and Information

Chapter 92

Glossary of Immune System Terms

acquired immunity: Immunity that develops during a person's lifetime.

active immunity: Immunity that develops after exposure to a disease-causing infectious microorganism or other foreign substance, such as following infection or vaccination.

adaptive immune response: Second line of the immune response that is specific to a given foreign molecule or pathogen and leads to an "immunological memory" after the first response to the molecule or pathogen.

adenoid: Small pad of infection-fighting tissue located near the eustachian tube.

agammaglobulinemia: Congenital or acquired absence of, or extremely low levels of, gamma globulin in the blood.

allergy: A condition in which the body has an exaggerated response to a substance (e.g. food or drug). Also known as hypersensitivity.

antibodies: Special proteins made by the body in response to antigens (foreign substances, e.g., bacteria or viruses). Antibodies bind with antigens on microorganisms to protect the body against infection.

This glossary contains terms excerpted from documents produced by several sources deemed reliable.

antigen: Any substance that is foreign to the body and triggers an immune response. Antigens include bacteria, viruses, and allergens, such as pollen.

antinuclear antibody (ANA): A type of antibody directed against the nuclei of the body's cells. Because these antibodies can be found in the blood of children with lupus and some other rheumatic disorders, testing for them can be useful in diagnosis.

antiviral: Any medicine capable of destroying or weakening a virus.

apoptosis: The deliberate, programmed death of a cell. Apoptosis is a normal biological process that helps the body stay healthy by eliminating old or damaged cells.

asplenia: Absence of a functioning spleen.

attenuated: A type of live vaccine containing viruses or bacteria too weak to cause disease, but strong enough to cause the body to make antibodies.

autoantibodies: Antibodies that attack one's own cells.

autoimmune disorder: A condition that occurs when the immune system mistakenly attacks and destroys healthy body tissue. Autoimmune disorders may be caused by drugs used to treat opportunistic infections.

B lymphocyte: A type of lymphocyte. B lymphocytes (B cells) produce antibodies to help the body fight infection.

basophil: A type of white blood cell that helps the body fight infection by triggering an inflammatory response to an antigen.

bone marrow: Soft tissue located within bones that produces all blood cells, including the ones that fight infection.

booster: An additional vaccine dose needed to "boost" (increase) antibody levels after protection begins to decrease.

C-reactive protein: A protein produced by the body during the process of inflammation. A positive blood test for the protein indicates the presence of inflammation in the body.

CD4+ T-cell: A type of lymphocyte; the main target in the body for infection by HIV.

chemokines: Small proteins secreted by cells to mobilize and activate infection-fighting white blood cells. Chemokines are involved in many immune and inflammatory responses.

cytokine: A family of proteins produced by cells, especially by immune cells. Cytokines act as chemical messengers between cells to regulate immune responses.

deoxyribonucleic acid (DNA): The building block of life contained in each of our cells that carries our genetic information.

enzyme: A protein that speeds up chemical reactions in the body.

eosinophils: Immune cells that have granules (small particles) with enzymes that are released during infections, allergic reactions, and asthma.

erythrocyte sedimentation rate (ESR): A blood test that signals the presence of inflammatory disease by measuring the speed at which red blood cells settle to the bottom of a test tube.

gene: A hereditary unit that is composed of a sequence of DNA and occupies a specific position or locus.

immune globulin: A protein found in the blood that fights infection. Also known as gamma globulin.

immune response: Actions of the immune system to defend the body against bacteria, viruses, or other substances that the body recognizes as foreign and harmful.

immune system: A complex network of specialized cells, tissues, and organs that recognize and defend the body from foreign substances, primarily disease-causing microorganisms such as bacteria, viruses, parasites, and fungi.

immune tolerance: A state of unresponsiveness to a specific antigen or group of antigens to which a person is normally responsive.

immunity: Protection against disease caused by infectious microorganisms or by other foreign substances. Immunity can be acquired through vaccination, by contracting the disease, or by transfer of antibodies produced by another person or animal.

immunized: The process of having induced immunity from receiving a vaccine, toxoid, antibody, or antitoxin.

immunodeficiency: Inability to produce an adequate immune response because of an insufficiency or absence of antibodies, immune cells, or both. Immunodeficiency disorders can be inherited, such as severe combined immunodeficiency; they can be acquired through infection, such as with HIV; or they can result from chemotherapy.

Immunoglobulin A (IgA): A class of immunoglobulin that is the second most common immunoglobulin in blood. It is the main immunoglobulin found in secretions, such as tears, saliva, colostrum, mucous membranes of the intestine, respiratory and reproductive tracts. IgA provides local defense against microorganisms as they try to infect mucous membranes.

immunosuppression: The artificial suppression of the immune response, usually through drugs, so that the body will not reject a transplanted organ or tissue.

immunosuppressive drugs: Drugs that suppress the immune response and can be used to treat autoimmune disease. Unfortunately, because these drugs also suppress normal immunity, they leave the body at risk for infection.

immunotherapy: Treatment of disease by stimulating the body's own immune system.

inflammation: A reaction of body tissues to injury or disease, typically marked by five signs: swelling, redness, heat, pain, and loss of function.

innate immune response: Initial immediate immune response that is not specific to a certain foreign molecule or pathogen.

innate immune system: The part of the immune system that is more primitive. It employs types of white blood cells called granulocytes and monocytes to destroy harmful substances.

interferon: Cytokines secreted by certain cells in response to an antigen, usually a virus. Interferon signals neighboring cells into action and inhibits the growth of malignant cells.

interleukin: One of a group of related proteins made by leukocytes (white blood cells) and other cells in the body. Interleukins regulate immune responses. Interleukins made in the laboratory are used as biological response modifiers to boost the immune system in cancer therapy.

Intravenous immunoglobulin (IVIG): A solution of antibodies prepared for injection into a person's vein. Intravenous immunoglobulin (IVIG) is composed of antibodies removed from the blood of healthy donors and then pooled together and purified. IVIG is approved for use in children infected with HIV to reduce the risk of serious bacterial infections.

live vaccine: Vaccine in which live virus is weakened through chemical or physical processes in order to produce an immune response without causing the severe effects of the disease.

lymph nodes: Lymph nodes play a crucial role in the immune system. When lymph is filtered through the lymph nodes, foreign substances are trapped and destroyed by the lymphocytes that line the walls of the lymph nodes.

lymphatic system: A network of organs, nodes, ducts, and vessels that produce and transport lymph from the body's tissues to the bloodstream. The lymphatic system helps to maintain fluid balance in the tissues and blood; to supply nutrients, oxygen, and hormones to cells; to transport fats, proteins, and white blood cells to the blood; and to fight infection and filter out foreign organisms and waste products.

lymphocyte: A type of white blood cell. Most lymphocytes can be classified as T lymphocytes (T cells), B lymphocytes (B cells), or natural killer cells. Lymphocytes are found in the blood, lymph, and lymphoid tissue and help the body fight infection.

lipoprotein: A compound molecule that contains both a protein and a lipid component.

macrophage: A type of white blood cell that fights infection by ingesting foreign substances, such as microorganisms and dead cells. Macrophages also act as antigen-presenting cells to stimulate other immune cells to fight infection.

mast cell: A type of white blood cell found in almost all tissues, particularly in the skin. Mast cells help the body fight infection by triggering an inflammatory response to an antigen.

monoclonal antibody: A type of protein made in the laboratory that can bind to substances in the body, including cancer cells. They can be used alone or to carry drugs, toxins, or radioactive substances directly to cancer cells.

monocyte: Type of mononuclear white blood cell; part of the body's immune system with several roles in the body's immune response.

natural killer cell: A type of lymphocyte. Natural killer cells contain enzymes that can kill other cells, especially tumor cells and cells infected by viruses.

neutropenia: A condition where there are lower-than-normal number of neutrophils (a type of white blood cell) in the blood. Moderate to severe neutropenia can increase the risk of bacterial and fungal infections. Neutropenia may occur as a result of HIV infection or use of some antiretroviral (ARV) drugs.

neutrophil: A type of white blood cell that fights infection by engulfing and killing foreign substances, such as bacteria.

passive immunity: Protection against disease through antibodies produced by another human being or animal. Passive immunity is effective, but protection is generally limited and diminishes over time (usually a few weeks or months). For example, maternal antibodies are passed to the infant prior to birth. These antibodies temporarily protect the baby for the first 4-6 months of life.

pathogen: Any disease-causing microorganism, such as a bacterium or virus.

persistent infection: Infection that lasts for long periods, and occurs when the primary infection is not cleared by the immune response to the exposure.

phagocytosis: Internalization or engulfment of particles or cells by specific cells (i.e., phagocytes), such as such as macrophages or neutrophils.

platelet: An irregularly shaped cell-like particle found in the blood. Platelets cause blood clots to form, which helps prevent bleeding.

rheumatoid factor (RF): An antibody that is present eventually in the blood of most people with rheumatoid arthritis. Not all people with rheumatoid arthritis test positive for rheumatoid factor, and some people test positive for rheumatoid factor, yet never develop the disease.

serum: The clear, yellowish liquid part of blood that remains after clotting. Serum is used for various laboratory tests.

spleen: An abdominal organ in the lymphatic system that filters the blood, removes infectious agents and uses them to activate cells called lymphocytes, removes worn-out red blood cells, and stores extra blood in the body.

stem cells: Cells made by the bone marrow that can differentiate into different kinds of blood cells, as needed by the body.

T-cells: T-cells are thymus-derived lymphocytes. T-cells are the major component of cell-mediated immunity.

thymus: A gland that lies in the upper chest area beneath the breastbone and plays an important role in the development of the immune system in early life. Its cells form a part of the body's normal immune system.

vaccination: Injection of a killed or weakened infectious organism in order to prevent the disease.

vaccine: A product that produces immunity therefore protecting the body from the disease. Vaccines are administered through needle injections, by mouth and by aerosol.

virus: A microorganism that can infect cells and cause disease.

Chapter 93

Glossary of Autoimmune Diseases

acquired immunodeficiency syndrome: A medical condition where the immune system cannot function properly and protect the body from disease. As a result, the body cannot defend itself against infections (like pneumonia).

Addison disease: A condition that occurs when the adrenal glands (a pair of glands situated on top of the kidneys) fail to secrete enough corticosteroid hormones.

alopecia areata: An autoimmune, often reversible disease in which loss of hair occurs in sharply defined areas usually involving the scalp or beard, but any area of the body where hair grows can be affected.

ankylosing spondylitis: An inflammatory form of arthritis that primarily affects the spine, leading to stiffening and possible fusion.

arthritis: Literally means joint inflammation. Arthritis causes joint swelling, pain, and stiffness.

celiac disease: A digestive disease that damages the small intestine and interferes with absorption of nutrients from food. When people with celiac disease eat foods containing gluten, their immune system responds by damaging the small intestine.

Crohn's disease: A chronic medical condition characterized by inflammation of the bowel.

This glossary contains terms excerpted from documents produced by several sources deemed reliable.

diabetes: A disease in which the body does not produce or properly use insulin, a hormone that is necessary to convert sugar, starches, and other food into energy.

graft-versus-host disease: A major complication of bone marrow transplantations and sometimes blood transfusions in which white blood cells called lymphocytes, which are found in the marrow or blood, attack tissues in the body into which they were transplanted.

Graves disease: An autoimmune disease of the thyroid gland that results in the overproduction of thyroid hormone. This causes such symptoms as nervousness, heat intolerance, heart palpitations, and unexplained weight loss.

Guillain-Barre syndrome: A rare neurological disease characterized by loss of reflexes and temporary paralysis. Muscle paralysis starts in the feet and legs and moves upwards to the arms and hands. Sometimes paralysis can result in the respiratory muscles causing breathing difficulties.

immune thrombocytopenic purpura: An autoimmune disorder in which the immune system destroys platelets. The destruction of platelets leads to abnormal blood clotting and easy or excessive bruising and bleeding. The exact cause of idiopathic thrombocytopenia purpura is unknown; however, the disorder may develop with a viral infection, including HIV.

inflammatory bowel disease: A general term for any disease characterized by inflammation of the bowel. Examples include colitis and Crohn's disease. Symptoms include abdominal pain, diarrhea, fever, loss of appetite and weight loss.

juvenile arthritis: A term often used to describe arthritis in children.

juvenile rheumatoid arthritis: A term used to describe the most common types of arthritis in children. It is characterized by joint pain, swelling, tenderness, warmth, and stiffness that lasts for more than 6 weeks and cannot be explained by other causes.

lupus: A disease characterized by inflammation of the connective tissue (which supports and connects all parts of the body). Chronic swelling of the connective tissue causes damage to the skin, joints, kidneys, nervous system and mucous membranes.

pernicious anemia: A potentially dangerous form of anemia, usually caused by an autoimmune process, which results in a deficiency of vitamin B12.

rheumatic diseases: Characterized by signs of inflammation (redness, heat, swelling, pain) and loss of function of joints, tendons, ligaments, bones, or muscles. Some rheumatic diseases can also involve internal organs.

rheumatoid arthritis: An autoimmune disease that targets primarily the membrane lining the joints, leading to pain, stiffness, swelling, and joint deformity.

scleroderma: An autoimmune disease characterized by abnormal growth of connective tissue in the skin and blood vessels. In more severe forms, connective tissue can build up in the kidneys, lungs, heart, and gastrointestinal tract, leading in some cases to organ failure.

severe combined immune deficiency: Included in a group of rare, life-threatening disorders caused by at least 15 different single gene defects that result in profound deficiencies in T- and B-lymphocyte function.

Sjögren syndrome: A condition in which the body's immune system attacks the moisture-producing glands, resulting in uncomfortable and sometimes damaging dryness of tissues, particularly those of the eyes and mouth.

systemic lupus erythematosus: A chronic autoimmune disease of the connective tissue that can attack and damage the skin, joints, blood vessels, and internal organs.

telangiectasia: A condition caused by the swelling of tiny blood vessels, in which small red spots appear on the hands and face. Although not painful, these red spots can create cosmetic problems.

type 1 diabetes: A condition in which the immune system destroys insulin-producing cells of the pancreas, making it impossible for the body to use glucose (blood sugar) for energy. Type 1 diabetes usually occurs in children and young adults.

uveitis: Inflammation of the inner eye that includes the iris, the tissue that holds the lens of the eye, and a network of blood vessels surrounding the eyeball called the choroid plexus.

vitiligo: A disorder in which the immune system destroys pigment-making cells called melanocytes. This results in white patches of skin on different parts of the body.

Chapter 94

Directory of Organizations with Immune Disorders Information

Government Organizations

National Cancer Institute (NCI)
Medical Center Dr.
BG 9609 MSC 97609609
Bethesda, MD 20892-9760
Toll-Free: 800-4-CANCER
(800-422-6237)
Toll-Free TTY: 800-332-8615
Website: www.cancer.gov
E-mail: cancergovstaff@mail.nih.gov

National Eye Institute (NEI)
31 Center Dr.
MSC 2510
Bethesda, MD 20892-2510
Phone: 301-496-5248
Website: www.nei.nih.gov
E-mail: 2020@nei.nih.gov

National Heart, Lung, and Blood Institute (NHLBI) Health Information Center
P.O. Box 30105
Bethesda, MD 20824-0105
Phone: 301-592-8573
Fax: 301-592-8563
Website: www.nhlbi.nih.gov
E-mail: nhlbiinfo@nhlbi.nih.gov

National Human Genome Research Institute (NHGRI)
31 Center Dr., MSC 2152, 9000 Rockville Pike
Bldg. 31, Rm. 4B09
Bethesda, MD 20892-2152
Phone: 301-402-0911
Fax: 301-402-2218
Website: www.genome.gov

Resources in this chapter were compiled from several sources deemed reliable, October 2016.

561

National Immunization Program (NIP)
NIP Public Inquiries
1600 Clifton Rd.
Mailstop E-05
Atlanta, GA 30333
Toll-Free: 800-232-2522
Website: www.cdc.gov/nip
E-mail: nipinfo@cdc.gov

National Institute of Allergy and Infectious Diseases (NIAID)
Office of Communications
5601 Fishers Ln.
MSC 9806
Bethesda, MD 20892-9806
Toll-Free: 866-284-4107
Phone: 301-402-1663
Toll-Free TDD: 800-877-8339
Fax: 301-402-0120
Website: www.niaid.nih.gov
E-mail: niaidnews@niaid.nih.gov

National Institute of Arthritis and Musculoskeletal and Skin Diseases (NIAMS)
Information Clearinghouse
1 AMS Cir.
Bethesda, MD 20892-3675
Toll-Free: 877-22-NIAMS
(877-226-4267)
Phone: 301-495-4484
TTY: 301-565-2966
Fax: 301-881-2731
Website: www.niams.nih.gov
E-mail: niamsinfo@mail.nih.gov

National Institute of Diabetes and Digestive and Kidney Diseases (NIDDK)
Information Clearinghouse
9000 Rockville Pike
Bethesda, MD 20892-3560
Toll-Free: 800-860-8747
Website: www.niddk.nih.gov

National Institute of Neurological Disorders and Stroke (NINDS)
P.O. Box 5801
Bethesda, MD 20824
Toll-Free: 800-352-9424
Phone: 301-496-5751
Website: www.ninds.nih.gov

NIH Clinical Center Patient Recruitment and Referral Center (for specific NIH clinical trials information)
10 Center Dr.
Bethesda, MD 20892
Toll-Free: 800-411-1222
Phone: 301-496-2563
TTY: 866-411-1010
Fax: 301-402-2984
Website: clinicalstudies.info.nih.gov/referring_patient.html
E-mail: prpl@mail.cc.nih.gov

National Kidney and Urologic Diseases Information Clearinghouse (NKUDIC)
3 Information Way
Bethesda, MD 20892-3580
Toll-Free: 800-891-5390
Phone: 301-654-4415
Website: www.ninds.nih.gov
E-mail: nkudic@info.niddk.nih.gov

Office of Rare Diseases (ORD)
6701 Democracy Blvd.
Ste. 1001, MSC 4874
Bethesda, MD 20892
Phone: 301-402-4336
Fax: 301-480-9655
Website: rarediseases.info.nih.gov
E-mail: ord@od.nih.gov

Private Organizations

A-T Children's Project
5300 W. Hillsboro Blvd., Ste. 105
Coconut Creek, FL 33073
Toll-Free: 800-5-HELP.A-T
(800-543-5728)
Phone: 954-481-6611
Website: www.atcp.org
E-mail: info@atcp.org

American Academy of Dermatology (AAD)
P.O. Box 4014
Schaumburg, IL 60168-4014
Toll-Free: 888-462-3376
Phone: 847-330-0230
Fax: 847-330-0050
Website: www.aad.org

American Academy of Orthopaedic Surgeons (AAOS)
9400 W. Higgins Rd.
Rosemont, IL 60018
Toll-Free: 800-346-AAOS
(800-346-2267)
Phone: 847-823-7186
Fax: 847-823-8125
Website: www.aaos.org

American Academy of Physical Medicine and Rehabilitation (AAPMR)
9700 W. Bryn Mawr Ave., Ste. 200
Rosemont, IL 60018-5701
Toll-Free: 877-227-6799
Phone: 847-737-6000
Website: www.aapmr.org
E-mail: info@aapmr.org

American Association for Clinical Chemistry (AACC)
900 Seventh St. N.W., Ste. 400
Washington, DC 20001
Phone: 202-857-0717
Toll Free: 800-892-1400
Fax: 202-887-5093
Website: www.aacc.org

American Association of Colleges of Osteopathic Medicine (AACOM)
5550 Friendship Blvd., Ste. 310
Chevy Chase, MD 20815
Phone: 301-968-4100
Fax: 301-968-4101
Website: www.aacom.org
E-mail: webmaster@aacom.org

American Autoimmune-Related Diseases Association, Inc. (AARDA)
22100 Gratiot Ave.
Eastpointe, MI 48021
Toll-Free: 800-598-4668
Phone: 586-776-3900
Fax: 586-776-3903
Website: www.aarda.org

American Behcet's Disease Association (ABDA)
P.O. Box 80576
Rochester, MI 48308
Website: www.behcets.com
E-mail: webmaster@behcets.com

American College of Rheumatology (ACR)
2200 Lake Blvd N.E.
Atlanta, GA 30319
Phone: 404-633-3777
Fax: 404-633-1870
Website: www.rheumatology.org

American Diabetes Association (ADA)
1701 N. Beauregard St.
Alexandria, VA 22311
Toll-Free: 800-DIABETES
(800-342-2383)
Website: www.diabetes.org
E-mail: askada@diabetes.org

American Federation for Medical Research (AFMR)
500 Cummings Center, Ste. 4550
Beverly, MA 01915
Phone: 978-927-8330
Fax: 978-524-8890
Website: www.afmr.org
E-mail: admin@afmr.org

American Liver Foundation (ALF)
39 Broadway, Ste. 2700
New York, NY 10006
Toll-Free: 800-465-4837
Phone: 212-668-1000
Fax: 212-483-8179
Website: www.liverfoundation.org
E-mail: support@liverfoundation.org

American Lung Association (ALA)
55 W. Wacker Dr., Ste. 1150
Chicago, IL 60601
Toll-Free: 800-LUNGUSA
(800-586-4872)
Website: www.lungusa.org
E-mail: info@lung.org

American Skin Association (ASA)
6 E. 43rd St., 28th Fl.
New York, NY 10017
Toll-Free: 800-499-SKIN
(800-499-7546)
Phone: 212-889-4858
Fax: 212-889-4959
Website: www.americanskin.org
E-mail: info@americanskin.org

American Thyroid Association (ATA)
6066 Leesburg Pike
Ste. 550
Falls Church, VA 22041
Phone: 703-998-8890
Fax: 703-998-8893
Website: www.thyroid.org
E-mail: thyroid@thyroid.org

Arthritis Foundation
1355 Peachtree St. N.E.
Ste. 600
Atlanta, GA 30309
Toll-Free: 844-571-4357
Phone: 404-872-7100
Website: www.arthritis.org

Celiac Disease Foundation (CDF)
20350 Ventura Blvd.
Ste. 240
Woodland Hills, CA 91364
Phone: 818-716-1513
Fax: 818-267-5577
Website: www.celiac.org

Celiac Support Association (CSA)
413 Ash St.
Seward, NE 68434
Toll-Free: 877-CSA-4CSA
(877-272-4272)
Phone: 402-643-4101
Fax: 402-643-4108
Website: www.csaceliacs.org
E-mail: celiacs@csaceliacs.org

Chediak-Higashi Syndrome Association (CHS)
1 South Rd.
Oyster Bay, NY 11771
Toll-Free: 800-789-9477
Phone: 516-922-4022
Website: www.chediak-higashi.org
E-mail: hpsnet@worldnet.att.net

Crohn's and Colitis Foundation of America (CCFA)
733 Third Ave.
Ste. 510
New York, NY 10017
Toll-Free: 800-932-2423
Website: www.ccfa.org
E-mail: info@ccfa.org

Gluten Intolerance Group (GIG)
31214 124th Ave. S.E.
Auburn, WA 98092
Phone: 253-833-6655
Fax: 253-833-6675
Website: www.gluten.net
E-mail: customerservice@gluten.org

Graves' Disease and Thyroid Foundation (GDATF)
P.O. Box 2793
Rancho Santa Fe, CA 92067
Toll-Free:877-643-3123
Fax: 877-643-3123
Website: www.gdatf.org
Email: info@gdatf.org

Guillain-Barré Syndrome
Foundation International
(GBS)
104 1/2 Forrest Ave.
Narberth, PA 19072
Phone: 610-667-0131
Fax: 610-667-7036
Website: www.guillain-barre.com

Immune Deficiency
Foundation (IDF)
110 West Rd., Ste. 300
Towson, MD 21204
Toll-Free: 800-296-4433
Phone: 800-296-4433
Fax: 410-321-9165
Website: www.primaryimmune.
org
E-mail: info@primaryimmune.org

International Pemphigus
Foundation (IPPF)
1331 Garden Hwy.
Ste. 100
Sacramento, CA 95833
Toll-Free: 855-473-6744
Phone: 916-922-1298
Website: www.pemphigus.org
E-mail: info@pemphigus.org

Jeffrey Modell Foundation
(JMF)
National Primary
Immunodeficiency Resource
Center
730 Third Ave.
New York, NY 10017
Phone: 212-819-0200
Website: www.info4pi.org
E-mail: info@jmfworld.org

Lupus Foundation of
America, Inc.
2121 K St. N.W.
Ste. 200
Washington, DC 20037
Toll-Free: 800-558-0121
Phone: 202-349-1155
Fax: 202-349-1156
Website: www.lupus.org
E-mail: info@lupus.org

Lupus Research Alliance
275 Madison Ave.
10th Fl.
New York, NY 10016
Toll-Free: 800-867-1743
Phone: 646-884-6000
Fax: 212-218-2448
Website: www.lupusny.org
E-mail: info@lupusresearch.org

Multiple Sclerosis
Foundation (MSF)
6520 N. Andrews Ave.
Ft. Lauderdale, FL 33309-2132
Toll-Free: 888-MSFOCUS
(888-673-6287)
Phone: 954-776-6805
Fax: 954-351-0630
Website: www.msfocus.org
E-mail: support@msfocus.org

Muscular Dystrophy
Association (MDA)
222 S. Riverside Plaza
Ste. 1500
Chicago, Il 60606
Toll-Free: 800-572-1717
Website: www.mdausa.org
E-mail: mda@mdausa.org

566

*Myasthenia Gravis
Foundation of America
(MGFA)*
355 Lexington Ave.
15th Fl.
New York, NY 10017
Toll-Free: 800-541-5454
Phone: 651-917-6256
Fax: 212-297-2159
Website: www.myasthenia.org

*The Myositis Association
(TMA)*
1737 King St.
Ste. 600
Alexandria, VA 22314
Toll-Free: 800-821-7356
Phone: 703-299-4850
Fax: 703-535-6752
Website: www.myositis.org
E-mail: TMA@myositis.org

*National Academy of
Sciences (NAS)*
500 Fifth St. N.W.
Washington, DC 20001
Phone: 202-334-2000
Website: national-academies.org

*National Adrenal Diseases
Foundation (NADF)*
505 Northern Blvd.
Great Neck, NY 11021
Phone: 516-487-4992
Website: www.nadf.us
E-mail: nadfsupport@nadf.us

*National Alopecia Areata
Foundation (NAAF)*
65 Mitchell Blvd., Ste. 200-B
San Rafael, CA 94903
Phone: 415-472-3780
Fax: 415-480-1800
Website: www.naaf.org
E-mail: info@naaf.org

*National Graves' Disease
Foundation (NGDF)*
P.O. Box 1969
Brevard, NC 28712
Phone: 904-278-9482
Fax: 904-278-9488
Website: www.ngdf.org
E-mail: nancy@ngdf.org

*National Kidney Foundation
(NKF)*
30 E. 33rd St.
New York, NY 10016
Toll-Free: 800-622-9010
Phone: 212-889-2210
Website: www.kidney.org
E-mail: info@kidney.org

*National Multiple Sclerosis
Society (NMSS)*
733 Third Ave.
6th Fl.
New York, NY 10017-3288
Toll-Free: 800-344-4867
Phone: 212-986-3240
Fax: 212-986-7981
Website: www.nmss.org
E-mail: nat@nmss.org

National Organization for Rare Disorders (NORD)
55 Kansas Ave.
Danbury, CT 06813-1968
Toll-Free: 800-999-6673
Phone: 203-744-0100
Fax: 203-263-9938
Website: www.rarediseases.org
E-mail: orphan@rarediseases. org

National Psoriasis Foundation (NPF)
S.W. 92nd Ave.
Ste. 300
Portland, OR 97223-7195
Toll-Free: 800-723-9166
Phone: 503-244-7404
Fax: 503-245-0626
Website: www.psoriasis.org
E-mail: getinfo@npfusa.org

National Sarcoidosis Resources Center (NSRC)
P.O. Box 1593
Piscataway, NJ 08855-1593
Phone: 732-463-0497
Fax: 732-463-0467
Website: nsrc-global.org

National Vitiligo Foundation, Inc. (NVFI)
11250 Cornell Park Dr.
Ste. 207
Cincinnati, OH 45242
Phone: 513-793-NVFI
(513-793-6834)
Fax: 513-793-6887
Website:
nationalvitiligofoundation. wildapricot.org
E-mail: info@nvfi.org

Platelet Disorder Support Association (PDSA)
8751 Brecksville Rd.
Ste. 150
Cleveland, OH 44141
Toll-Free: 87-PLATELET
(877-528-3538)
Phone: 440-746-9003
Fax: 844-270-1277
Website: www.pdsa.org
E-mail: pdsa@pdsa.org

Scleroderma Foundation
300 Rosewood Dr.
Ste. 105
Danvers, MA 01923
Toll-Free: 800-722-4673
Phone: 978-463-5843
Fax: 978-777-1313
Website: www.scleroderma.org
E-mail: sfinfo@scleroderma.org

Scleroderma Research Foundation (SRF)
220 Montgomery St.
Ste. 1411
San Francisco, CA 94104
Toll-Free: 800-441-CURE
(800-441-2873)
Phone: 415-834-9444
Fax: 415-834-9177
Website: www.srfcure.org

Sjögren's Syndrome Foundation (SSF)
6707 Democracy Blvd.
Ste. 325
Bethesda, MD 20817
Toll-Free: 800-475-6473
Phone: 301-530-4420
Fax: 301-530-4415
Website: www.sjogrens.org

Society for Investigative Dermatology (SID)
526 Superior Ave. E.
Ste. 340
Cleveland, OH 44114
Phone: 216-579-9300
Fax: 216-579-9333
Website: www.sidnet.org
E-mail: sid@sidnet.org

Spondylitis Association of America (SAA)
P.O. Box 5872
Sherman Oaks, CA 91413
Toll-Free: 800-777-8189
Phone: 818-892-1616
Fax: 818-892-1611
Website: www.spondylitis.org
E-mail: info@spondylitis.org

Index

Index